Dementia and Subjectivity / Demenz und Subjektivität

Daniela Ringkamp / Sara Strauß /
Leonie Süwolto (eds./Hrsg.)

Dementia and Subjectivity / Demenz und Subjektivität

Aesthetic, Literary and Philosophical Perspectives / Ästhetische, literarische und philosophische Perspektiven

PETER LANG
EDITION

Bibliographic Information published by the Deutsche Nationalbibliothek
The Deutsche Nationalbibliothek lists this publication in the Deutsche Nationalbibliografie; detailed bibliographic data is available in the internet at http://dnb.d-nb.de.

Library of Congress Cataloging-in-Publication Data
Names: Ringkamp, Daniela, editor.
Title: Dementia and subjectivity : Demenz und Subjektivität : aesthetic, literary and philosophical perspectives : Ästhetische, literarische und philosophische Perspektiven / Daniela Ringkamp, Sara Strauss, Leonie Suwolto (eds./Hrsg.).
Other titles: Demenz und Subjektivitat
Description: New York : Peter Lang, 2017. | Papers from a conference held at the University of Paderborn in November 2015. | Includes bibliographical references. | English or German.
Identifiers: LCCN 2017017075 | ISBN 9783631725399
Subjects: LCSH: Dementia–Patients–Congresses. | Dementia–In literature–Congresses.
Classification: LCC RC521 .D44338 2017 | DDC 616.8/31–dc23
LC record available at https://lccn.loc.gov/2017017075

Cover illustration: *Dealing With Dementia* © freshidea / Fotolia.com

ISBN 978-3-631-72539-9 (Print)
E-ISBN 978-3-631-72572-6 (E-PDF)
E-ISBN 978-3-631-72573-3 (EPUB)
E-ISBN 978-3-631-72574-0 (MOBI)
DOI 10.3726/b11287

Peter Lang Edition is an Imprint of Peter Lang GmbH.

Peter Lang – Frankfurt am Main · Bern · Bruxelles · New York · Oxford · Warszawa · Wien

This publication has been peer reviewed.

www.peterlang.com

Contents/Inhaltsverzeichnis

Introductory Reflections/ Einführende Beiträge

Daniela Ringkamp/Sara Strauss/
Leonie Süwolto (Magdeburg/Paderborn)

Introduction/Einleitung

The term 'de-mentia' derives from the Latin word '*mens*' for 'mind' and means nothing less than *to lose one's mind.* It assumes an understanding of the subject as an *animal rationale* and suggests that dementia can be defined primarily by a loss of cognitive abilities. That is why, for some authors, dementia may be seen as a kind of antonym to the dominant idea of man's intellectual efficiency and the idea of autonomy based mainly on reason and the capacity to judge.[1] In contrast to this image of human rationality forming the basis of hegemonic structures in society, dementia reveals *ex negativo* the normative standards of a meritocracy. The course of the disease, which amongst other symptoms involves the loss of memory and intellectual power and a fading ability to orientate oneself in space and time, poses a serious threat to a knowledge-based society which in our times especially values cognitive abilities and efficiency and establishes the dictum of lifelong learning. Hence, dementia is an ongoing challenge to the predominant idea of man.[2]

Dementia is known primarily for the loss of memory it causes during its course. Patients first start to forget things in their daily lives until eventually, well-known people become strangers to them. But dementia is not simply a synonym for memory disorder. It implies a variety of symptoms and dysfunctions. We know that dementia is a neurodegenerative disease that often starts years before the first symptoms are recognized by the patients themselves or the people around them. In most cases short-term memory is the first thing affected by the degenerative process. With time the progression of dementia causes impairments of almost all cognitive skills, like attention, comprehension, intellectual capacity, sense of direction, and the ability to communicate orally and in writing. People suffering from

1 See Körtner, Ulrich H. J. "Das Menschenbild der Leistungsgesellschaft und die Irritation Demenz." In: *Zeitschrift für medizinische Ethik: Wissenschaft, Kultur, Religion*, 58,1 (2012): 3–33, 4: "Gemessen an einem Menschenbild, das den Wert des Lebens an den kognitiven Leistungen unseres Gehirns bemisst, das in der Autonomie den höchsten Wert erkennt, die wiederum an unser kognitives Bewusstsein, unsere Einsichts- und Urteilsfähigkeit gebunden ist – gemessen an einem solchen Verständnis des Menschen erscheinen Menschen mit einer Demenz als unwürdige Greise."

2 See Körtner. "Das Menschenbild der Leistungsgesellschaft und die Irritation Demenz," 4.

dementia are severely limited in the ability to express themselves. Beyond the fact that a sense of time and space gets lost during the course of dementia, a change of social behaviour is seen in most cases: impulse and control disorders, impairments of mood, disturbed perceptions, and a disrupted relationship with reality are the main symptoms, which are often accompanied by feelings of fear, depression and restlessness.[3] As a consequence of these mental impairments late-stage dementia also leads to physical symptoms as the patients can no longer walk, may suffer from diseases or side effects of their immobility or lack of muscle control, and ultimately lose the ability to swallow food.[4]

Normally, the course of the disease is divided into three long-term phases starting with mild dementia, which usually implies light cognitive impairment, and progressing to moderate dementia, followed by severe dementia. Even in the second stage of the disease, the possibilities of independent living are gravely restricted, and in the last phase of severe dementia, patients need comprehensive care.[5] In a time of double-income households and changing family structures, relatives have to entrust the care of their patients to care facilities, which of course leads to serious social challenges concerning nursing capacities and financial issues.

In our greying society we have to face a rapidly increasing number of people suffering from dementia. The high proportion of old people in our society that is implied by the common expression *demographic change* has already led to the considerable number of "47 million people liv[ing] with dementia worldwide".[6] In Germany, for example, in addition to the current 1.5 million people diagnosed with dementia, 40,000 new occurrences of the disease are recorded every year. Here and in other European countries, such as the UK, the overall number of dementia patients is expected to double by 2050.[7] Dementia is therefore strongly linked with our image of old age because it serves as a metaphor for the ageing

---

3 See Kurz, Alexander, Freter, Hans Jürgen, Saxl, Susanna, Nickel, Ellen. *Demenz. Das Wichtigste. Ein kompakter Ratgeber*. Berlin: Deutsche Alzheimer Gesellschaft e.V., [2]2016, 6.

4 Alzheimer's Society. "The Later Stages of Dementia." <https://www.alzheimers.org.uk/info/20073/how_dementia_progresses/103/the_later_stages_of_dementia/2> (last access 17.02.2017).

5 Kurz et al. *Demenz. Das Wichtigste. Ein kompakter Ratgeber*, 19.

6 Rees, Glenn. "Foreword." In: Alzheimer's Disease International (ed.). *World Alzheimer Report 2016 – Improving Healthcare for People Living with Dementia*. London: Alzheimer's Disease International, 2016, i, i.

7 Kurz et al. *Demenz. Das Wichtigste. Ein kompakter Ratgeber*, 8; and Alzheimer's Society. "Introduction." In: *Dementia 2015 – Aiming Higher to Transform Lives*. London: Alzheimer's Society, 2015, 1–7, 1.

society and the threat it poses to a community based on a monetary intergenerational contract. Today almost every second person among those aged 90 is affected by dementia.[8]

In fact, the consequences of an increasing number of demented persons are measured and communicated to the public in economic terms and parameters. Like the forecasts of the looming pensions crisis, which are closely connected to the public discussion of the demographic collapse, the discourse of dementia follows an almost apocalyptic rhetoric.[9] Everyone is probably familiar with the predictions of the crisis in the healthcare sector, the surge in medical expenses and so on. Terms like these, which circulate constantly in the media, seem to cover the existential questions people who suffer from dementia are confronted with as well as the problems their families, friends and relatives are concerned with. Of course, society has to face several serious problems relating to nursing capacities. Yet when observing the public discourse about dementia, it is remarkable that Alzheimer's disease and other forms of dementia often carry a negative connotation and are regarded as an exclusively medical problem.[10] This is why major parts of the contemporary discourse on Alzheimer's disease refer to medical categories but ignore the many social, cultural and personal challenges of dementia, not only for society as a whole but also for the patients and their relatives, who often have to redefine their relationships.

The following collection of interdisciplinary essays, by contrast, tries to find another approach to dementia. It intends to respond to the demand for a more open discourse that involves multiple perspectives and moves the topic of dementia and its relevance for society as a whole into the centre of public and academic attention. As Aagje Swinnen and Mark Schweda explain,

> [c]ontrasting the dominance of naturalistic, neurobiological and biomedical discourses, dementia studies aims at a better understanding of dementia as a cultural phenomenon. [...] Understanding the multiple ways by which dementia, while biologically influenced,

---

8 See Kurz et al. *Demenz. Das Wichtigste. Ein kompakter Ratgeber*, 8.

9 See Freiburg, Rudolf, Kretzschmar, Dirk. "Einleitung: Grau-Werte." In: Rudolf Freiburg, Dirk Kretzschmar (eds.). *Alter(n) in Literatur und Kultur der Gegenwart*. Würzburg: Königshausen & Neumann, 2010, 1–30, 1.

10 See Wetzstein, Verena. "Alzheimer-Demenz – Entstehung eines Krankheitsbegriffes." In: Nationaler Ethikrat (ed.). *Altersdemenz und Morbus Alzheimer – Medizinische, gesellschaftliche und ethische Herausforderungen*. Berlin: Nationaler Ethikrat, 2006, 37–48, 38–39.

> is at the same time culturally constructed contributes to the fight against stigma and can improve the wellbeing of people with dementia and their caregivers.[11]

In understanding dementia as a cultural phenomenon, the authors in this volume emphasize the relation between subjectivity and intersubjectivity – between the conditions of experiencing dementia from a first-person perspective and from others. In doing so, the contributions also try to create awareness for the intertwined history of the philosophical concept of the subject, which might offer a different view on dementia sufferers. If we understand the subject from the viewpoint of the era of Enlightenment, for example, it may become apparent that the rationalism of the early Enlightenment had been replaced by the middle of the eighteenth century by movements concentrating on the subject's emotional determination. There has been a long development from the period of Romanticism, with its focus on the irrational and unconscious constitution of the subject, to its postmodern death, which sharpens our eyesight for alternative concepts of a ratio-centered understanding of subjectivity.[12] It can highlight the constructive character of subjectivity and thus disclose the rules of marginalizing and stigmatizing demented persons as rejects of a knowledge-based meritocracy. If constitutive aspects of human existence, like emotionality, irrationality, unconsciousness, dependency, passivity, loss, resignation and fragmentation, were reintegrated into concepts of subjectivity[13] – like they are in current research approaches – dementia sufferers would no longer be described in terms of deviation. Insights from philosophy and literary and cultural studies can contribute tremendously to this change of perspective.

The aim of this collection of articles from philosophy, literary studies, and cultural studies can be illustrated by several examples. For instance, at the beginning of his autobiographical report about his mother's disease, the journalist and author Jörn Klare asks her what it feels to suffer from dementia. "Undurchsichtig" – opaque, incomprehensible – she answers, with a clear voice that overrides the strangeness and insecurity she normally experiences when becoming aware of the symptoms of dementia.[14] With this, Klare's mother, who is in the second stage

---

11 Swinnen, Aagje, Schweda, Mark. "Popularizing Dementia. Public Expressions and Representations of Forgetfulness." In: Aagje Swinnen, Mark Schweda (eds.). *Popularizing Dementia. Public Expressions and Representations of Forgetfulness*. Bielefeld: transcript, 2015, 9–20, 11. Italics in the original.

12 See Körtner. "Das Menschenbild der Leistungsgesellschaft," 9.

13 See for example Körtner. "Das Menschenbild der Leistungsgesellschaft," 3.

14 Klare, Jörn. *Als meine Mutter ihre Küche nicht mehr fand. Vom Wert des Lebens mit Demenz*. Berlin: Suhrkamp, [2]2012, 46.

of the disease when she makes her statement, marks a mental condition which is not only barely available to herself from a subjective perspective but which also poses great challenges for her family and especially for her two sons. It is not only their mother but also themselves who have to find new ways of communicating and interacting with her. Dementia, it seems, not only alienates the affected patient from his or her former self, it also compels medical practitioners, nurses and the social environment to accept the disease and to respond to a person who may not have much in common with his or her former personality and character traits.

To explain his diseased mother's situation, Klare takes up the positions of medical experts as well as psychologists, philosophers, attorneys and nursing staff. The contributors to this volume also aim to investigate the mental condition of dementia sufferers from different perspectives. In contrast to Klare, however, they mainly refer to standpoints from literature, arts and the humanities. In doing so, the contributions will especially deal with first-person – subjective – and third-person – intersubjective – approaches to examine the mental state of the patients. This methodological directive implies two important aspects: First, the contributions focus predominantly on the mental and behavioural conditions of the patients and the consequences these conditions entail for their social and personal relationships. Secondly, the social and cognitive implications of dementia will primarily be explored not by medical and nursing issues but by perspectives from literature, philosophy and aesthetics, such as in movies or theatre or with regard to medical ethics. This extensive approach to dementia, which considers both the perspectives of the patients and their social environments, shows that an examination of the conditions and consequences of dementia on a mere neuromedical sphere – which is of course of fundamental importance – is not sufficient: Literary and philosophical examinations do not only point to important ethical questions which arise within the course of the disease; they also formally express the patients' decreasing ability to speak and to articulate themselves, they provide access to their experience, and they develop fictional and nonfictional strategies which represent ways of dealing with the challenges of dementia from first- and third-person perspectives.

In recent years, narrative representations of dementia have become increasingly important in literature, such as in autobiographical texts,[15] short stories and

---

15 See for example Bayley, John. *Iris: A Memoir of Iris Murdoch*. London: Duckworth, 1998; Geiger, Arno. *Der alte König in seinem Exil*. München: Hanser, 2011; Jens, Tilman. *Demenz. Abschied von meinem Vater*. Gütersloh: Gütersloher Verlagshaus, 2009.

other fictional and nonfictional texts.[16] This focus on dementia as one possibility for investigating mental pathologies in literature is accompanied by a series of cinematographic representations, such as *Away from Her* (2006), a cinematic adaptation of Alice Munro's short story "The Bear Came over the Mountain"; *The Iron Lady* (2011); and – probably the most influential one – *Still Alice* from 2014, for which Julianne Moore won an Academy as the female protagonist. The strategies and aims of literature as well as of the cinematic adaptations mentioned above are complex and multilayered. They provide outsiders with the ability to identify with persons suffering from dementia by portraying their subjective state, their living conditions under the constraints of decreasing mental capacities and disorientation, but also by pointing to the personality and the individual character of the patients, which are still fundamental bases of their identity. A further important subject in literary investigations is a critical examination of the treatment of dementia in society: As with other vulnerable groups, dementia sufferers are in danger of being marginalized. Their disease is often regarded as an unwanted loss of quality of life and – to some extent – is also demonized as a gruesome fate which destroys the core of human existence.

Beyond this, literature not only focuses on the representations and social handling of dementia but also aims at constructing aesthetic interpretations and counterfactual constellations, which introduce ways of interacting with dementia patients in situations that transcend medical responsibility and expertise. In doing so, arts and literature pay attention to patients' situations but also allow for considering the thoughts and concerns of persons from their social environment, who are in a position to find their own ways of dealing with the disease and interacting with the patient. The first-person perspective of the patient and the third-person perspective of relatives, friends and nursing staff are also reflected at a methodological level, such as in the use of fragmented speech and interior monologues and the verbalization of disruptive thoughts, which are visibly integrated in the typeface of the pages.

---

16 Draesner, Ulrike. "Ichs Heimweg macht alles allein." In: Clara Obermüller (ed.). *Es schneit in meinem Kopf. Erzählungen über Alzheimer und Demenz*. Zürich: Nagel & Kimche, 2006, 59–81; Farkas, Péter. *Acht Minuten*. München: Luchterhand Literaturverlag, 2011; Franzen, Jonathan. *The Corrections*. New York: Farrar Straus & Giroux, 2001; Franzen, Jonathan. "My Father's Brain." In: *The New Yorker* 10.09.2001, 80; McEwan, Ian. *Atonement*. London: Jonathan Cape, 2001; Munro, Alice. "The Bear Came over the Mountain." In: Alice Munro. *Hateship, Friendship, Courtship, Loveship, Marriage*. London: Chatto & Windus, 2001, 275–323; Suter, Martin. *Small World*. Zürich: Diogenes, 1999.

Some of the examples mentioned in literary representations also serve as starting points for philosophical reflections on dementia.[17] Even though philosophy's interest in dementia is especially pronounced in applied ethics with regard to questions of autonomy and care, challenges of dementia and Alzheimer's disease in general are also explored in philosophy of mind and philosophy of psychiatry. Contributions in this context often deal with questions concerning patients' change of identities, their attempts to maintain individual selves, and their struggles with the symptoms of the disease. Do the symptoms of dementia lead to the loss of personal identity, or should they be regarded as new character traits? What is the relation between previous thoughts and preferences and those wishes a patient articulates in a state of severe dementia? And, from a metaphysical perspective, what constitutes the self – is it the subjective mental state, the capacity for diachronic memory in the Lockean tradition, or, on the contrary, is it bodily integration, experiential interests and the emotional involvement of a person in his or her social environment? These aspects of identity theory initiate ethical investigations about the possibilities and limitations of the personal autonomy of dementia sufferers and of prolonged autonomy, nursing issues and adequate care. Even though many of these questions transcend the boundaries of philosophy, several approaches try to formulate conditions for and adequate treatment of these issues.[18] A central point of reference in these debates is the concept of personhood,

17 In the debate in Germany, Tilman Jens's report on his father, Walter Jens, and Arno Geiger's autobiographical novel are often seen as examples which show the implications of memory loss and changes of identity but which also adhere to the vulnerability and dignity of the patients.

18 Concerning the mental state of dementia patients see for example DeGrazia, David. *Human Identity and Bioethics*. Cambridge/New York: Cambridge University Press, 2005, 159–202; Dworkin, Ronald. "Autonomy and the Demented Self." In: *The Milbank Quarterly* 64,2 (1986): 4–16; Hughes, Julian C. *Thinking Through Dementia*. New York: Oxford University Press, 2011; McMillan, John. "Identity, Self, and Dementia." In: Julian C. Hughes, Stephen Louw, Stephen R. Sabat (eds.). *Dementia: Mind, Meaning, and the Person*. New York: Oxford University Press, 2006, 63–70; Lesser, Harry A. "Dementia and Personal Identity." In: Julian C. Hughes, Stephen Louw, Stephen R. Sabat (eds.). *Dementia: Mind, Meaning, and the Person*. New York: Oxford University Press, 2006, 55–61. Many of these authors also provide an examination of prolonged autonomy performed by dementia patients. Concerning the patient autonomy of dementia persons see Dresser, Rebecca. "Dworkin on Dementia: Elegant Theory, Questionable Policy." In: *The Hastings Center Report* 25,6 (1995): 32–38; Dworkin, Ronald. *Life's Dominion. An Argument About Abortion, Euthanasia, and Individual Freedom*. New York: Vintage Books, 1993, 218–42; Jaworska, Agnieszka. "Respecting the Margins of Agency:

understood both in an ontological and ethical framework. Whereas, on the one hand, dementia patients are regarded as "post-persons",[19] whose mental states are diminished, other perspectives claim a broad understanding of personhood which ignores rational competences and emphasizes emotional as well as experiential capacities, to which the social surrounding should respond.

The different approaches to dementia performed by literature, philosophy, aesthetics and cultural studies converge in several points, some of which have already been mentioned above. There are other aspects which must be noted in this context, such as narrative ethics: Accounts of narrative ethics are not only a frequently discussed strategy in literature as well as in personal identity theory, medical ethics and care – they are also analysed in some contributions in this volume as a possibility to strengthen the potential of dementia sufferers as independent actors. Whereas in contemporary research much attention has been paid to the interconnections between medical, psychological, palliative and nursing questions, comparatively little emphasis has been placed on the conjunctions between the different fields of arts, humanities and cultural studies. By considering topics from Austrian, German, Swiss, Hungarian, English, Canadian and American literature, from film studies and medical ethics, the following volume

---

Alzheimer's Patients and the Capacity to Value." In: *Philosophy and Public Affairs* 28,2 (1999): 105–38; Crayton, Harry. "From Childhood to Childhood? Autonomy and Dependence through the Ages of Life." In: Julian C. Hughes, Stephen Louw, Stephen R. Sabat (eds.). *Dementia: Mind, Meaning, and the Person*. New York: Oxford University Press, 2006, 277–86. Buchanan, Allen E., Brock, Dan W. *Deciding for Others. The Ethics of Surrogate Decision Making*. Cambridge/New York: Cambridge University Press, 1990, 165–89. For an insight into the German debate see Birnbacher, Dieter. "Patientenverfügungen und Advance Care Planning bei Demenz und anderen kognitiven Beeinträchtigungen." In: *Ethik in der Medizin*. Berlin/Heidelberg: Springer-Verlag, 2016. DOI 10.1007/s00481-016-0388-6; Schmidhuber, Martina. "Ethische Probleme der Patientenverfügung bei Demenzbetroffenen." In: *Ethica. Wissenschaft und Verantwortung* 22,2 (2014): 121–37; Sturma, Dieter. "Ethische Überlegungen zum Umgang mit demenziell erkrankten Personen." In: Olivia Dibelius, Wolfgang Maier (eds.). *Versorgungsforschung für demenziell erkrankte Menschen. Health Service Research for People with Dementia*. Stuttgart: Kohlhammer, 2011, 93–98; Hallich, Oliver. "Selbstbindung und medizinischer Paternalismus: Zum normativen Status von 'Odysseus-Anweisungen.'" In: *Zeitschrift für philosophische Forschung* 65,2 (2011): 151–72.

19 McMahan, Jeff. *The Ethics of Killing. Problems at the Margins of Life*. New York: Oxford University Press, 2002, 46. McMahan's position should not be conflated with Engelhardt's description of dementia patients as persons in a social sense. See Engelhardt, H. Tristram Jr. *The Foundations of Bioethics*. New York: Oxford University Press, 1996, 147.

aims to strengthen this alternative approach to dementia from an interdisciplinary and bilingual perspective.

The articles in this volume intend to offer new perspectives on questions which are highly relevant in the context of the arts and the humanities. The issues concern, among others, the personal identity of dementia patients, their familial relationships, the opportunities and restraints with regard to advance directives and patients' autonomy, the question of the legitimacy of paternalistic decisions, and the criticism of patients' stigmatization due to the disease. The common target that the authors in this volume pursue is to reflect on dementia from the perspectives of different disciplines. They aim at thinking beyond the boundaries of specific academic disciplines in order to bring philosophy and literary and cultural studies into a fruitful conversation about dementia and the challenges it entails for the individual and for society. These disciplines share an interest not only in the topic's relevance for society but also in its moral implications. Whereas analytic philosophy analyses ethical questions through abstractions, literature conducts ethical enquiries by means of exemplifying individual cases. Selected essays in applied philosophy, for example, examine how far traditional philosophical concepts, such as the concept of 'personhood' and its ethical implications, bear relevance for the discourse on dementia. In addition to analysing the aesthetic possibilities of representing subjective experiences of dementia, the articles on literary and cultural representations of the disease examine the potential of dementia narratives to inspire the reader to ethical reflections on moral and social challenges arising from dementia and Alzheimer's disease. It is through this combination of the abstract and the concrete that the essays intend to stimulate interdisciplinary discussions beyond the medical sphere. The volume thereby aims to contribute to a discourse on dementia that transcends the current debate, which is still strongly dominated by medical interests and insights.

Due to the volume's interdisciplinary approach to dementia, the following articles are thematically bundled into four topics. Some *introductory contributions* give insights into the articles' main focuses, questions and theoretical approaches. The second subject area concentrates on the intersection of *dementia and narrativity*. It examines how literary representations of the disease and its aesthetic strategies give insights into patients' subjective experiences, feelings and thoughts and how literature is able to create counterfactual knowledge about dementia and its sufferers, which undermines hegemonic perspectives on the disease and structures of marginalization resulting from this point of view. While the third part deals with *media representations of the disease*, which – especially in the last few years – have become an indispensable component of the discourse on dementia, the last part highlights fundamental *philosophical issues* arising from the controversy over dementia as a field of research.

The Contributions in this Volume

In her article "Lebensgeschichte und personale Identität bei Demenz", Martina Schmidhuber criticises classic concepts of personal identity in the tradition of John Locke: Accounts which emphasize the importance of reminiscence and of a rational understanding of one's previous life are incompatible with the symptoms of dementia. Declining mental abilities complicate the performance of those character traits which are, for Locke, necessary for ascribing the status of personhood to an individual. To face this, Schmidhuber points to the biography of the person concerned and to narrative aspects: By re-telling their life stories the diachronic identity of dementia patients can be maintained.

Against the background of long-established philosophical criteria to evaluate personhood, like rationality and self-consciousness, Johanna Zeisberg examines ethical reflections on the criteria of personhood in contemporary American, German and Hungarian fiction. In her essay "Verortungen des Selbst in Demenznarrationen der Gegenwart" she reflects on traditional views on personal identity and strategies of outlining alternative criteria that outlive advanced stages of dementia in novels, autobiographical narrations and short stories by Jonathan Franzen, Péter Farkas, Sibylle Knauss and Ulrike Draesner.

Bettina Rabelhofer's essay "Ich – das sind die Anderen. Erzählen von Demenz, Alter und Tod" is focused on the significance of intersubjectivity and the 'other's' role in conveying a demented person's point of view. Regarding examples from contemporary German-language literature, like Arno Geiger's popular autobiographical narration *Der alte König in seinem Exil*, she highlights the double transformation of the non-assimilated and non-symbolized mental contents the 'other' has to accomplish. While the real communication with the patient has to be managed mentally on the one hand, the content has to be transformed poetically through the aesthetic representation in literature. Rabelhofer assumes that the aesthetic representation of the neurodegenerative disease may be judged ambivalently. Though it intends to give insights into the demented person's imagination, it might be seen as an artistic exploitation of symbols that may remain inaccurate but are seized upon due to the need for expression.

In her contribution "Zum Verhältnis von Subjektivität und Sprache in Arno Geigers *Der alte König in seinem Exil*" Leonie Süwolto examines the difficulties the progressing speechlessness of dementia sufferers means to literary representations, especially from a narratological point of view. In terms of postcolonial theory she offers a critical approach to the role of narrators who often appear as translators of a demented person's enigmatic perspective in contemporary literature. The significance of translation can be judged critically because it stigmatises dementia sufferers as the 'others' of the predominant ratio-based subject. Regarding Arno Geiger's autobiographical text about his father's disease *Der alte König in seinem Exil* the methodological approach allows to unveil the hierarchical order of the demented subject and the narrator who serves as the mediator of an apparently unintelligible perspective. The simulated inner perspective of the demented protagonist in Geiger's text, which seems to overcome the hierarchical implications of translations, is clearly marked as a generous gesture of letting someone speak for him- or herself. Therefore it reinforces the hierarchical disparity between the patient and the mediator.

Against the background of narrative ethics Sara Strauss' contribution examines in how far innovative narrative techniques, such as a combination of traditional narrative situations with second person narrative situation and a fragmentation of the narrative, can imitate the disoriented mind of a dementia patient. By analysing Alice LaPlante's novel *Turn of Mind*, the article exemplifies how these narrative techniques create narrative empathy with the fictional characters and how literature is thereby able to stimulate the reader to ethical reflections on dementia and the challenges it poses to society.

Elaine Lux' essay elaborates on the importance of memory for a person's coherent narrative identity and on the challenges the loss of coherence resulting from memory loss poses to the artistic representation through narrative. Her analyses and comparisons of Alice Munro's short story "The Bear Came over the Mountain", Elie Wiesel's novel *The Forgotten* and Lisa Genova's novel *Still Alice* convey how these narratives meet the artistic challenges effectively. Moreover, in her analyses Lux does not only show how the authors narrate a story that the protagonists can no longer tell but also how, within the fictional world, family members of the dementia sufferers become agents who "treasure[ ] the narrative self for the memory-deprived person" (Lux, 117).

Alexander Schwieren's contribution draws comparisons between the focus on death and the dead during premodern times and contemporary society's preoccupation with old age and the elderly. In his article Alexander Schwieren analyses the use of metaphors of death and dying in contemporary literature about dementia. He thereby shows in how far dementia narratives relate to the (mental and imminent physical) absence of the dementia patient and thereby address the transience of human life.

Letizia Malottke's article "Lücken, Listen, Lexikonausschnitte. Die literarische Demenz-Darstellung in Max Frischs *Der Mensch erscheint im Holozän*" examines the literary treatment of dementia in Max Frisch's text. It focuses on the aesthetic and narratological dimensions of representing the neurodegenerative disease through fiction. Frisch creates a collage of quotations and text extracts from dictionary-documents to picture the protagonist's specific technique for retaining his knowledge and memory. His poetic strategy outlines vividly the desperate struggle of demented persons who fight against their fading memory while the specific narrative situation highlights the painful inner struggle of the story's protagonist as well.

In addition to these articles on the representation of dementia in literary texts, Jarmila Mildorf examines the representation of dementia in the media. Her article analyses the media coverage about Margaret Thatcher's illness as well as its representation in the movie *The Iron Lady*. From her analysis of the particular case of Margaret Thatcher's dementia and its representation in the media Mildorf is able to draw conclusions about the way in which the discourse on this topic is constructed in the media more generally. Thereby she convincingly argues that the stories reported and their metaphorical illustration "shape social perceptions and thus potentially perpetuate stereotypes and the stigma attached to dementia" (Mildorf, 161).

One of the most threatening effects of dementia is the experience of forgetting or losing one's self. In her contribution entitled "Selbst-Vergessen. Über den Umgang mit demenzbedingten Erfahrungen des Selbstverlusts", Katharina Bauer discusses concepts of coping with this experience. Based on the example of Arno Geiger's narrative about his father her paper suggests aiming at a joint re-interpretation of the patient's personality. With reference to Geiger's novel, Bauer indicates that the personality of dementia patients is conceived as a twofold concept which contains dialogic-poetic elements as well as social interactions. This literary interpretation is combined with philosophical analyses, especially with an examination of Michael Quante's and Harry Frankfurt's accounts on personhood. By integrating and modifying these concepts, Katharina Bauer argues that changes in character which dementia patients and their relatives are confronted with should be regarded as a change, but not as a loss of personality.

In her article "Dementia, Autonomy and Practical Selfhood" Daniela Ringkamp deals with the personhood of dementia patients and argues for a weaker sense of diachronic unity as a person-making characteristic which is mainly based on self-relations. Instead of memory achievements, which are often mentioned in traditional accounts of personal identity, the personhood of dementia patients should be constituted by volitions, which are – to a minimal degree – forward-looking and can still be performed in the later stages of the disease. The starting point for her analysis is Jeff McMahan's concept of time-relative interests. McMahan's approach does not only allow for a theoretical analysis of the personhood of dementia patients, but also concerns ethical implications concerning their decision-making in practical contexts.

Oliver Hallich's contribution "Dementia and the Principle of Precedent Autonomy" points to the justificatory role of advanced directives as a means of determining the interests of patients with dementia. In a detailed analysis of the underlying conditions of the 'dominance thesis', which supports the overridingness of previous critical interests, Hallich questions the moral binding force of these interests. In some – not in all – conflict cases, it is legitimate to disregard previous interests and to endorse experiential interests as an expression of the current wishes of the persons concerned. This conclusion is also compatible with some objections which point to the qualitative difference between critical and experiential interests or to an asymmetry of cognitive capacities, which is given in the distinct situations of previous and current decision-making. In sum, Hallich's limitation of the normative authority of precedent interests strengthens the experiential subjective status of patients with dementia.

In her article "Releasing Prisoners with Dementia: Could there be a Recollection Requirement for Expressivist and Communicative Justifications of Punishment?" Annette Dufner discusses a problem which increasingly concerns criminal law and ethics. In the case of offenders suffering from dementia a retrospective access to the crime which has been committed before the now demented person turned ill is often impossible. With reference to philosophical concepts of punishment Dufner holds that in these cases the offenders should not be penalized at all. Annette Dufner's contribution, like Sara Strauss' analysis of a literary example, pursues the question of dementia patients' responsibility for actions that they can no longer remember.

Acknowledgements

This volume goes back to the conference "Dementia and Subjectivity. Aesthetic, Literary and Philosophical Perspectives", which took place at the University of Paderborn in November 2015. Therefore we would like to say a few words of thanks to those institutions and people who contributed significantly to the success of the conference.

First of all we are greatly indebted to the Faculty of Arts and Humanities of the University of Paderborn, to its Kommission für Forschung und wissenschaftlichen

Nachwuchs as well as to the Universitätsgesellschaft Paderborn e.V. for their generous financial support, which made the event possible. Our thanks also go to the Deutscher Akademikerinnenbund e.V. (DAB) for their donation. In addition we express our gratitude to the Deutsche Alzheimer Gesellschaft e.V. for their support in terms of ideas and the provided information material.

Furthermore we like to express our appreciation to all the speakers for their inspiring speeches, the stimulating and fruitful discussions during the conference as well as for their contributions to this volume and the smooth cooperation during the preparation of this book.

We also would like to thank our colleague Lisa Ahrens, who kindly helped us with the organisation and realisation of the conference, as well as Sophie Andersen and Sahra Puscher for their assistance in preparing this volume.

Last but not least we would like to thank the Peter Lang Publishing Group especially Michael Rücker and Dr. Sebastian Schmitt for the professional cooperation during the development of this book.

Magdeburg and Paderborn, March 2017 — Daniela Ringkamp, Sara Strauss and Leonie Süwolto

References

Bayley, John. *Iris: A Memoir of Iris Murdoch*. London: Duckworth, 1998.

Birnbacher, Dieter. "Patientenverfügungen und Advance Care Planning bei Demenz und anderen kognitiven Beeinträchtigungen." In: *Ethik in der Medizin*. Berlin/Heidelberg: Springer-Verlag, 2016. DOI 10.1007/s00481-016-0388-6.

Buchanan, Allen E., Brock, Dan W. *Deciding for Others. The Ethics of Surrogate Decision Making*. Cambridge/New York: Cambridge University Press, 1990.

Crayton, Harry. "From Childhood to Childhood? Autonomy and Dependence through the Ages of Life." In: Julian Hughes, Stephen Louw, Stephen R. Sabat (eds.). *Dementia: Mind, Meaning, and the Person*. New York: Oxford University Press, 2006, 277–86.

DeGrazia, David. *Human Identity and Bioethics*. Cambridge/New York: Cambridge University Press, 2005.

Draesner, Ulrike. "Ichs Heimweg macht alles allein." In: Clara Obermüller (ed.). *Es schneit in meinem Kopf. Erzählungen über Alzheimer und Demenz*. Zürich: Nagel & Kimche, 2006, 59–81.

Dresser, Rebecca. "Dworkin on Dementia: Elegant Theory, Questionable Policy." In: *The Hastings Center Report* 25,6 (1995): 32–38.

Dworkin, Ronald. *Life's Dominion. An Argument About Abortion, Euthanasia, and Individual Freedom*. New York: Vintage Books, 1993, 218–42.

Dworkin, Ronald. "Autonomy and the Demented Self." In: *The Milbank Quarterly* 64,2 (1986): 4–16.

Farkas, Péter. *Acht Minuten*. München: Luchterhand Literaturverlag, 2011.

Franzen, Jonathan. *The Corrections*. New York: Farrar Straus & Giroux, 2001.

Franzen, Jonathan. "My Father's Brain." In: *The New Yorker* 10.09.2001.

Freiburg, Rudolf, Kretzschmar, Dirk. "Einleitung: Grau-Werte." In: Rudolf Freiburg, Dirk Kretzschmar (eds.), *Alter(n) in Literatur und Kultur der Gegenwart*. Würzburg: Königshausen & Neumann, 2010, 1–30.

Geiger, Arno. *Der alte König in seinem Exil*. München: Hanser, 2011.

Hallich, Oliver. "Selbstbindung und medizinischer Paternalismus: Zum normativen Status von 'Odysseus-Anweisungen.'" In: *Zeitschrift für philosophische Forschung* 65,2 (2011): 151–72.

Hughes, Julian C. *Thinking through Dementia*. New York: Oxford University Press, 2011.

Jaworska, Agnieszka. "Respecting the Margins of Agency: Alzheimer's Patients and the Capacity to Value." In: *Philosophy and Public Affairs* 28,2 (1999): 105–38.

Klare, Jörn. *Als meine Mutter ihre Küche nicht mehr fand. Vom Wert des Lebens mit Demenz*. Berlin: Suhrkamp, ²2012.

Körtner, Ulrich H. J. "Das Menschenbild der Leistungsgesellschaft und die Irritation Demenz." In: *Zeitschrift für medizinische Ethik: Wissenschaft, Kultur, Religion*, 58,1 (2012): 3–33.

Kurz, Alexander, Freter, Hans Jürgen, Saxl, Susanna, Nickel, Ellen (eds.). *Demenz. Das Wichtigste. Ein kompakter Ratgeber*. Berlin: Deutsche Alzheimer Gesellschaft e.V., ²2016.

Lesser, Harry A. "Dementia and Personal Identity." In: Julian Hughes, Stephen Louw, Stephen R. Sabat (eds.). *Dementia: Mind, Meaning, and the Person*. New York: Oxford University Press, 2006, 55–61.

McEwan, Ian. *Atonement*. London: Jonathan Cape, 2001.

McMillan, John. "Identity, Self, and Dementia." In: Julian Hughes, Stephen Louw, Stephen R. Sabat (eds.). *Dementia: Mind, Meaning, and the Person*. New York: Oxford University Press, 2006, 63–70.

Munro, Alice. "The Bear Came over the Mountain." In: Alice Munro. *Hateship, Friendship, Courtship, Loveship, Marriage*. London: Chatto & Windus, 2001, 275–323.

Rees, Glenn. "Foreword." In: Alzheimer's Disease International (ed.). *World Alzheimer Report 2016 – Improving Healthcare for People Living with Dementia.* London: Alzheimer's Disease International, 2016, i.

Schmidhuber, Martina. "Ethische Probleme der Patientenverfügung bei Demenzbetroffenen." In: *Ethica. Wissenschaft und Verantwortung* 22,2 (2014): 121–37.

Sturma, Dieter. "Ethische Überlegungen zum Umgang mit demenziell erkrankten Personen." In: Olivia Dibelius, Wolfgang Maier (eds.). *Versorgungsforschung für demenziell erkrankte Menschen. Health Service Research for People with Dementia.* Stuttgart: Kohlhammer, 2011, 93–98.

Suter, Martin. *Small World.* Zürich: Diogenes, 1999.

Swinnen, Aagje, Schweda, Mark. "Popularizing Dementia. Public Expressions and Representations of Forgetfulness." In: Aagje Swinnen, Mark Schweda (eds.). *Popularizing Dementia. Public Expressions and Representations of Forgetfulness.* Bielefeld: transcript, 2015, 9–20.

Wetzstein, Verena. "Alzheimer-Demenz – Entstehung eines Krankheitsbegriffes." In: Nationaler Ethikrat (ed.). *Altersdemenz und Morbus Alzheimer – Medizinische, gesellschaftliche und ethische Herausforderungen.* Berlin: Nationaler Ethikrat, 2006.

Martina Schmidhuber (Erlangen-Nürnberg)

Lebensgeschichte und personale Identität bei Demenz

Abstract: Philosophers discuss the question if people with dementia lose their personal identity. In traditional philosophy John Locke's definition of personal identity dominates, which emphasizes rationality, knowledge of past, present and future and self-consciousness. However, Locke's understanding of personal identity is not fruitful for people with dementia. I argue that personal identity is the biography of persons, also of persons with dementia. If we look at the biography of people with dementia, we can find out what is worthwhile and important for them.

Zu personaler Identität gibt es viele verschiedene philosophische Theorien, sowohl aus metaphysischer als auch aus praktischer Perspektive. So verschieden die Ansätze auch sein mögen, es eint sie die Fragestellung, was es denn ist, das die Person P zu Zeitpunkt 1 identisch sein lässt mit jener zum Zeitpunkt 2. Ist es ihre Erinnerung? Ihre Lebensgeschichte? Ihr Körper? Gedankenexperimente, die Körper- und Kopftransplantation zum Inhalt haben, versuchen, sich der Lösung, was die Identität von Personen ausmacht, zu nähern.[1]

Im folgenden Beitrag soll diese schwierige Frage auf Menschen mit Demenz angewandt werden: Gibt es etwas, das bei Menschen mit Demenz ihre personale Identität ausmacht, oder muss von einem Verlust der Identität aufgrund der Erkrankung ausgegangen werden? Zunächst wird im ersten Abschnitt kurz erläutert, was Demenz bedeutet bzw. welche Veränderungen mit dieser Erkrankung verbunden sind. Dann wird gezeigt, dass die klassischen philosophischen Überlegungen Menschen mit Demenz ihre Identität absprechen, weil diese sich auf Merkmale stützen, die Menschen mit Demenz nicht (mehr) aufweisen. Wie der Titel des Beitrags schon andeutet, werde ich argumentieren, dass personale Identität vor allem bei Demenz an die Lebensgeschichte geknüpft werden sollte.

1 Vgl. den Überblick zur Debatte von Gasser, Georg. "Einleitung: Zum Verhältnis von personaler Identität und praktischer Rationalität." In: Ders., Schmidhuber, Martina (eds.). *Personale Identität, Narrativität und Praktische Rationalität. Die Einheit der Person aus metaphysischer und praktischer Perspektive*. Münster: Mentis, 2013, 11–37.

I. Demenz – Ein Überblick

Alzheimer, benannt nach dem Entdecker der Krankheit, Alois Alzheimer (1864–1915), ist die häufigste Demenz-Form, die unabhängig von Bildung und Lebensstil jeden treffen kann. Vaskuläre Demenz ist die zweithäufigste Form der Erkrankung. Aber auch durch Alkoholmissbrauch, durch welchen das Gehirn geschädigt wird, kann eine Demenz verursacht werden. Ca. 60 Prozent der Menschen mit Demenz sind von Alzheimer betroffen.[2] Auch Mischformen sind möglich. Wenn im Folgenden von Demenz die Rede ist, ist damit die Alzheimer-Demenz gemeint, die aufgrund ihrer Häufigkeit hier im Zentrum stehen soll.

Die Alzheimer-Erkrankung wird vor allem mit Schmerz, Leid, dem Verlust der eigenen Persönlichkeit und der Abnahme von Lebensqualität in Verbindung gebracht. Alzheimer-Demenz ist eine Erkrankung, die von vielen als „Schreckgespenst" bezeichnet wird, von der jeder hofft, dass seine Angehörigen und er selbst von ihr verschont bleiben.[3] Nicht nur für die Erkrankten selbst, sondern auch für die (pflegenden) Angehörigen ist Alzheimer eine große Herausforderung und Belastung. Der nahestehende, an Demenz erkrankte Mensch verändert sich und kann sich immer weniger an die eigene Lebensgeschichte und die für ihn wichtigen Personen erinnern. Manchmal wird deswegen von einem Verlust der Identität gesprochen.[4]

Der Verlauf der Erkrankung wird grob in drei Stadien eingeteilt: (1) Im Frühstadium nimmt die Gedächtnisleistung kontinuierlich ab, Gegenstände werden verlegt, starke Stimmungsschwankungen fallen auf und die Orientierungsfähigkeit lässt nach. Die Probleme im Alltag werden vom Betroffenen selbst wahrgenommen, was ihn belastet und in weiterer Folge zu Depressionen führen kann.[5] (2) Im mittleren Stadium verstärken sich die Schwierigkeiten in der selbständigen

---

2 Maier, Wolfgang, Schulz, Jörg B., Weggen, Sascha, Wolf, Stefanie. *Alzheimer & Demenzen verstehen. Diagnose, Behandlung, Alltag, Betreuung.* Stuttgart: Trias, 2011, 23.

3 Der ehemalige britische Premierminister David Cameron bezeichnete beim G8-Demenzgipfel die Demenz als „die Pest des 21. Jahrhunderts". Vgl. Drzezga, Alexander, Sabri, Osama, Fellgiebel, Andreas. "Amyloid-Bildgebung: Reif für die Routine?" In: *Deutsches Ärzteblatt* 26 (2014): 1206–10, 1208.

4 Maier et al. *Alzheimer & Demenzen verstehen*, 110.

5 Vgl. zur Komorbidität von Demenz und Depression: Legal, Friederike, Preuss, Dirk. "Künstliche Intelligenz zur Überwachung von Verhalten? Ethische Erwägungen zu Detektionssystemen für demenzbedingte Veränderungsprozesse." In: Andreas Frewer, Lutz Bergemann, Martina Schmidhuber (eds.). *Demenz und Ethik in der Medizin. Standards zur guten klinischen Praxis.* Würzburg: Königshausen & Neumann, 2015, 23–48, 25.

Lebensführung. Im Alltag wird Hilfe zum Einkaufen, Kochen, Benutzen von Verkehrsmitteln, etc. benötigt, was beim Betroffenen angesichts seiner Hilflosigkeit Aggressionen auslösen kann.[6] (3) Im schweren Stadium verlieren Menschen mit Demenz ihre verbalen und motorischen Fähigkeiten, sodass sie gewaschen, gefüttert und angekleidet werden müssen. Vertraute Personen werden nicht mehr erkannt und/oder ihre Namen vergessen. Die Patienten werden oftmals bettlägerig und müssen künstlich ernährt werden.[7]

Die Erkrankung ist in jener Phase, in der der Betroffene merkt, dass er immer mehr vergisst, seine Orientierungsfähigkeit abnimmt und er mit seinem Alltag überfordert ist, besonders bedrückend. Er kann das Gefühl haben, sich selbst resp. seine Identität zu verlieren. Als „gnädige Schwelle" wird jener Punkt der Erkrankung bezeichnet, ab dem der Betroffene vergisst, dass er vergisst. Für die Angehörigen jedoch, die den Betroffenen in allen Phasen der Erkrankung begleiten, endet damit das Leid keineswegs. Bis hin zum letzten Stadium der Erkrankung ist der Verlauf für sie schmerzhaft.

Angesichts der Symptome und des Verlaufs der Erkrankung scheint es naheliegend, dass Menschen mit Demenz tatsächlich ihre Identität verlieren. Wie sehr es aber auf das Identitätsverständnis ankommt, das man zugrunde legt, soll im folgenden Abschnitt gezeigt werden.

II. Personale Identität im klassischen Philosophieverständnis

In der klassischen Philosophie hat John Locke (1632–1704) ein Verständnis von Identität vorgelegt, das den Begriff der Person voraussetzt. Eine Person zu sein impliziert nach Locke die Fähigkeit zum Selbst-Bewusstsein. Menschsein hingegen ist Locke zufolge nur an die Biologie des Körpers gebunden, es hat nichts mit mentalen Zuständen zu tun. Um nun Identität ausbilden zu können, muss man über Selbst-Bewusstsein im Sinne Lockes verfügen. Eine Person ist nach Locke ein „denkendes, verständiges Wesen, das Vernunft und Überlegung besitzt und sich selbst als sich selbst betrachten kann".[8] Die Person, die sich als rationales Wesen Gedanken über sich machen kann und auch will, ist aufgrund ihrer Erfahrung des „Sich-selbst-gleich-Bleibens"[9] identisch. Sie kann sich „zu verschiedenen Zeiten

---

6 Vgl. Maier et al. *Alzheimer & Demenzen verstehen,* 120.

7 Vgl. Maier et al. *Alzheimer & Demenzen verstehen,* 33–39.

8 Locke, John. *Versuch über den menschlichen Verstand.* Hamburg: Meiner, 1981, 419.

9 Locke. *Versuch über den menschlichen Verstand*, 420.

und an verschiedenen Orten“[10] als dieselbe denken. Das Selbst-Bewusstsein ermöglicht es ihr, sich als eine Einheit denken zu können.

Auf den ersten Blick scheint es durchaus sinnvoll und plausibel, Kriterien für personale Identität an Erinnerung, Gedächtnis und (Selbst-)Bewusstsein zu knüpfen. Wenn wir uns aufgrund unseres Gedächtnisses an die Vergangenheit erinnern, diese mit der Gegenwart verknüpfen können und uns dessen bewusst sind, scheint dies ein klares Indiz dafür zu sein, dass die frühere Person mit der gegenwärtigen identisch ist oder zumindest sehr viel mit dieser zu tun hat.

Auch Autoren anderer Disziplinen übernehmen dieses Verständnis wie selbstverständlich, etwa die Juristin Dorothea Magnus:

> Die Entscheidungsfähigkeit ist in jedem Fall dann ausgeschlossen, wenn der Betroffene sich in seiner Umgebung nicht mehr orientieren kann, ihm das Gefühl nach Zeit und Ort fehlt und er seine Identität nicht mehr kennt.[11]

Oder aus einem Beitrag zur Musiktherapie für Menschen mit Demenz:

> In der Betreuung demenziell Erkrankter sind emotionale Unterstützungsangebote besonders wichtig, die es den Patient*innen immer wieder ermöglichen, eine Verbindung zu sich selbst und ihrem sozialen Umfeld zu schaffen, stellt doch der Verlust der Erinnerung eine zentrale Bedrohung der eigenen Identität dar.[12]

Es wird deutlich, dass die Antwort auf die Frage, was bei Menschen mit Demenz ihre Identität ausmacht, vor allem damit zusammenhängt, wie man Identität versteht. Die locke'schen Fähigkeiten, die wir gesunden Personen durchaus zuschreiben und vermutlich auch als essentiell für ihre Identität anerkennen würden, gehen bei Menschen mit Demenz im Zuge der Erkrankung verloren. Sie sind sich ihrer selbst immer weniger bewusst. Es ist ab einem gewissen Zeitpunkt der Erkrankung auch nicht mehr möglich, sich in der Vor- oder Rückschau diachron zu verschiedenen Zeiten an verschiedenen Orten als dieselbe Person zu verstehen. Das zeigt sich vor allem daran, dass sich Menschen mit Demenz häufig plötzlich sehr gut an ihre Kindheit erinnern, viel davon erzählen und scheinbar in ihrer

---

10 Locke. *Versuch über den menschlichen Verstand*, 419.

11 Magnus, Dorothea. “Sterbehilfe und Demenz.” In: *Neue Zeitschrift für Strafrecht* 1,33 (2013): 1–6, 2.

12 Fröhlich-Güzelsoy, Leyla. “Musik- und Erinnerungstherapie bei demenziell erkrankten Patient*innen mit Migrationsgeschichte. Ethische Desiderate der Demenzbehandlung.” In: Andreas Frewer, Lutz Bergemann, Martina Schmidhuber (eds.). *Demenz und Ethik in der Medizin. Standards zur guten klinischen Praxis*. Würzburg: Königshausen & Neumann 2015, 73–95, 85.

Kindheit leben.[13] Wenn beispielsweise eine 85 Jahre alte Dame mit Demenz im Seniorenheim auf ihre Mutter wartet, macht dies deutlich, dass sie sich in ihre Kindheit zurückversetzt fühlt. Darüber hinaus ist es auch nicht mehr möglich, vernünftige Überlegungen und Entscheidungen von Menschen mit Demenz zu erwarten. Sie handeln impulsiv und haben auch nicht mehr die Fähigkeit, über Konsequenzen ihrer Handlungen nachzudenken. Vor allem das, was ein Leben lang unterdrückt wurde, und auch bestimmte gesellschaftliche Konventionen, an die man sich hielt, spielen teilweise keine Rolle mehr.[14]

Das Identitätsverständnis, das aus der klassischen Philosophie kommt, so lässt sich konstatieren, kann also nicht auf Menschen mit Demenz angewandt werden. Nun stellt sich die Frage, ob Identität auch so aufgefasst werden kann, dass dies nicht der Fall ist. Hängt Identität tatsächlich vor allem von Gedächtnisleistungen, Erinnerung und Rationalität ab?[15]

III. Lebensgeschichte als personale Identität

Wenn sich unsere Lebensumstände ändern, passen wir uns ihnen an. Ein Jobwechsel bedeutet häufig auch einen Wechsel des Wohnortes, das Ende einer Beziehung zwingt Menschen dazu, ihr Leben neu zu sortieren, ein unerfüllter Kinderwunsch verlangt eine Umorientierung im Privaten. Biografien sind permanent mit unvorhersehbaren Veränderungen verbunden, mit denen Menschen zurechtkommen müssen. So ist auch eine Krankheit ein solches Ereignis, das an Veränderungen geknüpft ist. Das Leben muss neu ausgerichtet und geplant werden. Aber genau

---

13 Martin Suter arbeitet dieses Thema in seinem Roman *Small World* auf und verknüpft damit eine Kriminalgeschichte, die sich in der Kindheit des von Demenz Betroffenen abgespielt hat: Suter, Martin. *Small World*. Zürich: Diogenes, 1999.

14 Zum Beispiel Frauen, die besonders auf ihre Figur achteten, essen plötzlich leidenschaftlich gerne (vgl. Zander-Schneider, Gabriela. *Sind Sie meine Tochter? Leben mit meiner demenzkranken Mutter*. Reinbek bei Hamburg: rororo, 2011, 31.) Auch hinsichtlich Sexualität und Sprache (Kraftausdrücke) ist dies bei Menschen mit Demenz zu beobachten. Vgl. auch Birnbacher, Dieter. "Patientenverfügungen und Advance Care Planning bei Demenz und anderen kognitiven Beeinträchtigungen." In: *Ethik in der Medizin:* Berlin/Heidelberg: Springer-Verlag, 2016. DOI 10.1007/s00481-016-0388-6

15 Vgl. dazu die Debatte zwischen Ronald Dworkin und Rebecca Dresser, die Oliver Hallich in diesem Band darstellt und meine Überlegungen in: "Gedächtnis und Erinnerung als Bedingungen personaler Identität? Überlegungen am Beispiel von Demenzbetroffenen." In: Danièle Moyal-Dharrock, Volker A. Munz, Annalisa Coliva (eds.). *Geist, Sprache und Handlung. Beiträge zum 36. Internationalen Ludwig Wittgenstein-Symposium*, Neulengbach 2013, 353–55.

diese Veränderungen, die wir nicht beeinflussen können, sind auch ein Teil der Identität einer Person. Nicht nur die Ziele, die eine Person selbst festlegt, sagen etwas über sie aus, sondern auch das, was ihr im Leben widerfährt und wie sie damit umgeht.[16] Die Biografie der Person, ihre ganze Lebensgeschichte macht ihre Identität aus. Die Person ist mit sich selbst identisch, weil sie diese eine individuelle Lebensgeschichte hat.

Dieses Verständnis von Identität ist ein narratives: Menschen erzählen die Geschichte ihres Lebens, in der kleinere und größere Veränderungen vorkommen. Ebenso kann es aufgrund bestimmter Ereignisse Brüche geben. So ist dies bei Demenz insbesondere der Fall, wie die Biografie von Walter Jens exemplarisch zeigt. Der einst berühmte Rhetorikprofessor, der sich als Mann des Wortes und der Sprache verstand, verlor genau diese Fähigkeiten aufgrund der Erkrankung. Er konnte sich nur noch auf eine kindliche Art und Weise verbal ausdrücken und verlernte, zu lesen und zu schreiben. Dennoch ist auch dies Teil seiner Lebensgeschichte, die als ganze betrachtet werden muss:

> The narrative approach can be understood as a way of retrieving and continuing a person's preferences, but it also challenges us to look at a person's life as a whole, and make an over-all assessment of that life.[17]

Menschen entwickeln sich in ihrer Persönlichkeit im Laufe des Lebens. Persönlichkeit entsteht erst durch Veränderungen und diese müssen in die Biografie eingebaut werden; dabei spielt auch die Sozialisation des Individuums eine maßgebliche Rolle.[18] Hier ist es also wesentlich, den Unterschied zwischen der Identität der Person und der Identität der Persönlichkeit zu berücksichtigen. Die Person bleibt in ihrer numerischen Identität „dieselbe von der Wiege bis zur Bahre",[19] wie Dieter Birnbacher dies auf den Punkt bringt. Die Persönlichkeit verändert sich aber im Laufe des Lebens der Person aufgrund ihrer Erlebnisse, Widerfahrnisse und Erfahrungen. Eine Person, deren Persönlichkeit sich nicht verändern würde, würde sich nicht weiterentwickeln.

---

16 Vgl. dazu auch Schmidhuber, Martina. *Der Prozess personaler Identitätsbildung und die Rolle von Institutionen. Eine philosophisch-anthropologische Untersuchung*. Münster: LIT, 2011.

17 Schermer, Maartje. "In Search of 'the Good Life' for Demented Elderly." In: *Medicine, Health Care and Philosophy* 6 (2003): 35–44, 40.

18 Vgl. Quante, Michael. *Person*. Berlin: de Gruyter, 2012, 176.

19 Vgl. Birnbacher. "Patientenverfügungen und Advance Care Planning bei Demenz und anderen kognitiven Beeinträchtigungen." In: *Ethik in der Medizin:* DOI 10.1007/s00481-016-0388-6

Eine Erkrankung wie die Demenz verändert die Persönlichkeit sicher auf drastische Weise, aber dadurch geht die personale Identität von Menschen mit Demenz nicht verloren. Die Persönlichkeitsveränderung ist meistens für die Angehörigen am schmerzhaftesten, weil sie die Person mit der Persönlichkeit aus früheren Zeiten kennen und vermissen.

Menschen sind keine rein rationalen Wesen. Es scheint jedoch nicht unüblich zu sein, das individuelle Leben nach rationalen Maßstäben zu planen, von der Karriere bis zur Familie. Allerdings kann es aufgrund nicht beeinflussbarer äußerer Umstände auch anders als geplant verlaufen und auch das ist dann Teil der individuellen Identität, die den Menschen prägt.

Diese Rationalisierung von Menschen und die Betonung, dass es sich dabei um etwas Wünschenswertes handelt, ist bereits früh in der Geschichte der Philosophie erkennbar, wie in der Stoa bei Epiktet. Hier gilt der Geist als das Wesentliche im Menschen, die lange Beschäftigung mit körperlichen Dingen kennzeichnet hingegen den „Unedlen“:

> Es ist das Merkmal einer gemeinen Natur, wenn einer bei körperlichen Dingen lange verweilt, z.B. lange turnt, lange ißt, lange trinkt, lange abseits geht, lange beim Weibe bleibt. Solches sollte man vielmehr nur nebenher tun; auf den Geist dagegen verwende man seine ganze Sorgfalt.[20]

Aufgrund dieser Ratio-Zentrierung, die in der westlichen Gesellschaft prägend ist, wird häufig vergessen, dass Menschen darüber hinaus auch körperliche Wesen sind. Nicht nur das, was Menschen aus rationalen Gründen entscheiden, macht sie aus, sondern auch das, was sie fühlen resp. was ihre körperlichen Bedürfnisse sind. Besonders drastisch zeigt sich dies in Fällen von Essstörungen, bei welchen die (häufig) jungen Mädchen ihre Identität am eigenen Körper festmachen. Die Gestaltbarkeit des Körpers mittels Verweigerung der Nahrungsaufnahme vermittelt das trügerische Gefühl der Kontrolle über sich selbst: „Der Körper wird damit zum Dreh- und Angelpunkt im Ringen um eine eigene Identität.“[21]

Menschen bestehen also nicht nur aus ihren mentalen Zuständen wie Rationalität und Erinnerungsvermögen, sondern haben auch eine leibliche Wahrnehmung und Gefühle. Im Zustand der Demenz, wenn die intellektuellen Fähigkeiten immer mehr in den Hintergrund treten, zeigt sich die leibliche Beschaffenheit besonders deutlich. Nahrungsaufnahme, menschliche Nähe, das Streicheln von

20 Epiktet. *Das Buch vom geglückten Leben.* Köln: Anaconda Verlag, 2005, 53.

21 Stahr, Ingeborg. “Frauen-Körper-Identität im Kontext gesellschaftlicher Modernisierung.” In: Doris Janshen (ed.). *Blickwechsel. Der neue Dialog zwischen Frauen- und Männerforschung.* Frankfurt/Main: Campus-Verlag, 2000, 81–105, 84.

Tieren, etc. werden für viele Menschen mit Demenz immer wichtiger. Einige Autoren warnen davor, ein Leben mit Demenz als schönes Leben jenseits des intellektuellen Tunnelblicks zu verstehen, weil nur noch leiblicher Genuss im Vordergrund steht.[22] Das kann und soll hier auch gar nicht geschehen, denn niemand kann sich vorstellen, wie es sich anfühlt, dement zu sein, wenn er es nicht selbst ist. Nachvollziehbar ist jedoch, dass der Leib der Person mit Demenz Teil ihrer Identität bleibt:

> In regard to this question an anthropology of the bodily existence of human beings argues that the bodily presence of a person with dementia, his or her bodily acting, confronts us with a personal identity which morally binds us to respect the desires of these persons. Even though the mental capabilities vanish, the self of the person remains. What vanishes is one aspect of his or her bodily identity, but the other aspects remain and in those we are still confronted with the identity of the person.[23]

Personen sind darüber hinaus üblicherweise in ein soziales Umfeld eingebettet. Andere Menschen prägen das Leben des Einzelnen von Anfang an. In besonders vulnerablen Situationen des Lebens ist man stärker auf andere angewiesen, wie etwa im Kindesalter, während einer Krankheit oder im hohen Alter.[24] Der Austausch mit und die Unterstützung von anderen beeinflusst auch die Lebensgeschichte. Stets gibt es im Leben Personen, die einen besonders geprägt haben, das kann bewusst oder unbewusst geschehen. Diese nahestehenden Personen sind es auch, die die individuelle Lebensgeschichte zu Ende erzählen können, wenn zum Beispiel keine Patientenverfügung vorhanden ist und man sich die Frage stellt, ob der Mensch mit Demenz im schweren Stadium noch künstlich ernährt werden soll. Selbst wenn der von Demenz Betroffene mit einer Patientenverfügung, die immer wieder als wichtiges Instrument zur Selbstbestimmung betont wird, vorgesorgt hat, ist er stets auf die Interpretation der aktuellen Situation und der Patientenverfügung durch andere angewiesen.[25]

---

22 Vgl. Coors, Michael. "A Dementalized Body? Reconsidering the Human Condition in the Light of Dementia." In: *Geriatric Mental Health Care* 1 (2013): 34–38, 38.

23 Coors. "A Dementalized Body? Reconsidering the Human Condition in the Light of Dementia," 38.

24 So konstatieren Hughes und Baldwin: "In the case of people with dementia, [...] the need for *being with* becomes more acute." Hughes, Julian C., Baldwin, Clive. *Ethical Issues in Dementia Care. Making Difficult Decisions.* London: Jessica Kingsley Publishers, 2006, 82. Kursivsetzung im Original.

25 Vgl. Schmidhuber, Martina. "Die Rolle der Patientenverfügung für Menschen mit Demenz." In: *Lebendige Seelsorge* 1 (2015): 49–54, 53.

Die Anforderungen im Pflegealltag übersteigen oft die psychischen und physischen Möglichkeiten der pflegenden Angehörigen. Depressionen, Angst, angespannte Beziehungen zu anderen Familienmitgliedern und ein allgemeines Gefühl der Überforderung können die Folge sein.[26] Studien zeigen jedoch, dass Angehörige die kognitiven Defizite weniger belasten, als die emotionalen Veränderungen.[27] Die Herausforderung bei diesem Verständnis von Identität mit Blick auf Demenz ist deshalb, die Erkrankung als Teil der Lebensgeschichte anzusehen. Es scheint „einfacher" bzw. emotional weniger belastend, die Person mit Demenz als eine andere anzusehen, weil sie nicht mehr an die Person, die man einmal liebte, erinnert. Dabei handelt es sich jedoch weiterhin um dieselbe Person, mit einer aufgrund der Erkrankung stark veränderten Persönlichkeit, wie oben erläutert wurde. Aggressivität, verzweifelte Hilflosigkeit und Gewalt haben auch Walter Jens verändert, der im schlimmsten Fall seine Frau schlug.[28] Inge Jens versuchte sich immer wieder klar zu machen, dass es nicht ihr Mann ist, der sie schlägt, sondern dies durch seine Krankheit hervorgerufen wird. Tilman Jens erzählt: „Meine Mutter sagt verstörend direkt: *Er ist nicht mehr der Mann, den ich liebte.*"[29] Trotz dieser starken Persönlichkeitsveränderung ist es aber immer noch Walter Jens mit seinem Leib und seiner Vergangenheit, der sich nun wegen der Demenzerkrankung, die auch zu seiner Lebensgeschichte gehört, so verhält.

Die personale Identität eines Menschen ist also nichts, was rein von den rationalen Fähigkeiten abhängt. Sowohl der Einfluss von außen, von anderen Menschen, als auch die eigene Leiblichkeit prägen die je individuelle Geschichte. Solange man mitten im Leben steht und dieses scheinbar völlig selbstbestimmt gestaltet, werden die Einflüsse und andere Faktoren nicht so bewusst wahrgenommen. Man denkt, selbst Erzähler der eigenen Geschichte zu sein. Erst in vulnerablen Situationen wird die Abhängigkeit, in der Menschen stehen, deutlich spürbar.[30]

---

26 Vgl. Wetzstein, Verena. *Diagnose Alzheimer. Grundlagen einer Ethik der Demenz.* Frankfurt/Main: Campus, 2005, 203.

27 Vgl. Füsgen, Ingo. *Demenz. Praktischer Umgang mit der Hirnleistungsstörung.* München: Vieweg Verlag, 1995, 96.

28 Vgl. Jens, Tilman. *Demenz. Abschied von meinem Vater.* Gütersloh: Goldmann Verlag, 2009, 10.

29 Jens. *Demenz*, 10. Hervorhebung im Original.

30 U.a. Judith Butler betont immer wieder die grundsätzliche menschliche Vulnerabilität. Vgl. dazu die hilfreiche Darstellung von Butlers Begriff der Vulnerabilität von Pistrol, Florian. "Vulnerabilität. Erläuterungen zu einem Schlüsselbegriff im Denken Judith Butlers." In: *Zeitschrift für Praktische Philosophie* 3,1 (2016): 233–72.

IV. Die Geschichte durch individuell abgestimmte Pflege weitererzählen

Macht man sich diese Abhängigkeit bewusst, ist es auch denkbar, dass während der Demenzerkrankung andere Menschen die Lebensgeschichte des Betroffenen weitererzählen, den Menschen mit Demenz in seiner weiteren Lebensgeschichte begleiten. Dafür ist es erforderlich, die Fürsorge und Pflege an die individuelle Person anzupassen, sie mit ihren Bedürfnissen und Wünschen ernst zu nehmen, aber auch Brüche in der Biografie anzuerkennen und darauf einzugehen. Es reicht nicht aus, die Biografie des Betroffenen zu kennen, weil sich Vorlieben und Wertungen im Laufe der Erkrankung, wie auch bei gesunden Menschen, ändern können. Darüber hinaus ist es erforderlich, die Besonderheit der leiblichen Äußerungen und den meist zunehmenden Wert der menschlichen Nähe zu berücksichtigen.

Erfahrungsberichte von pflegenden Angehörigen können diese Besonderheiten der Fürsorge von Menschen mit Demenz besonders eindrücklich schildern. Deshalb sollen im Folgenden exemplarisch Erlebnisse von Angehörigen zeigen, wie sich die Identität von Menschen mit Demenz mit besonderer Rücksicht auf den sensiblen Umgang mit Brüchen, Erinnerungsarbeit, Leiblichkeit und In-Beziehung-Sein in ihrer Lebensgeschichte wahrnehmen und unterstützen lässt.

Gabriela Zander-Schneider, die ihre demenzkranke Mutter zu Hause pflegte, hat die Herausforderungen, Schwierigkeiten und eigenen Grenzen in ihrem Erfahrungsbericht *Sind Sie meine Tochter? Leben mit meiner alzheimerkranken Mutter* niedergeschrieben. Sie ist anfangs angesichts der Veränderungen im Verhalten und den neuen Vorlieben ihrer Mutter irritiert. So scheint diese, die stets auf ihre Figur achtete, nun das Essen besonders zu genießen. Im gemeinsamen Urlaub stellt Zander-Schneider fest, dass ihre Mutter große Freude an den Mahlzeiten im Hotel hat, sich bei allen Speisen am Buffet bediente und sich auch mehrmals hintereinander Gerichte holte. Sie schien plötzlich nicht mehr die figurbewusste Frau zu sein, die peinlich genau auf Kalorien achtet, sondern vielmehr zu genießen. Das Erstaunlichste für Zander-Schneider war jedoch, dass ihre Mutter immer wieder eine riesige Portion Eis aß, obwohl diese eigentlich kein Eis mochte.[31]

Hier zeigen sich zwei wesentliche Elemente: Zum einen wird deutlich, dass der leibliche Genuss im Augenblick eine große Rolle zu spielen scheint. Das Genießen von Speisen wurde ein wichtiger Aspekt im Leben der Mutter. Es steht nicht mehr die schlanke Figur im Vordergrund, sondern der Genuss im Moment. Zum anderen gibt es einen Bruch bzw. eine Veränderung der Vorlieben. Das früher

31 Vgl. Zander-Schneider, *Sind Sie meine Tochter?*, 31.

verschmähte Eis scheint aktuell besonders zu schmecken. Freilich könnte man auch deuten, dass sie sich das Eis zugunsten ihres Gewichts nie gönnte und deshalb vorgab, es nicht zu mögen. Wie oben bereits erläutert, brechen auch manchmal nicht zugelassene Vorlieben erst während der Erkrankung durch.

Ein weiterer Bruch zeigt sich bei Zander-Schneiders Mutter, als sie versucht, dieser eine besondere Freude zu machen, indem sie sie ermuntert, am duftenden Flieder zu riechen.

> ‚Mutter, komm, riech doch auch mal.' Ich weiß, dass sie solche Gerüche immer gemocht hat, weiß aber auch, dass der Verlust des Geschmacks- und Geruchssinns zu Alzheimer dazugehören kann. Mutter steht neben mir und schaut mir zu. So stecke ich selbst demonstrativ die Nase noch einmal tief in den Flieder hinein. ‚Komm, probier es mal.' – ‚Ja', sagt sie und lacht mich verständnislos an. Es hat keinen Zweck. Sosehr ich ihr auch eine Freude machen will, sie versteht nicht, was ich meine.[32]

Diese verwehrte Möglichkeit, ihrer Mutter mit Dingen, die sie einst mochte, Freude zu bereiten, ist eine nicht leicht hinzunehmende Veränderung und Herausforderung.

Andererseits können es aber genau jene Dinge sein, die sich das ganze Leben lang in der Biografie als wesentlich gezeigt haben, die nun auch noch während der Demenz als identitätsstiftend aufgefasst werden. Das erlebt Zander-Schneider, als sie mit ihrem Bruder die Mutter im Seniorenheim besucht und ihre Mutter mitten im Raum tanzt. Sie tanzt alleine zur Musik, dreht sich im Kreis und hält die Arme in die Luft. Zander-Schneider und ihr Bruder denken dabei an die vielen Feste, die ihre Eltern früher im eigenen Haus veranstaltet haben, bei denen sie genauso getanzt hat.[33]

Ein weiterer wichtiger Autor zum Thema Alzheimer-Demenz ist der Österreicher Arno Geiger. Er hat die Erkrankung seines Vaters im Buch *Der alte König in seinem Exil* niedergeschrieben. Geiger, der seinen Vater pflegte, erlebt, dass es Dinge in dessen Leben gibt, die ihn nach wie vor prägen und ihm auch Sicherheit geben. So war sein Vater lange Ministrant, bis ins Erwachsenenalter hinein. Selbst im Alter konnte er noch die lateinische Messe auswendig, die er manchmal am Küchentisch gelesen hat. Noch während der Demenzerkrankung konnte er sie auswendig:

32 Zander-Schneider, *Sind Sie meine Tochter?*, 195.

33 Vgl. Zander-Schneider, *Sind Sie meine Tochter?*, 209–10.

> Das war so tief in ihn eingeschrieben, all diese rituellen, liturgischen Sätze, Formeln, die Lieder, die Gesänge. Ich glaube, dass man derlei mitnimmt und dass Wiederholung Vertrauen schafft, weil das richtige Wort wieder kommt, alles an seinem Platz, eine geordnete Welt.[34]

Die Tätigkeit als Ministrant schien für den Vater ein wichtiger Teil seiner Identität zu sein.

Sinnliche Erlebnisse scheinen auch Menschen, die ihr Leben sehr intellektualistisch gestaltet haben, im Zuge der Demenz immer wichtiger zu werden. Der Intellektuelle Walter Jens legt plötzlich kindliches Verhalten an den Tag, genießt Essen wie nie zuvor und das Streicheln von Tieren, gegen die er früher allergisch war.[35]

V. Schlussüberlegungen

Identität nicht als starres und unveränderbares Konstrukt, sondern im Sinne einer Lebensgeschichte als Ganzes zu verstehen – das ist die spezielle Herausforderung bei Demenz. Häufig wird ganz im Sinne der traditionellen Philosophie argumentiert, dass nur derjenige, der sich zu verschiedenen Zeiten an verschiedenen Orten als derselbe denken kann, eine Identität hat. Es wurde gezeigt, dass diese Auffassung von Identität zu kurz greift, weil es zur Lebensgeschichte von Personen gehört, dass darin auch Brüche vorkommen, sowohl beabsichtigte als auch unbeabsichtigte. Darüber hinaus ist auch der Leib ein Teil der Identität, mit dem Menschen sich non-verbal äußern und so anderen etwas vermitteln.

Im Umgang mit Menschen mit Demenz ihre Biografie zu berücksichtigen, aber auch im Blick zu haben, dass sich Vorlieben und Bedürfnisse ändern können, dass es Brüche gibt, ist die besondere Herausforderung.

Bei Menschen mit Demenz spielen Gefühle, die Verbundenheit mit anderen und Nähe eine besonders große Rolle. Dies wird u.a. in filmischen Darstellungen

---

34 Garhammer, Erich, Geiger, Arno. "Sehnsucht nach einem Zuhause, in dem wir genug sind. Ein Gespräch mit Arno Geiger." In: *Lebendige Seelsorge* 1 (2015): 2–10, 7.

35 Auch im Roman *Mein Leben ohne Gestern* von Lisa Genova, der unter dem englischen Originaltitel *Still Alice* mit Julianne Moore verfilmt wurde, wird das sinnliche Erleben der an Demenz erkrankten Harvard-Professorin betont: „Sie sah über das dunkle Wasser hinaus. Ihr Körper, kräftig und gesund, hielt sie Wasser tretend an der Oberfläche, kämpfte mit jedem Instinkt um ihr Leben. Na schön, sie konnte sich nicht erinnern, heute Abend mit John gegessen zu haben oder was er gesagt hatte, wohin er noch wollte. Und es konnte gut sein, dass sie sich morgen früh nicht mehr an diese Nacht erinnern würde, aber in diesem Augenblick fühlte sie sich nicht verzweifelt. Sie fühlte sich lebendig und glücklich." Genova, Lisa. *Mein Leben ohne Gestern.* Köln: Bastei Lübbe, 2009, 162.

besonders deutlich, wie etwa in *Still Alice*. Die ehrgeizige Harvard-Professorin Alice, die den Versuch ihrer jüngsten Tochter, Schauspielerin zu werden, sehr skeptisch sieht, wird im Zuge ihrer Demenzerkrankung zu einer sanften Frau, die sich dann gerade dieser Tochter besonders nahe fühlt. Es ist, auch angesichts der Zunahme der Demenzerkrankungen in unserer Gesellschaft, Zeit, Abstand von den ratio-zentrierten Überlegungen der personalen Identität zu nehmen und uns mehr darauf zu besinnen, was Personen in ihrer Identität wirklich ausmacht. In diesem Sinne gab schon Arthur Schopenhauer zu Bedenken:

> Je älter wir werden, desto spurloser geht Alles vorüber. Hohes Alter, Krankheit, Gehirnverletzung, Wahnsinn, können das Gedächtniß ganz rauben. Aber die Identität der Person ist damit nicht ganz verloren gegangen. [...] Im Herzen steckt der Mensch, nicht im Kopf.[36]

Bibliographie

Birnbacher, Dieter. "Patientenverfügungen und Advance Care Planning bei Demenz und anderen kognitiven Beeinträchtigungen." In: *Ethik in der Medizin*. Berlin/Heidelberg: Springer-Verlag, 2016. DOI 10.1007/s00481-016-0388-6.

Coors, Michael. "A Dementalized Body? Reconsidering the Human Condition in the Light of Dementia." In: *Geriatric Mental Health Care* 1 (2013): 34–38.

Drzezga, Alexander, Sabri, Osama, Fellgiebel, Andreas. "Amyloid-Bildgebung: Reif für die Routine?" In: *Deutsches Ärzteblatt* 26 (2014): 1206–10.

Epiktet. *Das Buch vom geglückten Leben*. Köln: Anaconda Verlag, 2005.

Fröhlich-Güzelsoy, Leyla. "Musik- und Erinnerungstherapie bei demenziell erkrankten Patient*innen mit Migrationsgeschichte. Ethische Desiderate der Demenzbehandlung." In: Andreas Frewer, Lutz Bergemann, Martina Schmidhuber (eds.). *Demenz und Ethik in der Medizin. Standards zur guten klinischen Praxis*. Würzburg: Königshausen & Neumann, 2015.

Füsgen, Ingo. *Demenz. Praktischer Umgang mit der Hirnleistungsstörung*. München: Vieweg Verlag, 1995.

Garhammer, Erich, Geiger, Arno. "Sehnsucht nach einem Zuhause, in dem wir genug sind. Ein Gespräch mit Arno Geiger." In: *Lebendige Seelsorge* 1 (2015): 2–10.

Gasser, Georg. "Einleitung: Zum Verhältnis von personaler Identität und praktischer Rationalität." In: Ders., Schmidhuber, Martina (eds.). *Personale Identität, Narrativität und Praktische Rationalität. Die Einheit der Person aus metaphysischer und praktischer Perspektive*, Münster: Mentis, 2013, 11–37.

36 Schopenhauer, Arthur. *Die Welt als Wille und Vorstellung*. Stuttgart: Reclam, 1987, 314–15.

Genova, Lisa. *Mein Leben ohne Gestern.* Köln: Bastei Lübbe, 2009.

Hughes, Julian C., Baldwin, Clive. *Ethical Issues in Dementia Care. Making Difficult Decisions.* London: Jessica Kingsley Publishers, 2006.

Legal, Friederike, Preuss, Dirk. "Künstliche Intelligenz zur Überwachung von Verhalten? Ethische Erwägungen zu Detektionssystemen für demenzbedingte Veränderungsprozesse." In: Andreas Frewer, Lutz Bergemann, Martina Schmidhuber (eds.). *Demenz und Ethik in der Medizin. Standards zur guten klinischen Praxis.* Würzburg: Königshausen & Neumann 2015, 23–48.

Locke, John. *Versuch über den menschlichen Verstand.* Hamburg: Meiner, 1981.

Magnus, Dorothea. "Sterbehilfe und Demenz." In: *Neue Zeitschrift für Strafrecht* 1,33 (2013): 1–6.

Maier, Wolfgang, Schulz, Jörg B., Weggen, Sascha, Wolf, Stefanie. *Alzheimer & Demenzen verstehen. Diagnose, Behandlung, Alltag, Betreuung.* Stuttgart: Trias, 2011.

Pistrol, Florian. "Vulnerabilität. Erläuterungen zu einem Schlüsselbegriff im Denken Judith Butlers." In: *Zeitschrift für Praktische Philosophie* 3,1 (2016): 233–72.

Quante, Michael. *Person.* Berlin: de Gruyter, 2012.

Schermer, Maartje. "In Search of 'the Good Life' for Demented Elderly." In: *Medicine, Health Care and Philosophy* 6 (2003): 35–44.

Schmidhuber, Martina. *Der Prozess personaler Identitätsbildung und die Rolle von Institutionen. Eine philosophisch-anthropologische Untersuchung.* Münster: LIT, 2011.

Schmidhuber, Martina, "Gedächtnis und Erinnerung als Bedingungen personaler Identität? Überlegungen am Beispiel von Demenzbetroffenen." In: Danièle Moyal-Dharrock, Volker A. Munz, Annalisa Coliva (eds.). *Geist, Sprache und Handlung. Beiträge zum 36. Internationalen Ludwig Wittgenstein-Symposium.* Neulengbach, 2013, 353–55.

Schmidhuber, Martina. "Die Rolle der Patientenverfügung für Menschen mit Demenz." In: *Lebendige Seelsorge* 1 (2015): 49–54.

Schopenhauer, Arthur. *Die Welt als Wille und Vorstellung.* Stuttgart: Reclam, 1987.

Stahr, Ingeborg. "Frauen-Körper-Identität im Kontext gesellschaftlicher Modernisierung." In: Doris Janshen (ed.). *Blickwechsel. Der neue Dialog zwischen Frauen- und Männerforschung.* Frankfurt/Main: Campus-Verlag, 2000, 81–105.

Suter, Martin. *Small World.* Zürich: Diogenes, 1999.

Wetzstein, Verena. *Diagnose Alzheimer. Grundlagen einer Ethik der Demenz.* Frankfurt/Main: Campus, 2005.

Zander-Schneider, Gabriela. *Sind Sie meine Tochter? Leben mit meiner demenzkranken Mutter.* Reinbek bei Hamburg: rororo, 2011.

Dementia and Narrativity/Demenz und Narrativität

Johanna Zeisberg (Graz)

Verortungen des Selbst in Demenznarrationen der Gegenwart

Abstract: Neurodegenerative dementias gradually destroy cerebral capacities and challenge long-established philosophical criteria of personhood like rationality and self-consciousness. When dealing with dementia, contemporary literature initiates an ethical reflection on traditional views on personal identity and outlines alternative criteria that outlive even the latest stages of dementia.

I. Ein ethisches Dilemma fortgeschrittener Demenz

Der bekannte ehemalige Rhetorikprofessor und Gelehrte Walter Jens hat 1995 gemeinsam mit dem Theologen Hans Küng ein Buch über menschenwürdiges Sterben geschrieben. Darin plädiert er für die Möglichkeit, seinem Leben – zur Not auch durch fremde Hilfe – selbstbestimmt ein Ende setzen zu dürfen, wenn die geistige und körperliche Autonomie durch eine irreversible Krankheit gefährdet seien.[1] Einige Jahre später zeigten sich bei ihm die ersten Symptome der bis heute unheilbaren Alzheimer-Demenz.

In einem Interview mit der Zeitschrift *stern* hat Inge Jens die krankheitsbedingten Veränderungen ihres Ehemanns prägnant formuliert:

> Den Mann, den ich liebte, gibt es nicht mehr. [...] Was Sie wahrscheinlich kaum realisieren können, ist, was es heißt, dass der Mann, der aussieht, als wenn er der Ihre wäre, der Ihre nicht mehr ist. [...] Die Krankheit hat ihn zu einem anderen Menschen gemacht. Damit muss ich umgehen.[2]

In seinem Buch *Demenz. Abschied von meinem Vater* spielt Walter Jens' Sohn Tilman Jens das ethische Dilemma durch, das sich aus dem früher geäußerten Wunsch des Vaters und seiner von Inge Jens beschriebenen krankheitsbedingten

1 Jens, Walter, Küng, Hans. *Menschenwürdig Sterben - Ein Plädoyer für Selbstverantwortung.* München: Piper, 1995. Für Walter Jens' sehr eindringliches Resümee vgl. bes. ibid., 124–26.

2 Luik, Arno. "Walter Jens' Ehefrau Inge im Interview." In: *Stern* 10.06.2008. <http://www.stern.de/kultur/buecher/walter-jens--ehefrau-inge-im-interview--die-krankheit-hat-ihn-zu-einem-anderen-menschen-gemacht--3093172.html> (letzter Zugriff 28.02.2017).

Wesensveränderung ergab. Konkret musste sich die Familie die Frage stellen, ob der kaum wiederzuerkennende, demente Ehemann und Vater, den man nun nicht mehr nach seiner rational abwägenden Meinung fragen konnte, wohl noch immer die für einen solchen Fall einst erhoffte Sterbehilfe in Anspruch nehmen wollen würde. Denn nach einer anfänglich besonders leidvollen Periode, die noch vom Bewusstsein der eigenen geistigen Zerrüttung geprägt war, schien der Kranke nun einigermaßen zufrieden, phasenweise sogar auch glücklich zu sein. Und als er einmal in einem kurzen Moment geistiger Klarheit feststellte, er habe nun genug vom Leben, und sich die Familie bereits auf die versprochene Sterbehilfeleistung einzurichten begann, ergänzte er nach einer kleinen Pause ‚lächelnd', wie es bei Tilman Jens heißt: „‚Aber schön ist es doch.'"[3] Mit diesem Nachsatz war für die Familie die Angelegenheit abgeschlossen:

> […] aber schön ist es doch: Redet so einer, der zum Sterben entschlossen ist? Meine Mutter, mein Bruder und ich sind uns einig, das Mandat, ihm aktiv beim Sterben zu helfen, ist in dieser Sekunde erloschen. Ein Zwar-ist-es-schrecklich-aber-schön-ist-es-manchmal-noch-immer ist keine Grundlage, um einen schwerkranken Mann aus der Welt zu schaffen.[4]

II. Frage nach der Identität der Person

Ohne hier auf die Diskussionen über die gesetzliche Bewilligung von Sterbehilfe eingehen zu wollen,[5] möchte ich das Augenmerk auf eine diesem Dilemma zugrundeliegende, ganz zentrale philosophische Fragestellung lenken, deren lebensweltliche Relevanz sich erst in existenziellen Grenzsituationen wie der geschilderten offenbart.

Wenn man überlegt, ob der früher geäußerte Wunsch nach Sterbehilfe auch für den kranken Walter Jens noch gilt, dann steht eigentlich zur Diskussion, ob und inwiefern der Gesunde und der Kranke dieselbe Person sind. Man fragt also nach den (diachronen) Identitätskriterien des Personseins. Denn diese werden, wenn man an Inge Jens' Äußerungen denkt, durch die Auswirkungen der Demenz enorm

3 Jens, Tilman. *Demenz. Abschied von meinem Vater*. Gütersloh: Gütersloher Verlagshaus, 2009, 133.

4 Jens. *Demenz*, 133.

5 Gesetzlich ist die Form aktiver Sterbehilfe (Tötung auf Verlangen), die in einem Fall wie dem von Walter Jens wohl nötig wäre, in Deutschland nach § 216 des Strafgesetzbuches (StGB) nach wie vor verboten.

strapaziert, sie verlieren – auch über den philosophischen Diskurs hinaus – an Selbstverständlichkeit.[6]

Der primäre Ort der diskursiven Verhandlung personaler Identität ist die Philosophie. Bereits in der Antike finden sich erste Überlegungen, was die Essenz, das Bleibende des Menschen im Verlauf seiner Lebenszeit ausmacht.[7] Spätestens aber seit John Lockes viel zitierter Begriffsbestimmung der Person als „denkendes, verständiges Wesen, das Vernunft und Überlegung besitzt und sich selbst" durch die Zeit hinweg „als sich selbst betrachten kann",[8] zählt diese „mit enormer Intensität geführte Diskussion um die Bedingungen personaler Identität" zu den „festgefahrenste[n] und verworrenste[n] Debatte[n] der neuzeitlichen Philosophie".[9] Was im Falle von Walter Jens traurige Wirklichkeit geworden ist – ein Intellektueller mit Patientenverfügung, der an Demenz erkrankt, im Krankheitszustand aber nicht durchwegs unglücklich wirkt – kursiert denn auch in einschlägigen philosophischen Texten über personale Identität als hypothetisches Fallbeispiel eines Extrems, an dem sich die jeweiligen Positionen abarbeiten.[10]

---

6 Ein ähnlicher Konflikt wurde jüngst bezüglich möglicher 'gruppennützlicher' Medikamententests an Demenzkranken ausgetragen – vgl. hierzu den Feuilletonartikel von Becker, Kim Björn. "Autonomie und Alzheimer. Darf man an Dementen Medikamente testen? Eine ethische Debatte, die an Grundfragen rührt." *Süddeutsche Zeitung* 29.06.2016 – und im November 2016 vom Deutschen Bundestag zugunsten solcher Tests entschieden, vgl. die diesbezügliche Meldung des Bundesministeriums für Gesundheit vom 11.11.2016, Bundesministerium für Gesundheit. "Deutscher Bundestag verabschiedet Viertes Gesetz zur Änderung arzneimittelrechtlicher und anderer Vorschriften." https://www.bundesgesundheitsministerium.de/ministerium/meldungen/2016/4-amg-novelle-verabschiedet.html. (letzter Zugriff 25.01.2017).

7 Zu solchen Überlegungen in Platons „Symposion" und „Alkibiades" vgl. Meuter, Norbert. Stichwort ‚Identität'. In: Petra Kolmer, Armin G. Wildfeuer (eds.). *Neues Handbuch philosophischer Grundbegriffe*: *Vol. 2*. Freiburg i.Br.: Karl Alber Verlag, 2011, 1199–1215, 1202–03.

8 Locke, John. *Versuch über den menschlichen Verstand: Vol. 1* (1689). Hamburg: Felix Meiner Verlag, 1981, 419.

9 Quante, Michael. "Warum (und in welchem Sinne) gibt es keine personale Identität?" In: *Deutsche Zeitschrift für Philosophie* 56,4 (2008), 555–67, 555.

10 Vgl. hierzu u.a. Dworkin, Ronald. *Die Grenzen des Lebens. Abtreibung, Euthanasie und persönliche Freiheit.* Deutsch v. Susanne Höbel et al. Reinbek bei Hamburg: Rowohlt, 1994; McMahan, Jeff. *The Ethics of Killing, Problems at the Margins of Life.* Oxford/New York: Oxford University Press, 2002, 502–3 und für den dt. Sprachraum Rippe, Klaus Peter. "Demenz, Ethik und die Konstruktion des Selbst." In: Brigitta Annette Weinhardt, Joachim Weinhardt (eds.). *Naturwissenschaften und Theologie 2*. Stuttgart: Verlag W. Kohlhammer, 2013, 163–95.

Für die Einlösung des vorgängigen Sterbewunsches plädieren vor allem die Philosophen, die Personsein – wie John Locke – allein über Verstandeskriterien definieren. In ein argumentatives Patt geraten sie jedoch mit all jenen Positionen, für die ganz andere Kriterien über die Identität einer Person entscheiden.[11]

Betrachtet man die trotz äußerst differenzierter Analysen[12] kaum auflösbaren Widersprüche der philosophischen Diskussion, scheint das Herausfordernde der Frage nach validen diachronen Identitätskriterien darin zu liegen, dass man eine allgemeingültige Antwort darauf nicht unter Anwendung einer angemessenen Methode finden und sie dann *ad acta* legen kann. Stattdessen beruht jede mögliche Antwort unausweichlich auf einer Vorentscheidung, einer anfänglichen Setzung – nämlich dessen, was man unter einer Person versteht, und was für die Identitätsfeststellung relevante Elemente sind. Daher gibt es nicht nur eine mögliche Antwort, sondern viele.

Angesichts der möglichen Folgen dieser Antwort ist ihre Offenheit allerdings prekär. Denn für welche Setzung auch immer wir uns entscheiden: Sie wird Konsequenzen für unseren Umgang mit uns selbst, vor allem aber auch mit anderen haben. Die Frage nach den Identitätskriterien des Personseins ist eine solche, die auf jene Ebene, in der sie gestellt wird, zurückwirkt. Sie ist auf irritierende Weise selbstbezüglich, da sie auch jenes Selbst, von dem sie ausgeht, zur Verhandlungssache erklärt. Ihre Beantwortung betrifft auch die Fragenden, reicht über die Ebene des Diskurses hinaus hinein in die Praxis. Sie wird, gerade auch was den Umgang mit anderen angeht, zu einer Handlungsforderung. Insofern ist die Frage nach den Identitätskriterien der Person eine ethische Fragestellung.

III. Identitätsangebote in der Literatur

Mit der ethischen Fragestellung nach den Identitätskriterien des Personseins beschäftigt sich neben der Philosophie auch die Literatur. Seit einigen Jahrzehnten erscheinen regelmäßig und in allen Teilen der Welt Romane, Essays und Erzählungen, die mit oder ohne autobiographischen Hintergrund im Zentrum oder am Rande des Geschehens Figuren enthalten, die an einer dementiellen Erkrankung leiden. Wie ich im Folgenden an vier Beispielen zeigen möchte, erproben viele von ihnen in direkter Auseinandersetzung mit der neurodegenerativen Krankheit im experimentellen Raum der Fiktion alternative Vorstellungen personaler

---

11 Wie z.B. ein Mensch zu sein, einen Leib zu haben, ein soziales Wesen zu sein usw.

12 Eine solche Analyse ist Michael Quante zu verdanken, der den verworrenen Diskussionsstand der Identitätsdebatte höchst differenziert und kritisch portraitiert. Vgl. dazu Quante, Michael. *Person*. Berlin/Boston: De Gruyter, [2]2012.

Identität, die geeignet sind, von den Symptomen der Demenz unangetastet zu bleiben. Indem die Texte den Blick auf einen konkreten sozialen Anlass und auf die Motivationen der Identitätszuschreibungen lenken, geben sie darüber hinaus Aufschluss über den oben skizzierten, spezifischen Status der Identitätsfrage.

Der Wille in Jonathan Franzens „Das Gehirn meines Vaters" (2002)

In seinem autobiographisch motivierten Essay „Das Gehirn meines Vaters" (2002) spricht Jonathan Franzen über sein Erleben der Alzheimererkrankung seines Vaters. Einleitend führt er die Zumutung vor Augen, die eine rein neurologisch-medizinische Beschreibung der Erkrankung und ihrer Symptome für die Einzigartigkeit und Identität des betroffenen Menschen bedeutet:

> Ich erinnere mich, wie ich [...] mit dem Autopsiebericht ins Schlafzimmer ging, mich dort hinsetzte und ihn las. *Das Gehirn* (so begann er) *wog 1255g und wies eine parasagittale Atrophie mit Erweiterung der Sulci auf.* Ich erinnere mich, wie ich Gramm in Pfunde und Pfunde in die vertrauten vakuumverpackten Äquivalente in einer Supermarktfleischtruhe umrechnete. Ich erinnere mich, dass ich, statt weiterzulesen, den Bericht zurück in den Umschlag schob. (Franzen. „Das Gehirn meines Vaters," 13; Hervorhebung im Original)

Franzen schildert sein langes „Widerstreben", den Begriff ‚Alzheimer' auf seinen Vater anzuwenden, und erklärt es aus dem Bedürfnis,

> [...] das Besondere des Earl Franzen vor dem Allgemeinen eines benennbaren Befunds zu schützen. Befunde haben Symptome; Symptome verweisen auf die organische Grundlage von allem, was wir sind. Sie verweisen auf das Gehirn als Klumpen Fleisch. Und wo ich eigentlich akzeptieren sollte, ja, das Gehirn ist ein Klumpen Fleisch, bewahre ich mir offenbar einen blinden Fleck, über den ich dann Geschichten lege, die die seelenartigeren Aspekte des Ichs betonen. Meinen leidenden Vater als Bündel organischer Symptome zu sehen würde mich dazu verleiten, den *gesunden* Earl Franzen (und mich) ebenfalls in symptomatischen Kategorien zu sehen – unsere geliebte Persönlichkeit auf eine endliche Reihe neurochemischer Koordinaten zu reduzieren. Wer will schon so eine Lebensgeschichte? (Franzen. „Das Gehirn meines Vaters," 26; Hervorhebung im Original)

Expliziter als die meisten anderen Texte führt Franzens literarischer Essay vor Augen, dass es in erster Linie das zentrale Bedürfnis der Angehörigen ist, in den Handlungen und Äußerungen der Kranken noch Spuren ihres einzigartigen Charakters und ihrer einstigen Persönlichkeit zu sehen. In einer Passage reflektiert er über „eine der Grundeigenschaften des Verstandes [...], dass er aus Bruchstücken unbedingt ein Ganzes machen will" (Franzen. „Das Gehirn meines Vaters," 21), und vergleicht diese Verstandesfähigkeit mit dem anatomisch wirklich vorhandenen „blinden Fleck in unserem Sehfeld" (ibid.), der unser Gehirn auch nicht an der Wahrnehmung einer nahtlosen, vollständigen Welt zu hindern imstande ist:

> In gleicher Weise neigte ich wohl dazu, über das Schweigen und die Absencen meines Vaters hinwegzugehen und ihn als denselben alten, gänzlich ganzen Earl Franzen zu sehen. Ich brauchte ihn weiterhin als Akteur in der Geschichte meiner selbst. (Franzen. „Das Gehirn meines Vaters," 22)

Dieses Bedürfnis wird besonders deutlich in Franzens Schilderung der Abschiedsszene bei seinem letzten Besuch:

> Da sah er [der Vater, JZ] zu mir auf und sagte [...]: ‚Danke fürs Kommen. Schön, dass du dir Zeit genommen hast, mich zu besuchen.' Höflichkeitsfloskeln? Ein Fenster zu seinem eigentlichen Ich? Ich habe wohl kaum die Wahl, an welche der beiden Deutungen ich glauben soll. (Franzen. „Das Gehirn meines Vaters," 40)

Für Franzen zählt vor allem die enorme Willensstärke des Vaters, die sich bis zum Schluss durch die Krankheit hindurch bemerkbar macht. Wie im Dialog mit den oben referierten philosophischen Positionen fragt sich der Autor, „ob Erinnerung und Bewusstsein tatsächlich ein so sicheres Anrecht darauf haben, der Hort der Individualität zu sein" (Franzen. „Das Gehirn meines Vaters," 37), da er selbst auch nach Verlust dieser Fähigkeiten im Leben des Vaters unablässig ‚Sinn findet' (vgl. ibid.). Diesen findet er in erster Linie in einer Interpretation der Äußerungen und Handlungen des Vaters als ein Ausdruck seines anhaltenden enormen Willens: „Vor allem anderen staune ich über das offenkundige Fortbestehen seines *Willens*." (Franzen. „Das Gehirn meines Vaters," 37–38; Hervorhebung im Original) Der Sohn fühlt sich „außerstande, *nicht* zu glauben" (Franzen. „Das Gehirn meines Vaters," 38; Hervorhebung im Original), dass die Versuche des Vaters, die Krankheit so gut es geht zu verbergen, und die Verweigerung der Nahrungsaufnahme kurz vor seinem Tod Ausdruck seines ganz individuellen Willens gewesen seien:

> Noch immer liebte ich, ganz spezifisch und individuell, den Mann, der da in dem Bett gähnte. Und wie konnte ich aus dieser Liebe nicht Geschichten bilden – Geschichten eines Mannes, dessen Wille intakt genug geblieben war, dass er das Gesicht wegdrehte, wenn ich versuchte, ihm den Mund mit einem feuchten Lappen abzuwischen? Noch auf meinem Totenbett werde ich darauf beharren, dass mein Vater entschlossen war, so gut er konnte und auf seine eigene Weise zu sterben. (Franzen. „Das Gehirn meines Vaters," 44)

Das leibliche Selbst in Péter Farkas' *Acht Minuten* (2007)

Ein philosophischer Versuch, der Infragestellung des Selbst der Erkrankten zu begegnen, geht auf leibesphänomenologische Ansätze zurück. Thomas Fuchs, Philosoph und Psychiater an der Universität Heidelberg, kritisiert das

„zerebrozentrische[]"[13] Personenbild der Gegenwart, das Ursprung der Infragestellung der Identität der Demenzkranken sei. Dem will er, geschult durch Leibesphänomenologen wie Merleau-Ponty und Waldenfels, „eine andere Auffassung von Personalität"[14] entgegenstellen: „Danach ist Selbstsein wesentlich verkörpert; es realisiert und reproduziert sich fortwährend in unseren leiblichen Handlungen und in unserem zwischenleiblichen Austausch mit anderen."[15] Fuchs unterscheidet den von uns beobachtbaren Körper, den wir haben, von dem Leib, der wir sind.

Dieser unser Leib habe, so Fuchs, ein eigenes Gedächtnis: das sogenannte ‚implizite' oder auch ‚Leibgedächtnis', das sich aus einer Geschichte leiblicher Erfahrungen zusammensetzt, die sich in unseren Gewohnheiten des wahrnehmenden, fühlenden und handelnden Umgangs mit der Welt niedergeschlagen hat. Dieses Leibgedächtnis „weist auf eine Kontinuität der Person hin, die nicht in ihrem (sic!) expliziten Erinnerungs- und Wissensbeständen verankert ist, sondern in einer im habituellen Leib sedimentierten Erfahrung."[16]

Von einer solchen verbleibenden, identitätskonstituierenden Leiblichkeit des demenzkranken Menschen scheint der Roman *Acht Minuten* des ungarischen Schriftstellers Péter Farkas zu erzählen. Im Mittelpunkt des Romans steht ein gemeinsam gealtertes Ehepaar, das in unterschiedlichen Stadien an Demenz leidet. Geschildert wird der Alltag des dementen Paares, für dessen eigenwilliges Gelingen allein der Mann zuständig ist, da sich die Frau bereits in einem sehr späten Stadium der Krankheit befindet. Der Text setzt schon mit einer außergewöhnlichen Fokussierung auf Leiblichkeit ein:

> Die alte Frau nahm mit Zeigefinger und Daumen ein Stückchen Butter, hob es vor die Augen und betrachtete es erstaunt. Der alte Mann berührte sanft ihr Handgelenk. [...] Während sie mümmelte, blinzelte sie ihn dankbar an. Eine starke, warme Strömung flutete durch den Körper des alten Mannes. Von der Oberfläche der Haut bis in die Tiefen des Fleisches. Die Flut riss sein Ich, sein Körpergefühl in einem einzigen Aufwallen mit sich; und alles das, was einstens er gewesen war, wurde jetzt zur Überflutung selbst. (Farkas. *Acht Minuten*, 5)

---

13 Fuchs, Thomas. "Das Leibgedächtnis in der Demenz." In: Andreas Kruse (ed.). *Lebensqualität bei Demenz? Zum gesellschaftlichen und individuellen Umgang mit einer Grenzsituation im Alter*. Heidelberg: AKA, 2010, 231–42, 231. Ein entscheidender Anstoß für eine leibesphänomenologische Demenzforschung findet sich auch bei Kontos, Pia C. "Embodied Selfhood. An Ethnographic Exploration of Alzheimer's Disease." In: Annette Leibing, Lawrence Cohen (eds.). *Thinking about Dementia. Culture, Loss, and the Anthropology of Senility*. New Brunswick et al.: Rutgers University Press, 2006, 195–217.

14 Fuchs. *Das Leibgedächtnis*, 231.

15 Fuchs. *Das Leibgedächtnis*, 231–32.

16 Fuchs. *Das Leibgedächtnis*, 232.

Anzeichen eines über den eigenen Körper vermittelten Erhalts des Selbst durchziehen den gesamten Text. Während der alten Frau die konkreten Erinnerungen irgendwann „einfach *weggeblieben*" seien,

> so bewahrte der Körper der alten Frau unerschütterlich die in den geleerten Requisitenkammern unbemerkt gespeicherten Erinnerungen weiter auf. Allerdings wurden diese nicht mehr von ihrem Gehirn abgerufen, mit der dazu passenden Dramaturgie und Choreographie, sondern von ihren Nerven und Instinkten. Statt des Bewusstseins erinnerten sich ihre Nase, der Gaumen, die Zungenspitze, Ohren und Augen und vor allem die Haut. (Farkas. *Acht Minuten*, 6–7)

Und während die seltenen Besucher die alte Frau „einfach für dement" halten, weiß der alte Mann die in die Leiblichkeit der Frau versunkene Welt nach gemeinsamen Erinnerungen zu „kartographieren" und so eine Kommunikation mit ihr auch in ihren apathischsten Zuständen zu ermöglichen:

> Bei der Vermessung der Oberflächenformen ging er nach dem Prinzip des Echolots vor und vermochte mit dieser Methode selbst in Zeiten der tiefsten Apathie mit der alten Frau zu kommunizieren. (Farkas. *Acht Minuten*, 8)

Der alte Mann beobachtet, wie das Ich der alten Frau allmählich zerfällt. Er „erkannte immer seltener, wer das war, der in der ersten Person Einzahl sprach, wenn zum Beispiel die alte Frau sagte: Ich habe Hunger." (Farkas. *Acht Minuten*, 61) Irgendwann aber versteht er, dass sich ihr Körper „restlos mit dem von den Empfindungen direkt gereizten Punkt" identifiziert: „Das heißt, wenn die alte Frau hungrig war, so wurde sie zu einem hungrigen Magen, wenn sie Durst hatte, zu einer dürstenden Kehle" (Farkas. *Acht Minuten*, 64).

In Farkas' Roman ist das, was bleibt, ein berührbarer, aber auch berührungsfähiger Körper. Der alte Mann und die alte Frau, die keines Namens mehr bedürfen, da sie ganz Leib geworden sind, leben in ihren Berührungen, in der Harmonie, aber auch in der Nacktheit und Gebrochenheit ihrer in den Körpern aufgespeicherten lebenslangen Vertrautheit.

Doch wie in Franzens Essay der Sohn für den Vater steht auch bei Farkas der Mann für den Identitätserhalt seiner Frau ein:

> Nur der alte Mann maß die Zeit, und nur er suchte in ihr unaufhörlich den Inhalt, den er ‚Ich' nennen konnte. Er befürchtete, wenn er das nicht mehr tun würde, würde er auch die alte Frau verlieren. (Farkas. *Acht Minuten*, 64)

Externe Speicherung des Selbst in Sibylle Knauss' *Das Liebesgedächtnis* (2015)

Eine in neueren Demenznarrationen populäre, recht pragmatisch anmutende Möglichkeit, die eigne Identität trotz der Krankheit zu bewahren, ist die externe Speicherung dessen, was man ist und war, in Medien, die den eigenen Gedächtnisverlust überdauern.[17] In dem ersten weltweit breit rezipierten Alzheimer-Roman *The Notebook* (1996) vom US-amerikanischen Bestsellerautor Nicholas Sparks ist es das titelgebende Notizbuch des Ehemanns, in dem dieser – auf die Bitte seiner an Alzheimer erkrankten Frau hin – ihre gemeinsame Lebens- und Liebesgeschichte festgehalten hat.

Während es hier der gesunde Partner ist, der die gemeinsamen Erinnerungen im heute fast schon altmodisch anmutenden externen Identitätsspeicher eines Notizheftes festschreibt, so ist es in Sibylle Knauss' neuerem Roman *Das Liebesgedächtnis* (2015) die Kranke selbst, die bei den ersten Anzeichen ihrer ererbten Krankheit folgenden Entschluss fasst:

> Wie unwesentlich das Gedächtnis ist, erkenne ich daran, dass man es problemlos auslagern kann. Man kann seine Inhalte speichern auf einer Festplatte. Und das ist es, was ich mir vornehme. Sicher. Beständig. Jederzeit abrufbar. Auf diesem Speicherplatz können sie sogar überleben, wenn ich schon gestorben bin. Doch so viel verlange ich gar nicht. Keine informationstechnologisch erschlichene Unsterblichkeit. Ich möchte vielleicht nur manchmal, solange ich lebe, darauf zurückgreifen. Nachlesen, wie es war. Und selbst, wenn ich irgendwann auch vergessen haben sollte, dass es ihn gibt, diesen Ort, an dem meine Erinnerungen aufbewahrt sind, dann hört er doch nicht auf, zu existieren. Das ist tröstlich. Denn er ist nicht virtuell! Eine Festplatte ist Hardware, Ding unter Dingen, metallisch beschichtetes Glas. (Knauss. *Das Liebesgedächtnis*, 43–44)

Dieses externe Speichermedium kommt in einem kurz darauf angestellten Vergleich mit dem Gehirn deutlich besser weg. Denn „[m]it Entsetzen" stellt sich die Protagonistin dagegen ihr

> vegetatives Speichermedium vor, eine weiche graue Masse, verklumpt von Plaques, in Zersetzung begriffen, bedroht von Tumoren, von Gefäßen versorgt, deren Ablagerungen die Neigung zu Schlagflüssen begünstigen, das Ganze notdürftig geborgen in sprödem Knochenmaterial, das bei jedem Treppensturz brechen kann. Dagegen mein Notebook

17 Die Auslagerung des Selbst auf solcherlei identitätserhaltende Medien findet sich als durchaus ernstgemeinte Option theoretisch fundiert bei Leibing, Annette. "Divided Gazes. Alzheimer's Disease, the Person within, and Death in Life." In: Annette Leibing, Lawrence Cohen (eds.). *Thinking about Dementia. Culture, Loss, and the Anthropology of Senility*. New Brunswick et al.: Rutgers University Press, 2006, 240–68, 260.

> und seine Festplatte! Hart. Härter. Am härtesten. Hardware. Es ist ja wohl nicht die Frage, welches Speichermedium mehr Vertrauen verdient. (Knauss. *Das Liebesgedächtnis*, 44)

Dieser zunächst erleichternden Idee folgt jedoch sogleich die schwierige Frage: „Was vertraue ich ihm an?“ (Knauss. *Das Liebesgedächtnis*, 44) Was sind eigentlich die Informationen, die sie ganz persönlich ausmachen? Die Protagonistin entscheidet sich – analog zu Sparks' Roman – dafür, ihr Liebesgedächtnis festzuhalten. Um das eigene Ich vor dem Zugriff anderer zu schützen, sichert sie die Datei mit einem Passwort. Dass sie hierfür den Namen „Chateaubriand“ (Knauss. *Das Liebesgedächtnis*, 47) wählt, den des Autors der *Mémoires d'outre-tombe* (1848), also der Erinnerungen von jenseits des Grabes, verweist auf den prekären Status des dementen Ichs.

Wie schon bei Franzen, Farkas und Sparks ist es auch in Knauss' Roman das menschliche Gegenüber, welches das Ich bewahrt – hier in der Verwaltung und Bewahrung des als Identitätsspeicher genutzten elektronischen Speichermediums. In einem finalen Wechsel der Perspektive hören wir am Ende des Textes den Geliebten am Bett der Kranken:

> Du liest darin. Du liest den Anfang. Du liest hier und da ein paar Sätze. Du suchst nach etwas. Und manchmal verzweifelst du, weil du nicht finden kannst, was du suchst. Mehrmals schon hast du im Zorn alles gelöscht, dem alten Zorn, der dich immer befallen hat, wenn dir etwas nicht gelang, und ich fand dich mit leerem Blick einen leeren Bildschirm anstarrend vor. Hab keine Angst. Es ist nichts verloren. Ich habe jedes Mal, wenn ich zu dir komme, eine Kopie dabei. Du glaubst doch nicht, dass ich zulasse, dass du dein Liebesgedächtnis verlierst? Es ist auch meins, und ich möchte es mit dir teilen, solange wir leben. (Knauss. *Das Liebesgedächtnis*, 189)

Das inkommensurable Subjekt in Ulrike Draesners „Ichs Heimweg macht alles alleine“ (2006)

Auch Ulrike Draesners Erzählung „Ichs Heimweg macht alles alleine“ wirft implizit die Frage nach dem Verbleib des Subjekts angesichts der dementiellen Erkrankung eines Menschen auf. Dabei versucht sie jedoch weder, eine gleichbleibende Konstante der Persönlichkeit trotz der Krankheit zu ermitteln, noch unterzieht sie die dementiellen Veränderungen textintern einer ästhetischen Revision.[18] Stattdessen lässt sich bei Draesner beobachten, wie sich das von Aphasie gezeichnete, nurmehr

18 Eine solche Revision liefert zum Beispiel Arno Geigers *Der alte König in seinem Exil*. Hier ‚erschreibt‘ der Sohn seinem an Demenz erkrankten Vater eine neue, ästhetische Identität. Vgl. hierzu Zeisberg, Johanna. “Demenz und Literatur zwischen Ethik und Ästhetik.” In: Corina Caduff, Ulrike Vedder (eds.). *Gegenwart schreiben. Zur deutschsprachigen Literatur 2000–2015*. München: Wilhelm Fink, 2017, 105–13.

brüchig ,erzählende' und zugleich erzählte Subjekt in der formalen Zweiteilung des Texts in Innen- und Außenperspektive – der ein poetologisch raffiniertes, unentwirrbares Widerspiel von Innen- und Außenraum, Haus und Garten korrespondiert – eigentlich erst entfaltet. Statt also eines notwendig reduzierenden Versuchs, des krankheitsbedingt entschwindenden Subjekts in irgendeiner Form habhaft zu werden, hält dieser literarische Text die potentiell tragische Differenz zwischen Innen- und Außensicht nicht nur aus, sondern erweist sie letztlich als den Raum, in dem sich das Subjekt allererst konstituiert.[19]

Draesners Erzählung ist in zwei Hälften geteilt. Eingangs befindet sich der Leser unmittelbar in dem sprachlich bereits stark beeinträchtigten Bewusstseinsstrom der dementen Protagonistin Sarah. Die fortgeschrittenen aphatischen Störungen mit assoziativen Laut- und Bedeutungsverschiebungen, Wortfindungsstörungen, eingestreuten Kinderliedzeilen, Neologismen sowie einer aufgelösten Syntax erschweren das Verständnis dessen, was das hier präsentierte Ich, das von sich zwar als ,Ich', aber in der dritten Person spricht, gerade durchlebt. Umso deutlicher ist jedoch, dass dieses Ich mit „leichtem Vergessensgefühl" mit und um sich selber ringt: „Schafe, will ich denken, aber ich denkt Rauch, ich wischt das Fenster frei, es ist so glatt, durchsichtig, als wäre es nicht da, und manchmal ist ich nicht da"; „ich kann nicht mit allem kämpfen" (Draesner. „Ichs Heimweg macht alles alleine," 59, 62 u. 67). Währenddessen irrt dieses Ich scheinbar allein – „ich ist jetzt immer allein" (Draesner. „Ichs Heimweg," 67) – in einem Haus umher, wacht jeden Morgen, so meint es, auf wundersame Weise in einem neuen Bett ein Stockwerk höher auf und befindet sich auf der angestrengten Suche nach einem Mann namens Hans, den es sehnsüchtig vermisst. Diese Suche treibt das Ich, wie man erst später erfährt, eines Morgens bis aufs Dach des Hauses, von wo aus es dem nunmehr selbst bange suchenden Hans „aus vier Meter Höhe" in die Arme rutscht, ihn dabei umwirft und – ohne ihn weiter zu beachten – ins Haus zurückgeht.

In der zweiten Hälfte berichtet eben jener Hans, der, wie man nun erfährt, Sarahs Partner ist und ein pensionierter Physiker, unbeholfen von Sarahs Erkrankung, dem nur schwer zu bewältigenden Alltag und seiner Angst, von der Krankheit angesteckt, infiziert, auch körperlich beeinträchtigt zu werden. Dabei ringt er mit der Sprache und dem Erzählen, das ihm als an Fakten, Zahlen und Maße gewohnten Physiker, wie er betont, äußerst schwer falle. Konsequent, angesichts seiner anfänglichen Feststellung, dass ,schön nur das sei', „was sich

19 Insofern geschieht Identität hier tatsächlich eher im Zwischenraum zwischen den beteiligten Subjekten. Vgl. dazu die auf eine postmoderne Identitätskonzeption zielende sozialwissenschaftliche Studie von Röttgers, Kurt. *Identität als Ereignis. Zur Neufindung eines Begriffs*. Bielefeld: transcript, 2016.

erzählt" (Draesner. „Ichs Heimweg," 70), verläuft sein Bericht zunächst stockend, inkohärent und sprunghaft bis zu dem Moment, wo er mit der Erzählung jenes oben geschilderten morgendlichen Zwischenfalls auf dem Dach beginnt, um den die Erzählung insgesamt kreist und in dem sich für ihn ein letztes Mal und so „lebendig [...] wie vielleicht nie zuvor" (Draesner. „Ichs Heimweg," 81) jenes „Wir" vollzieht, von dem auch die demente Protagonistin anfangs noch weiß und weiß, dass sie es weiß (vgl. Draesner. „Ichs Heimweg," 59), wie es im Text heißt.

Nicht nur Sarahs Identität scheint sich in den aphatischen Bedeutungsfetzen allmählich aufzulösen. Durch die Konfrontation mit seiner erkrankten Frau wird Hans einerseits in seiner Identität als Physiker in Frage gestellt, da sich sein Wissen angesichts der Krankheit als gänzlich machtlos erweist. Andererseits wird aber auch seine Identität als Partner existenziell erschüttert, da Sarah ihn nicht mehr als ihren Hans erkennt: „Manchmal nennt sie mich Augustin. Ich verabscheue diesen Namen." „[S]ie greift meine Finger wie ein kleines Kind, das seine Puppe umklammert. Puppe Augustin." (Draesner. „Ichs Heimweg," 77 u. 79)

Neben die solcherart ‚ver-rückte' Selbstwahrnehmung beider Protagonisten tritt die veränderte Wahrnehmung des jeweils anderen. Hans reflektiert in diesem Sinne über die für ihn rätselhafte Verwandlung der erkrankten Sarah, über sein „universales Paradox", wie er sie nennt:

> Sie ist langsam geworden, sehr langsam, zumindest außen, wo ich sie sehen, hören kann, und was in ihrem Inneren vor sich geht, weiß ich nicht. Meist denke ich, das ist wie bei uns auch, außen schnell, innen schnell, außen langsam, innen langsam, aber dann lächelt sie manchmal so unvermutet, verschmitzt, oder sagt etwas, das meinen Gedanken weit voraus ist. Was in ihr vorgeht, ist mir ein Rätsel, und immer öfter habe ich das Gefühl, dass sie sich ausdehnt! [...] Doch eben während ihre geistigen Fähigkeiten und ihr Mitteilen nach außen abnehmen, habe ich das mir unbegreifliche, aber unabweisbare Gefühl, dass sie immer umfassender wird. (Draesner. „Ichs Heimweg," 72–73)

Doch nicht nur Sarah wächst über Hans hinaus. Denn dass Ichs titelgebender „Heimweg" zum Fluchtpunkt jederzeit nicht das so oft erwähnte Haus, sondern letztlich Hans hat, zeigt sich in der dem Ich häufig unterlaufenden lautlichen Verschmelzung von Hans und Haus zu „Hanshaus" (Draesner. „Ichs Heimweg," 62): „Hans, flüstert ich, Hans, Haus, sei mir nicht böse" (Draesner. „Ichs Heimweg," 67). Auf der ständigen Suche nach Hans – „ich ist wo-ist-Hans?" (Draesner. „Ichs Heimweg," 67) – erscheint dem Ich das verlorene Gesicht ihres Geliebten zuletzt hoch oben in den Wolken: „da hat der Mond hinter dem Hügel gelacht und ist hervorgekommen, hinter der Wolke, das Gesicht von Hans, hat ich in die Wange gekniffen, da hat ich ein Gesicht gehabt" (Draesner. „Ichs Heimweg," 68).

Diese beidseitige Suchbewegung ist letztlich zum Scheitern verurteilt. In der einzigen Berührung des Paares, die im Text stattfindet, reißt die vom Dach ihm entgegenrutschende Sarah Hans zu Boden. Während Sarah dabei verzweifelt Hans' Gesicht in den Wolken sucht, feiert Hans diesen Moment als den lebendigsten, den sie je hatten, und als das ungeahnte Telos des einstigen Kaufs des gemeinsamen Hauses, dessen Bestimmung er nun als erfüllt ansieht und es daher zum Kauf anbietet.

Durch die dargebotene Doppelperspektive führt Draesner in ihrer Erzählung vor, dass das, was das Subjekt ausmacht, nur durch eine Polyphonie der Stimmen, die sich ihm von innen und außen gleichermaßen nähern, tentativ zu erfassen ist. Zugleich zeigt sie damit, dass der eigentliche Umfang des Subjekts weder in der eigenen Stimme, noch in der äußeren Beschreibung vollständig aufgeht, sondern sich in der Differenz überhaupt erst konstituiert, über jede Bestimmung hinauswächst, „sich ausdehnt", „immer umfassender" wird, wie es im Text heißt. Dies spiegelt sich in der Erzählung virtuos in der immer undurchschaubarer werdenden Topographie des gemeinsamen Ferienhauses, die mit dem verschobenen Ich-Erleben der Protagonistin Sarah korrespondiert: „Es war leicht hereinzukommen, keine Schwelle oder – doch, eine Tür, aber erst als ich sich umdrehte, da war ich schon drin" (Draesner. „Ichs Heimweg," 59).

Die Vorstellungen vom ‚Subjekt' werden in Draesners Erzählung somit auch über die Krankheit hinaus einer kritischen Revision unterzogen, aus der es nicht als ‚vermessen' und eingeordnet, sondern als existenziell inkommensurable, mehrstimmig sich konstituierende Größe hervorgeht.

IV. Verortungen des sich selbst vergessenden Selbst

Identität ist nichts Gegebenes, sondern wird geformt. Und an dieser Formung ist nicht nur das Ich, sondern sind ganz entscheidend in gesunden, insbesondere aber auch in Phasen der Krankheit die Mitmenschen beteiligt. So lasse sich, Robert Spaemann zufolge, eine „einzige Person in der Welt [...] nicht denken. [...] Personalität kann es [...] nur als eine Vielheit von Personen geben".[20] Denn die Bestimmung personaler Identität kann im ethischen Sinne keine analytische Erkenntnisleistung sein, sondern sie ist ein „Akt der Anerkennung bestimmter Verpflichtungen gegen denjenigen, den man so bezeichnet".[21] Die für den Anerkennungsakt nötige ursprüngliche Setzung regelt die Inklusions-, aber eben

20 Spaemann, Robert. *Personen. Versuche über den Unterschied zwischen ‚etwas' und ‚jemand'*. Stuttgart: Klett-Cotta, 1996, 49.

21 Spaemann. *Personen*, 26. Für die Validität seiner Argumentation nicht notwendig scheint mir Spaemanns theologische Pointe, derzufolge Personen als Schöpfungen Gottes per se ein solcher Anerkennungsanspruch zukommt (vgl. dazu Spaemann. *Personen*, 252–53).

auch die Exklusionsmechanismen, die zur Ausgrenzung bestimmter Gruppen von Menschen führen.

Literarische Texte können aufgrund ihrer potentiell polyphonen Struktur ein Experimentierfeld von Identitätskonzepten sein. Sie können darüber hinaus aber auch, und das ist die vielleicht noch größere Leistung, ein Ort sein, um den der Identitätsbestimmung zugrundeliegenden Akt der Setzung zu demaskieren, dessen Ergebnis zu relativieren und zu einer immer wieder von Fall zu Fall neu zu beginnenden Aufgabe umzuformulieren: der verantwortungsvollen Verortung des sich selbst vergessenden Selbst durch die Stimme des anderen, die bleibt. Dass dies kein Akt reiner Barmherzigkeit gegenüber den Erkrankten ist, davon zeugen alle hier genannten literarischen Texte. Denn mindestens gleichermaßen ist es ein nahezu existenzielles Bedürfnis der Angehörigen, die den anderen, wie es Jonathan Franzen formuliert hat, „weiterhin als Akteur in der Geschichte“ ihrer selbst (Franzen. „Das Gehirn meines Vaters,“ 22) benötigen.

Bibliographie

Becker, Kim Björn. “Autonomie und Alzheimer. Darf man an Dementen Medikamente testen? Eine ethische Debatte, die an Grundfragen rührt.” In: *Süddeutsche Zeitung* 29.06.2016.

Bundesministerium für Gesundheit. “Deutscher Bundestag verabschiedet Viertes Gesetz zur Änderung arzneimittelrechtlicher und anderer Vorschriften.” https://www.bundesgesundheitsministerium.de/ministerium/meldungen/2016/4-amg-novelle-verabschiedet.html (letzter Zugriff 08.03.2017)

Draesner, Ulrike. “Ichs Heimweg macht alles alleine.” In: Klara Obermüller (ed.). *Es schneit in meinem Kopf. Erzählungen über Alzheimer und Demenz.* München/Wien: Nagel & Kimche, 2006, 59–81.

Dworkin, Ronald. *Die Grenzen des Lebens. Abtreibung, Euthanasie und persönliche Freiheit.* Deutsch v. Susanne Höbel et al. Reinbek bei Hamburg: Rowohlt, 1994.

Farkas, Péter. *Acht Minuten* (2007). Aus dem Ungar. v. György Buda. München: btb, 2013.

Franzen, Jonathan. “Das Gehirn meines Vaters” (2002). In: Ders. *Anleitung zum Alleinsein. Essays.* Übers. v. Eike Schönfeld. Reinbek bei Hamburg: Rowohlt, 2007, 13–46.

Fuchs, Thomas. “Das Leibgedächtnis in der Demenz.” In: Andreas Kruse (ed). *Lebensqualität bei Demenz? Zum gesellschaftlichen und individuellen Umgang mit einer Grenzsituation im Alter.* Heidelberg: AKA, 2010, 231–42.

Jens, Tilman. *Demenz. Abschied von meinem Vater.* Gütersloh: Gütersloher Verlagshaus, 2009.

Jens, Walter, Küng, Hans. *Menschenwürdig Sterben – Ein Plädoyer für Selbstverantwortung.* München: Piper, 1995.

Knauss, Sibylle. *Das Liebesgedächtnis.* Tübingen: Klöpfer & Meyer, 2015.

Kontos, Pia C. "Embodied Selfhood. An Ethnographic Exploration of Alzheimer's Disease." In: Annette Leibing, Lawrence Cohen (eds.). *Thinking about Dementia. Culture, Loss, and the Anthropology of Senility.* New Brunswick et al.: Rutgers University Press, 2006, 195–217.

Leibing, Annette. "Divided Gazes. Alzheimer's Disease, the Person within, and Death in Life." In: Annette Leibing, Lawrence Cohen (eds.). *Thinking about Dementia. Culture, Loss, and the Anthropology of Senility.* New Brunswick et al.: Rutgers University Press, 2006, 240–68.

Locke, John. *Versuch über den menschlichen Verstand: Vol. 1* (1689). Hamburg: Felix Meiner Verlag, 1981.

Luik, Arno. "Walter Jens' Ehefrau Inge im Interview." In: *Stern* 10.06.2008. http://www.stern.de/kultur/buecher/walter-jens--ehefrau-inge-im-interview--die-krankheit-hat-ihn-zu-einem-anderen-menschen-gemacht--3093172.html (letzter Zugriff 28.02.2017).

McMahan, Jeff. *The Ethics of Killing. Problems at the Margins of Life.* Oxford/New York: Oxford University Press, 2002.

Meuter, Norbert. "Stichwort 'Identität'." In: Petra Kolmer, Armin G. Wildfeuer (eds.). *Neues Handbuch philosophischer Grundbegriffe: Vol. 2.* Freiburg i.Br.: Karl Alber Verlag, 2011, 1199–1215.

Quante, Michael. "Warum (und in welchem Sinne) gibt es keine personale Identität?" In: *Deutsche Zeitschrift für Philosophie* 56,4 (2008), 555–67.

Quante, Michael. *Person.* Berlin/Boston: De Gruyter, ²2012.

Rippe, Klaus Peter. "Demenz, Ethik und die Konstruktion des Selbst." In: Brigitta Annette Weinhardt, Joachim Weinhardt (eds.). *Naturwissenschaften und Theologie 2.* Stuttgart: Verlag W. Kohlhammer, 2013, 163–95.

Röttgers, Kurt. *Identität als Ereignis. Zur Neufindung eines Begriffs.* Bielefeld: transcript, 2016.

Spaemann, Robert. *Personen. Versuche über den Unterschied zwischen ‚etwas' und ‚jemand'.* Stuttgart: Klett-Cotta, 1996.

Zeisberg, Johanna. "Demenz und Literatur zwischen Ethik und Ästhetik." In: Corina Caduff, Ulrike Vedder (eds.). *Gegenwart schreiben. Zur deutschsprachigen Literatur 2000–2015.* München: Fink, 2017, 105–13.

Bettina Rabelhofer (Graz)

Ich – das sind die Anderen. Erzählen von Demenz, Alter und Tod

Abstract: The focus of the article is on the 'other'. This 'other' is the one who has to accomplish the (double) transformation of the non-assimilated and non-symbolized mental contents (mentally in the real communication with the person suffering from dementia and 'poetically' in a second semiotic transformation through the aesthetic / aisthetic representation in literature). The therapeutic agent of narrative, thereby, may have an ambivalent function.

Die Aushandlung von Subjektivität ist schon von jeher in Selbst- und Fremdzuweisungen verstrickt. Demenz unterbricht personale Kontinuität und Kohärenz in so radikaler Weise, dass die Innenseite des Bewusstseins kaum noch intersubjektiv ‚übersetzt' werden kann, und sie spricht, gleich der Psychose, damit auch dem Basistheorem einer bürgerlichen Anthropologie Hohn, der die Selbstbestimmung des Subjekts als oberster Wert gilt.

In naturwissenschaftlich ausgerichteten Theoriegebäuden wird der Blick auf die organische Verursachung von Demenz geschärft, während psychischen, biographischen oder sozialen Faktoren nur ausgestaltende Funktion zukommt.[1] Die Risse im Selbstgefüge der Person, verursacht durch unabwendbare Entgleisungen im Hirnstoffwechsel, scheinen, stärker noch als die psychotischen Symptome geisteskranker Menschen, die cartesianische Existenzbehauptung des ‚Cogito ergo sum' zu erschüttern. Wie der Psychotiker trägt auch der Demente die Erfahrung der Existenzunsicherheit als radikale Möglichkeit einer Zerstörung des Selbst in sich, die „zu einem Zeichen und zu einem Bild eines anderen ‚möglichen Selbst' des modernen Individuums werden"[2] kann. Während Schizophrenien die

1 Vgl. Drerup, U. "Psychoanalytische Aspekte der Demenz." In: Rolf Dieter Hirsch (ed.). *Psychotherapie bei Demenzen*. Heidelberg/Berlin: Springer, 1994, 35–46, 36.

2 Leferink, Klaus. "Sympathie mit der Schizophrenie – Die Moderne und ihre psychische Krankheit." In: Manfred Zaumseil, Klaus Leferink (eds.). *Schizophrenie in der Moderne – Modernisierung der Schizophrenie. Lebensalltag, Identität und soziale Beziehungen von psychisch Kranken in der Großstadt*. Bonn: Edition Narrenschiff im Psychiatrieverlag, 1997, 27–81, 29. Leferink zitiert hier Markus, Hazel Rose, Nurius, Paula. "Possible Selves." In: *American Psychologist* 41 (1986): 954–69.

„Denormalisierungsangst"[3] einer Kultur intensivieren, scheinen Demenzen immer auch an Tod und Weltverlust gebunden und radikalisieren so den psychotischen ‚Abwandlungsprozess der Weltverdeckung' zum medikalisierten ‚Abbauprozess,'[4] an dessen Ende Subjektivität vielleicht nicht einmal mehr als Verlustmasse verhandelt, sondern in einem allerletzten Punktum überhaupt annulliert wird.

Subjektivität bzw. deren Konkursmasse als Forschungsgegenstand zu konstituieren bedeutet, die interdiskursive Aufmerksamkeit auf ein Phänomen zu richten, das das bürgerliche Ideal des ‚anthropologischen Normalfalls' konterkariert, symbolische Ordnungen unterläuft, kulturell austarierte Koordinaten ins Wanken bringt und damit die Grundlagen unseres Selbstverständnisses in Frage stellt. „Eine Krankheit hat Hochkonjunktur im westlichen Kulturbetrieb", schreibt Ulrich Stock, „und diese Krankheit ist der Kultur völlig entgegengesetzt":

> Die Krankheit heißt Alzheimer. Kultur heißt: lernen, bewahren, hinzufügen, lehren. Alzheimer heißt: alles vergessen. Diese Krankheit zerstört das Individuum bis auf den Grund, sie schleift die letzte Bastion der säkularen Gesellschaft, das Ich. Sie ist ein negatives Faszinosum […]. Sie ist ein Angriff auf das Einzige, dessen ich mir bis eben noch sicher war: Ich denke, also bin ich.[5]

Störungen der Person sind natürlich nicht unbedingt kulturgebundene Syndrome, sondern eben eine universelle Möglichkeit des Menschseins. Wohl aber wird die defekte Subjektivität, und wäre sie auch noch so sehr Naturphänomen, gesellschaftlich sanktioniert und anhand kultureller Parameter codiert und interpretiert, zumal derjenige, der ohne eigene Erzählfäden lebt, angewiesen ist auf den *Anderen*, um im kulturellen Netz der Repräsentation überhaupt noch mit Bedeutung aufgefangen zu werden.

Demenz als chronische oder fortschreitende Beeinträchtigung höherer kortikaler Funktionen „einschließlich Gedächtnis, Denken, Orientierung, Auffassung, Rechnen, Lernfähigkeit, Sprache und Urteilsvermögen",[6] ist eine „Krankheit der

---

3 Link-Heer, Ursula. "Doppelgänger und multiple Persönlichkeiten. Eine Faszination der Jahrhundertwende." In: Christina von Braun, Gabriele Dietze (eds.). *Multiple Persönlichkeit. Krankheit, Medium oder Metapher?* Frankfurt am Main: Neue Kritik, 1999, 32–59, 34.

4 Vgl. Drerup. "Psychoanalytische Aspekte der Demenz," 36.

5 Stock, Ulrich. "Vergessen erzählen. Alzheimer bedroht die alternde Gesellschaft. Mehr und mehr wird die Krankheit auch in Film und Literatur Thema. Was macht die Kunst mit der Demenz?" In: *Die Zeit* 10.4.2008. Zit. n. Seidler, Miriam. *Figurenmodelle des Alters in der deutschsprachigen Gegenwartsliteratur*. Tübingen: Narr, 2010, 414.

6 Dilling, Horst, Freyberger, Harald J. (eds.). *Taschenführer zur ICD-10-Klassifikation psychischer Störungen*. Bern: Huber, 2010, 24.

Person" und das heißt, dass „die Krankheit dem Subjekt nicht als etwas Äußerliches, ein ihr ‚zukommendes Merkmal' oder Prädikat zukommt, sondern etwas ist, das die Person in ihrem Innersten trifft". Im Unterschied zu ‚normalen' Krankheiten sind Demenzen wie Psychosen Störungen, „die unmittelbar die Bedeutungen treffen, die Personen haben".[7] Wenn sich Bedeutungen nicht mehr selbst herstellen lassen, prallt auch die sozialphilosophische Konstruktion einer selbstbewussten, verantwortungsvollen ‚Person' als Kürzel für die Einheit von intaktem Geist und akkordiert handelndem Körper auf die psychiatrische Konzeption einer ‚Krankheit' des Geistes: Der ‚Geisteskranke' lässt sich begriffslogisch nicht mehr als kranke ‚Person' denken. Entweder ist er geisteskrank oder aber eine ‚Person'.

Wer nicht mehr kohärent von sich selbst erzählen, seine eigene Unvernunft wahrnehmen und sich so doch wieder zur Vernunft bringen kann, dem droht in letzter Konsequenz die Vertreibung aus dem Paradies der Intersubjektivität in die bizarren Niederungen desemantisierten, leeren Sprechens. Beschreiben lässt sich all das nur von außen: Wer im Niemandsland lebt, schreibt nicht mehr. So wie der Tod ist auch der Selbstverlust in der Demenz ein existentielles Radikal, das jeder Selbstnarration spottet und so einzig erzähllogische Unmöglichkeit demonstriert. Wenn Literatur diese Einbrüche des ‚Realen' (Lacan) einer Repräsentationsform zugänglich machen will, hat sie es mit nicht-repräsentierten Erfahrungen zu tun, die sie in einen Zustand der ästhetischen ‚Transformation' und ‚Evokation' zu bringen versucht. In ihrem Bestreben, der inadäquaten Berichterstattung über sich selbst poetisch das Wort zu erteilen, macht sie sich nicht nur als Kontrastereignis zu Fortschrittsoptimismus und narzisstischer Selbstbespiegelung der Epoche bemerkbar, sondern stellt gleichzeitig einen Selbstverständigungsprozess über den Möglichkeitsraum von Identität auf höchst symbolischer und metaphorischer Ebene zur Verfügung.

Literarischen Niederschlag findet die Auseinandersetzung mit der Krisenhaftigkeit des Bewusstseins zumeist in (autobiographischen) Narrationen, die nicht nur die mutmaßliche Innenseite der erkrankten Subjektivität ästhetisch verarbeiten, sondern im Akt exzentrischen Sprechens ebenso die eigene Verstrickung in die Beziehung mit dem Patienten aufarbeiten. Demenz setzt so einen autobiographischen Selbstvergewisserungsprozess in Gang, der danach trachtet, die mehr und mehr schwindende Fähigkeit, sich selbst zu erzählen, und den damit

7 Leferink, Klaus. "Die Person und ihre Krankheit. 'Mangelnde Einsicht' als Identitätsstrategie bei Menschen mit chronischer Schizophrenie." In: Matthias C. Angermeyer, Manfred Zaumseil (eds.). *Verrückte Entwürfe. Kulturelle und individuelle Verarbeitung psychischen Krankseins.* Bonn: Edition Das Narrenschiff im Psychiatrie-Verlag, 1997, 206–61, 252.

verbundenen Ich-Verlust zu kompensieren: Je stummer der Patient wird, desto gesprächiger werden die Umstehenden. Mit dem Verlust der Selbstbiographie des und der an Demenz Erkrankten verbindet sich auch der Verlust einer identitätsstiftenden Erzählung über ein gemeinsam verbrachtes Leben innerhalb der Familie oder Partnerschaft: Das vermeintlich unhintergehbare Koordinatensystem von Geburtsdaten, Namen, verwandtschaftlichen Beziehungen und Identitätszuschreibungen in der eigenen biographischen Entwicklung innerhalb des Familiensystems wird destabilisiert und durch den Einbruch idiosynkratischer Welt- und Zeitverknüpfungen schwer erschüttert. Als kompensatorischer Gestus der Fremdreferenz und „Alternative zu ökonomisch gefärbten, rational ausgerichteten und szientistisch strukturierten Diskursen kann das ‚andere', idiosynkratische Sprechen alter Männer und Frauen", so Rudolf Freiburg und Dirk Kretzschmar in der Einleitung ihres Sammelbandes zu *Alter(n) in Literatur und Kultur der Gegenwart*, „durchaus einen Charme entwickeln, der sich zu einer veritablen Poetizität von Texten verdichten mag".[8] Die Katastrophe des Alterns wird zum ästhetischen Krankheitsgewinn:

> Die wie auch immer derangierte Sicht der Welt atmet den Geist der Poesie und lässt noch in vermeintlich sinnlosen Kollokationen ein Stück Weisheit oder oxymoraler Erkenntnis aufblitzen. Die ‚andere' Welt des alten Menschen, die vor allem dann an Eigenartigkeit gewinnt, wenn sie aufgrund von Demenzsymptomen jenseits des leicht zu Kommunizierenden anzusiedeln ist, verströmt den Zauber des Enigmatischen, der in seiner Obskurität Wahrheiten mehr andeutet als ausformuliert.[9]

Wenn hier die ‚andere' Welt des alten Menschen, die die Ordnungsstrukturen des ‚Normalen' und Gewohnten aufhebt, geradezu zelebriert wird, so bekommt man abseits dieser ‚zauberhaften Welt des Enigmatischen' im realen Umgang mit dem und der Demenzkranken doch eine Ahnung davon, dass die im „Geist der Poesie" Sprechende nicht nur Künstlerin, sondern eben auch Patientin ist, die aus der Not fehlschlagender Symbolbildung heraus poetisch wird. Und man bekommt eine Ahnung davon, was es heißt, sich frei sprachhandelnd zu bewegen, und, jenseits dekonstruktivistischer Einwände, zumindest für die Alltagshermeneutik tauglich zu sein. Wenn die Symbolbildung nicht funktioniert, dann funktioniert beinahe gar nichts mehr: „Die sozialen Beziehungen sind schwer gestört, das Denken ist

---

8 Freiburg, Rudolf, Kretzschmar, Dirk. "Einleitung: Grau-Werte." In: Rudolf Freiburg, Dirk Kretzschmar (eds.) in Zusammenarbeit mit Josef Guggenberger. *Alter(n) in Literatur und Kultur der Gegenwart*. Würzburg: Königshausen und Neumann, 2012 (= Focus: Gegenwart. Vol. 2), 1–29, 17.

9 Freiburg, Kretzschmar. "Einleitung: Grau-Werte," 17.

gestört, die Sprache ist gestört, das Träumen ist gestört. Dann ist die Basisfunktion der Persönlichkeit gestört, dann können keine normalen Träume mehr geträumt werden, und wir befinden uns in den Katastrophen eines psychotischen Prozesses, am Rande eines seelischen Todes".[10]

Die literarisch induzierte Allianz von Poetik und Pathologie ist eine zweischneidige, – lassen die anarchischen Sprachdemontagen des Dadaismus und Surrealismus und die onomatopoetischen Lautgedichte der Wiener Gruppe als poetische Kunstsprachen Lautsymphonien, Assoziationscluster und Neologismen aufleben, die formalästhetisch primärprozesshaften Konstruktionsprinzipien, wie sie die Psychose generiert, Tribut zollen, so unterscheidet sich deren Kommunikationszusammenhang jedoch von jenem psychisch destabilisierter und aus ihrer Selbstgewissheit geworfener Menschen radikal. Bei ihnen handelt es sich um einen Gestus des Verstummens und um Spielarten von Kommunikationsinsuffizienz, die von den Verweigerungsmöglichkeiten des Literaten grundsätzlich verschieden sind: Rezipient und Produzent teilen keine Metaebene, auf der die Angriffe auf Syntax und Objektbeziehungen besprechbar wären.[11]

Der an Demenz Erkrankte ist nicht mehr in der Lage, die Tiefendimension von Bedeutungsverbindungen zu erfassen, er ersetzt sie durch eine Ausweitung der horizontalen Dimension. So bewegt er sich auf verqueren, in pragmatisch-persönlichen, durch Erfahrung gewonnenen Assoziationsketten, mitunter aber auch auf enzyklopädisch ausgetretenen Pfaden.

Kreativität, wie sie durch einen Krankheitsprozess hervorgerufen wird, unterscheidet sich jedoch nicht von der Kreativität Gesunder. Alfred Bader[12] hat mit Blick auf die Psychose das Terrain der Kreativität mit der Metapher des „Zaubergartens" belegt. – Dem Schizophrenen sei es vergönnt, sich dauernd im poetischen Zaubergarten aufzuhalten, wobei gerade die Permanenz seines Aufenthaltes das existentiell Bedrohliche ausmache, dann nämlich, wenn sich die Pforten

---

10 Beland, Hermann. "Sprache – Ödipus – Symbol." In: Heidi Möller, Wolfgang Hegener (eds.). *Psychotherapie – Profession oder Wissenschaft*. Symposion zur Ehrung von Frau Prof. Dr. Eva Jaeggi. Forschungsbericht aus der Abteilung Psychologie im Institut für Sozialwissenschaften der Technischen Universität Berlin, Nr. 2000-1, 18–26, 24. <http://psydok.sulb.uni-saarland.de/volltexte/2004/337/pdf/ber200001.pdf> (letzter Zugriff 28.2.2017).

11 Vgl. Gorsen, Peter. "Kunst und Krankheit. Zur Ästhetik der Grenzüberschreitung im 20. Jahrhundert." In: Peter Gorsen. *Kunst und Krankheit. Metamorphosen der ästhetischen Einbildungskraft.* Frankfurt: Europäische Verlagsanstalt, 1980, 99–212, 149–50.

12 Vgl. Bader, Alfred. "Zugang zur Bildnerei der Schizophrenen vor und nach Prinzhorn." In: *Confinia Psychiatrica* 15 (1972): 101–15.

des Gartens zum Verlassen nicht mehr öffnen; der Gesunde hingegen erwirke sich Einlass nur unter Anstrengung, könne aber seine Zelte auch nach eigenem Gutdünken wieder abbrechen.[13] Der Demente steht vor versperrter Pforte und hat das Feld der Kommunikation außerhalb des Zaubergartens geräumt.

Bei gesunden Menschen ist die regressive Vernachlässigung des Rationalen zugunsten des spontan Emotionalen und der darauffolgenden Neuordnung, Synthese und Integration vorübergehend:

> Des Weiteren besteht eine Affinität der erstgenannten Dimension [i.e. der regressiven Vernachlässigung des Rationalen, B.R.] zum primären Denkprozess (S. Freud) und zur Funktionsweise des Gehirns während des Traums oder bei phantasievoller künstlerischer Tätigkeit. Die zweite Dimension [die darauffolgende Neuordnung, Synthese und Integration, B.R.] ist dagegen sekundärprozesshaft, sie ist wichtig für die wissenschaftliche Tätigkeit und die Erfassung und Auseinandersetzung mit der Realität.[14]

Wenn der durch Demenz Beeinträchtigte die Realität der anderen nicht mehr intersubjektiv teilen kann und sein Sprechen mit der sprachlichen Wiedergabe und Interpretation empirischer Wahrnehmungen kollidiert, so stellt er doch die präsentische Geschehenslogik seiner eigenen, rational entbundenen Welt einem explizit deklarativen Modus des Benennens und Erinnerns gegenüber. Arno Geiger beschreibt in seinem Buch *Der alte König in seinem Exil* das Zusammenleben mit seinem demenzkranken Vater als ein Einrichten in einer Welt ohne objektiven Wahrheitsanspruch:

> Der tägliche Umgang mit ihm glich jetzt immer öfter einem Leben in der Fiktion. Wir richteten uns in all den Erinnerungslücken, Wahnvorstellungen und Hilfskonstruktionen ein, mit denen sein Verstand sich gegen das Unverständliche und die Halluzinationen wappnete. Der einzig verbliebene Platz für ein Miteinander, das sich lohnte, war die Welt, wie der Vater sie wahrnahm. Wir sagten so oft wie möglich Dinge, die seine Sicht bestätigten und ihn glücklich machten. Wir lernten, dass die Scheinheiligkeit der Wahrheit manchmal das Allerschlimmste ist. Sie brachte die Sache nicht weiter und diente allen schlecht. Einem Demenzkranken nach den herkömmlichen Regeln sachlich korrekte Auskunft zu geben, ohne Rücksicht darauf, *wo er sich befindet*, heißt versuchen, ihm eine

---

13 Vgl. Navratil, Leo. "Psychopathologie und Sprache." In: Winfried Kudszus (ed.). *Literatur und Schizophrenie. Theorie und Interpretation eines Grenzgebiets*. Tübingen: Niemeyer, 1977. (= Deutsche Texte. Vol. 45), 113–34, 121 bzw. Abraham, Werner. *Linguistik der uneigentlichen Rede. Linguistische Analysen an den Rändern der Sprache.* Tübingen: Stauffenburg, 1998. (= Stauffenburg-Linguistik.), 322.

14 Mentzos, Stavros. "Psychose und Kreativität." In: Stavros Mentzos, Alois Münch (eds.). *Psychose und Literatur*. Göttingen: Vandenhoeck und Ruprecht, 2004. (= Forum der psychoanalytischen Psychosentherapie. Vol. 11), 11–22, 14–15.

> Welt aufzuzwingen, die nicht die seine ist. (Geiger. *Der alte König in seinem Exil*, 117–18; Hervorhebung im Original)

In der „Privatlogik" des Vaters drückt sich das Aufzwingen der fremd gewordenen Weltsicht wohl so aus: „‚Außerdem wirkt es sich ungünstig aus, dass ihr mir ständig ins Wetter pfuscht.'" (Geiger. *Der alte König*, 52) Der Sohn kämpft lange Zeit noch für die „Aufrechterhaltung des gesunden Menschenverstands" (Geiger. *Der alte König*, 59): „Anstatt ihm [i.e. dem Vater; B.R.] die Angst zu nehmen, indem ich sagte, dass ich ihn beschützen und die *anderen* verjagen werde, versuchte ich ihn abzulenken. Ohne Erfolg. Er fühlte sich weiterhin bedroht und schaute reaktionsbereit mit eingezogenem Kopf nach links und nach rechts." (Geiger. *Der alte König*, 105) Später, als der Sohn anerkennt, dass die Brücke in die Welt des Vaters zunehmend nur mehr in eine Richtung befahrbar ist, macht es ihm nichts mehr aus, dass die „objektive Wahrheit" „unter die Räder" kommt: „[E]s kümmerte mich nicht, denn sie war wertlos. Gleichzeitig gewann ich zunehmend Freude daran, wenn meine Erklärungen in den Bereich der Fiktion abgleiten durften, es gab dabei nur den eigenen Maßstab: Je beruhigender für den Vater, desto besser." (Geiger. *Der alte König*, 118) Und in der Tat: „Sein Zustand änderte sich rapide, abhängig davon, in wie guten Händen er sich befand." (Geiger. *Der alte König*, 104) Für die Umstehenden heißt das, das Maß an eigener Geistesgegenwärtigkeit im Gleichklang mit dem Verlust an operationalem Denken auf Seiten des demenzkranken Gegenübers zu erhöhen:

> Die Ansprüche, die an uns gestellt wurden, waren ausgesprochen komplex, und so traurig es für meinen Vater war, dass sein Gehirn abbaute, für seine Angehörigen galt, dass Widrigkeiten den Verstand *schärfen*. Gespräche mit ihm waren eine gute Gymnastik gegen das eigene Einrosten. Sie erforderten ein beträchtliches Maß an Einfühlungsvermögen und Phantasie, denn im besten Fall gelang es durch ein richtiges Wort und eine richtige Geste, die Unruhe für einige Zeit zu beseitigen. (Geiger. *Der alte König*, 118–19; Hervorhebung im Original)

Die Anstrengung um das richtige Wort und die richtige Geste setzt Intuition voraus. Der Psychoanalytiker Wilfred Bion hat aus seiner Erfahrung mit psychotischen Menschen heraus ein Modell des Denkens entwickelt, das auf einer Theorie der Intuition, die Bion der Poesie entnommen hat, fußt. Es bedarf hier eines ‚träumenden' Anderen, der sich als Behältnis – Bion verwendet den Begriff des *containing*[15] – für die nicht assimilierten und nicht symbolisierten seelischen

---

15 Bion arbeitet das Beziehungsmodell des 'container/contained' im 28. Kapitel aus, für das sein Buch *Learning from Experience* berühmt geworden ist. Bion, Wilfred R. *Learning from Experience*. London: Heinemann, 1962.

Inhalte zur Verfügung stellt. Dabei muss auch jenen Elementen Platz gegeben werden, die vorbegrifflich sind,[16] um wieder neuen psychischen Raum in der Beziehung zum Gegenüber zu schaffen, das aufgrund seiner zerbrechenden Fähigkeit, die kognitiv und emotional zerfallenden Gestalten zu integrieren, bindungslos nach einer vertrauten Basis Ausschau hält.

Seine Theorie des Denkens versteht Bion als Voraussetzung für die Theorie des Sprechens in der Psychoanalyse. Die Psychoanalytikerin nimmt, so wie einst die Mutter bei ihrem Baby, Zeichen unterschiedlichster Äußerungen, die nicht symbolisiert werden können, – in Bions Sprache präverbale Beta-Elemente –, auf und repräsentiert diese in ihrem eigenen inneren Raum, gibt sie ‚entgiftet' und symbolisiert – in Bions Sprache als Alpha-Elemente – an ihr Kind zurück. Das Gegenüber muss also der Alpha-Funktion fähig sein, um den nicht symbolisierten Anteilen des Patienten psychischen Raum zu geben und namenlose Bedrohung in erträglich gemachte Angst zu verwandeln. Intuition entsteht nach Bion von Beginn des Lebens an. Die ‚Rêverie' der Mutter als ‚träumerisches Ahnungsvermögen'[17] ist gleichzusetzen mit der Alpha-Funktion, die sich in die präverbalen Erlebnis-Zustände des Säuglings einfühlen kann.

Fasst man das Phänomen der Demenz in Begriffen der Objektbeziehungstheorie, so stellt der verstehende Andere im Universum von beziehungszerstörenden Attacken auf Worte und Objektbeziehungen Verbindungen wieder her. Diese Verbindungen folgen jedoch einer präsentischen Logik, die die Möglichkeiten affektiver Resonanz nutzt und nicht dem Was, sondern dem Wie das Wort redet. Die akustische Therapeutik des Zuhörens und die leibliche des Präsentseins eröffnen einen Resonanzraum, in dem sich vor allem primäre Beziehungserfahrungen, wie sie sich in der Interaktion des Menschen mit dem ersten Objekt seiner Liebe, zumeist der Mutter, manchmal auch des Vaters, einschreiben. In der Psychoanalyse wird dem sinnlich-gestischen Austausch zwischen Säugling und primärer Bezugsperson eine bedeutende Rolle bei den Abstimmungs- und Spiegelungsprozessen

---

16 Vgl. dazu Bion, Wilfred R. *Cogitations*. London: Karnac Books, 1992, 133: "The problem is to give an answer VERBALLY about objects in a PRE-VERBAL state."

17 ‚Rêverie' wurde von Erika Krejci als „träumerische Gelöstheit" und von Hans A. Thorner als „träumerisches Ahnungsvermögen" übersetzt. Vgl. Warsitz, Rolf-Peter. "Zeichen indirekter Symbolisierung in poetischer Sprache. Variationen der psychoanalytischen Grundregel nach Wilfred R. Bion und Julia Kristeva." In: *Psyche* 68 (2014), Sonderheft: *Suche nach Repräsentanz. Neuere Arbeiten zu seelischen Transformationsprozessen*, 840–65, 852.

in der Beziehungsregulierung beigemessen.[18] Psychoanalytische Theorien der Wahrnehmung gehen davon aus, dass die Prozesse der sinnlichen Interaktion primär sind und vorerst die Sprache in ihrer Beziehung strukturierenden Funktion außer Kraft setzen.[19] So hört das Kind nicht so sehr auf die Worte der Mutter als auf ihre emotionale Freundlichkeit. Die Symbolkraft der Sprache als eines Übergangsobjekts kommt erst dort zum Tragen, wo getrennt wird.

Wenn nun die Sprache den Zustand der Trennung nicht mehr symbolisch beheben kann, geht auch jegliches Gefühl des Vertrautseins verloren und die Unmöglichkeit, sich geborgen zu fühlen, wird begleitet von einem Gefühl der Irritation und des Zweifels, das dem Nicht-zu-Hause-Sein eher Glauben schenkt als der empirischen Tatsache von Adresse, Hausnummer und Mobiliar.

Der demenzkranke August Geiger, der nach und nach aus Intersubjektivität und Sprache exilierte König, erkennt eines Tages sein eigenes Haus nicht mehr und möchte umso mehr nach Hause:

> ‚Das ist dein Haus!'
> ‚Nein, das ist nicht mein Haus', erwiderte er.
> ‚Dann sag mir, wo du wohnst.'
> Er nannte die korrekte Straße mit Hausnummer.
> Triumphierend zeigte Helga auf das Hausnummernschild neben der Eingangstür und fragte:
> ‚Und, was steht hier?'
> Er las die zuvor genannte Adresse vor.
> Helga fragte:
> ‚Was schließen wir daraus?'
> ‚Dass jemand das Schild gestohlen und hier angeschraubt hat', erwiderte der Vater trocken – was eine etwas phantastisch anmutende Deutung war, die aber keineswegs jede Schlüssigkeit vermissen ließ.
> ‚Warum sollte jemand unser Hausnummernschild klauen und an sein Haus schrauben?', fragte Helga empört.
> ‚Das weiß ich auch nicht. Die Leute sind halt so.'
> Das stellte er mit Bedauern fest, gleichzeitig zeigte er nicht den geringsten Anflug von Skepsis angesichts der Unwahrscheinlichkeit seiner Argumentation.

---

18 Zum Folgenden vgl. Leikert, Sebastian. "Die kinästhetische Semantik. Der Wahrnehmungsakt und die ihm korrespondierende Form der psychischen Organisation." In: *Psyche* 65 (2011): 409–38.

19 Vgl. Leikert. *Die kinästhetische Semantik*, 418. Leikert bezieht sich auf die Konzepte der Wahrnehmungsidentität (Freud), des Zärtlichkeitsstadiums (Ferenczi), der Grundstörung (Balint), des Empfindungs-Objekts (Tustin), des Haut-Ichs (Anzieu), des Verwandlungsobjekts (Bollas) und der autistisch-berührenden Position (Ogden).

> Zu einer anderen Gelegenheit antwortete er auf meine Frage, ob er denn seine eigenen Möbel nicht erkenne.
> ‚Doch, jetzt erkenne ich sie!'
> ‚Das will ich auch hoffen', sagte ich ein wenig von oben herab. Aber da schaute er mich enttäuscht an und erwiderte:
> ‚Du, das ist gar nicht so leicht, wie du denkst. Auch andere Leute haben solche Möbel. Man weiß nie.' (Geiger. *Der alte König*, 53–54)

Man weiß nie, ob man wirklich zu Hause ist. Empirische Wahrheitsbeweise können die Heimatlosigkeit nicht aufheben, wohl aber gelingt das in geglückten Augenblicken dem Containment des Anderen:

> ‚Ich gehe jetzt nach Hause', sagte er einmal, als er müde war, noch länger zu warten, dass ihn jemand mitnahm.
> ‚Gehst du mit oder bleibst du hier?'
> ‚Ich bleibe hier.'
> […]
> ‚Hast du mir eine Adresse? Oder eine andere Anweisung? Ich meine, du müsstest mir nur sagen, geh die obere Straße entlang, bis du das Haus siehst.'
> Die Art und Weise, wie er um Unterstützung bat, ging mir zu Herzen, ich sagte:
> ‚Ich habe es mir überlegt, ich komme mit. Wenn du noch eine halbe Stunde wartest, bis ich mit Tippen fertig bin, gehen wir gemeinsam.'
> ‚Wohin?', fragte er.
> ‚Heim', sagte ich. ‚Mich zieht es auch heim.'
> […]
> ‚Und du würdest tatsächlich mitgehen?'
> ‚Ja, sicher.'
> ‚Das würdest du tun?'
> Ich nahm seine Hand, drückte sie kurz:
> ‚Sehr gerne sogar.'
> Das war eine Antwort nach seinem Geschmack. Sogleich strahlte er über das ganze Gesicht, griff ebenfalls nach meiner Hand und sagte:
> ‚Danke!' (Geiger. *Der alte König*, 96–98)

Die affektive Resonanz im Anderen entspringt nicht einem kognitiv reduzierten Wahrnehmungsprozess, sondern einer Aufnahmefähigkeit und -bereitschaft für das elementare Bedürfnis nach Gehalten- und Verstanden-Werden.

Die erste Sozialisation eines Menschenkindes erfolgt im sensorisch-kinästhetischen Interaktionsraum der Mutter-Kind-Dyade. Alfred Lorenzer spricht in diesem Zusammenhang von einem „nicht-sprachlich organisierte[n], sinnlich-organismische[n] Verhaltenssystem, das er als „*Grundsystem* der Persönlichkeit mit eigenen Regeln" beschreibt:

> Dieses System wird nun in der weiteren Entwicklung Schritt für Schritt ersetzt durch ein anderes. Indem die Interaktionsformen, die Erlebnisniederschriften, an Sprachsymbole gebunden werden im Vorgang der Einführung von Sprache, werden die Interaktionsformen zu „symbolischen Interaktionsformen". Die verhaltensbestimmenden Erlebnisentwürfe werden damit doppelt registriert: Sie stehen einerseits im alten sinnlich-organismischen Regulationssystem, sie werden über die sprachliche Verfügung aber auch ins Sprachsystem einbezogen, und das heißt, sie geraten unter die Reglementierung der sprachlich organisierten Handlungsregeln und der in Sprache eingelassenen Handlungsnormen. Individuelle sinnliche Praxis wird so zu sprachsymbolisch vermittelter Praxis.[20]

Als basales Beziehungsmuster aus der Frühzeit menschlicher Individuation schließt das Erleben, dem die sprachsymbolisch vermittelte Praxis abhandenkommt, an den aisthetischen Erfahrungsraum der archaischen Mutterbeziehung an. Damit wird auch die Sprache versinnlicht und zu einem ästhetischen Phänomen, indem sie sich den Regeln einer kinästhetischen Semantik unterwirft. August Geiger wird in der Demenz zum Sprachspieler und Sänger:

> Beim Singen veränderte er scherzhaft die Texte. Auch beim Reden nahm sein Einfallsreichtum zu. Die Verschmitztheit, die er früher gehabt hatte, wurde wieder sichtbar, es war wie bei der Schönheit eines überwucherten Gartens, der ein wenig ausgelichtet war. ‚Bei diesen Dingen habe ich zum Teil auch mitgemacht', sagte er. ‚Aber bitte das Wort *zum Teil* nicht allzu groß aufzufassen, es ist sehr klein zu verstehen.'
> Diese Ausdrucksweise beeindruckte mich, ich fühlte mich in Berührung mit dem magischen Potential der Wörter. James Joyce hat von sich gesagt, er habe keine Phantasie, überlasse sich aber einfach den Offerten der Sprache. So kam es mir auch beim Vater vor. Aus *zukünftig* machte er *kuhzünftig*, das *Ende des Lateins*, das ich bekundete, konterte er, er selber befinde sich *nicht am Ende des Lateins, sondern am Ende des Daseins*. Dabei betonte er die Wörter so, dass die lautliche Verwandtschaft unüberhörbar war. (Geiger. *Der alte König*, 101; Hervorhebung im Original)

Die Poesie der Worte, ja, auch das Glück des Singens – „Singen ist lustiger, demente Menschen singen gern. Singen ist etwas Emotionales, ein Zuhause außerhalb der greifbaren Welt." (Geiger. *Der alte König*, 14) – öffnen einen intermediären Raum des Spiels und der Sprache, die erst dort zum poetischen Phänomen wird, wo sie versinnlicht wird: „Erst wenn die Sprache einen Rhythmus findet und ein Spiel mit Klangfarben und Lautähnlichkeiten ausbildet, wird sie poetisch. Sie gewinnt also genau dort poetische Qualität, wo sie nicht allein sprachlich-lexikalische, sondern

20 Lorenzer, Alfred. "Die Analyse der subjektiven Struktur von Lebensläufen und das gesellschaftlich Objektive." In: Dieter Baake, Theodor Schulze (eds.). *Aus Geschichten lernen. Zur Einübung pädagogischen Verstehens*. München: Juventa, 1984, 129–45, 137–38; Hervorhebung im Original.

zusätzlich musikalisch-kinästhetische Ordnungen in sich aufnimmt."[21] In diesem Sinne ist auch die Poesie die Ursprache des Menschengeschlechts und die Sätze des August Geiger hätte auch „ein Held von Franz Kafka oder Thomas Bernhard" (Geiger. *Der alte König*, 114) gesagt haben können. Die poetische Sprache in ihrer Primärprozesshaftigkeit ähnelt der Sprache des Traums. ‚Rêverie' auf Seiten des Zuhörenden bezieht sich so auch immer auf eine Performanz der Zeichengebung, hält sich als ein Lauschen auf das am Leben, was an Sprachofferten sich mit dem Eigenen verbindet und im statu nascendi ‚verdaut' werden kann. So hält der verstehende und fühlende Andere den Übergangsraum des Spiels und der Kreativität offen und träumt jenseits eines kognitiven Eros einen Traum oder auch Albtraum mit. Das der poetischen bzw. aisthetischen Funktion entlehnte Träumen nennt Bion mit den Worten des englischen Lyrikers John Keats „negative capability", die Fähigkeit nämlich, „das Ungewisse, die Mysterien, die Zweifel zu ertragen, ohne alles aufgeregte Greifen nach Fakten und Verstandesgründen".[22] Diese Fähigkeit, das Ungewisse zu ertragen und auch dem Bedrohlichen ein Behältnis zur Verfügung zu stellen, fordert dem Sohn als dem schreibenden Anderen eine doppelte Verwandlungsleistung ab – zum einen in der realen Kommunikation mit dem demenzkranken Vater und ‚poetisch' in einer zweiten semiotischen Transformation durch die ästhetische/aisthetische Repräsentation in der Literatur.

Dem Therapeutikum des Erzählens mag dabei durchaus eine ambivalente Funktion zukommen: Denkbar ist, dass die diskursive Strategie des Erzählers als Schutzschild fungiert, die Gefahr, die Tod und Selbstverlust für jegliches Gefühl der Stabilität darstellen, abzuwehren und im *Anderen* unterzubringen, ihm gleichsam das ‚Tödliche' im ästhetischen Akt wieder ‚zurückzuerstatten'. Damit wird Erzählen auch zur eigenen Überlebensstrategie.

Bibliographie

Abraham, Werner. *Linguistik der uneigentlichen Rede. Linguistische Analysen an den Rändern der Sprache.* Tübingen: Stauffenburg, 1998 (= Stauffenburg-Linguistik).

Bader, Alfred. "Zugang zur Bildnerei der Schizophrenen vor und nach Prinzhorn." In: *Confinia Psychiatrica* 15 (1972): 101–15.

21 Leikert. *Die kinästhetische Semantik*, 429.

22 Keats, John. *Werke und Briefe*. Übersetzt von Christa Schuenke. Stuttgart: Reclam, 1995, 334. Brief vom 21.12.1817 [an seinen Bruder] bzw. Bion, Wilfred R. *Aufmerksamkeit und Deutung*. Übers. von Elisabeth Vorspohl. Frankfurt am Main: Brandes und Apsel, 2006 [1970], 143.

Beland, Hermann. "Sprache – Ödipus – Symbol." In: Heidi Möller, Wolfgang Hegener (eds.). *Psychotherapie – Profession oder Wissenschaft*. Symposion zur Ehrung von Frau Prof. Dr. Eva Jaeggi. Forschungsbericht aus der Abteilung Psychologie im Institut für Sozialwissenschaften der Technischen Universität Berlin, Nr. 2000–1, 18–26. <http://psydok.sulb.uni-saarland.de/volltexte/2004/337/pdf/ber200001.pdf> (letzter Zugriff 28.2.2017).

Bion, Wilfred R. *Aufmerksamkeit und Deutung*. Übers. von Elisabeth Vorspohl. Frankfurt am Main: Brandes und Apsel, 2006 [1970].

Bion, Wilfred R. *Cogitations*. London: Karnac Books, 1992.

Bion, Wilfred R. *Learning from Experience*. London: Heinemann, 1962.

Dilling, Horst, Freyberger, Harald J. (eds.). *Taschenführer zur ICD-10-Klassifikation psychischer Störungen*. Bern: Huber, 2010.

Drerup, U. "Psychoanalytische Aspekte der Demenz." In: Rolf Dieter Hirsch (ed.). *Psychotherapie bei Demenzen*. Heidelberg/Berlin: Springer, 1994, 35–46.

Freiburg, Rudolf, Kretzschmar, Dirk. "Einleitung: Grau-Werte." In: Rudolf Freiburg, Dirk Kretzschmar (eds.) in Zusammenarbeit mit Josef Guggenberger. *Alter(n) in Literatur und Kultur der Gegenwart*. Würzburg: Königshausen und Neumann, 2012 (= Focus: Gegenwart. Vol. 2), 1–29.

Geiger, Arno. *Der alte König in seinem Exil*. München: Hanser, 2011.

Gorsen, Peter. "Kunst und Krankheit. Zur Ästhetik der Grenzüberschreitung im 20. Jahrhundert." In: Peter Gorsen. *Kunst und Krankheit. Metamorphosen der ästhetischen Einbildungskraft*. Frankfurt: Europäische Verlagsanstalt, 1980, 99–212.

Keats, John. *Werke und Briefe*. Übersetzt von Christa Schuenke. Stuttgart: Reclam, 1995.

Leferink, Klaus. "Die Person und ihre Krankheit. 'Mangelnde Einsicht' als Identitätsstrategie bei Menschen mit chronischer Schizophrenie." In: Matthias C. Angermeyer, Manfred Zaumseil (eds.). *Verrückte Entwürfe. Kulturelle und individuelle Verarbeitung psychischen Krankseins*. Bonn: Edition Das Narrenschiff im Psychiatrie-Verlag, 1997, 206–61.

Leferink, Klaus. "Sympathie mit der Schizophrenie – Die Moderne und ihre psychische Krankheit." In: Manfred Zaumseil, Klaus Leferink (eds.). *Schizophrenie in der Moderne – Modernisierung der Schizophrenie. Lebensalltag, Identität und soziale Beziehungen von psychisch Kranken in der Großstadt*. Bonn: Edition Das Narrenschiff im Psychiatrieverlag, 1997, 27–81.

Leikert, Sebastian. "Die kinästhetische Semantik. Der Wahrnehmungsakt und die ihm korrespondierende Form der psychischen Organisation." In: *Psyche* 65 (2011): 409–38.

Link-Heer, Ursula. "Doppelgänger und multiple Persönlichkeiten. Eine Faszination der Jahrhundertwende." In: Christina von Braun, Gabriele Dietze (eds.). *Multiple Persönlichkeit. Krankheit, Medium oder Metapher?* Frankfurt am Main: Neue Kritik, 1999, 32–59.

Lorenzer, Alfred. "Die Analyse der subjektiven Struktur von Lebensläufen und das gesellschaftlich Objektive." In: Dieter Baake, Theodor Schulze (eds.). *Aus Geschichten lernen. Zur Einübung pädagogischen Verstehens.* München: Juventa, 1984, 129–45.

Markus, Hazel Rose und Paula Nurius. "Possible Selves." In: *American Psychologist* 41 (1986): 954–69.

Mentzos, Stavros. "Psychose und Kreativität." In: Stavros Mentzos, Alois Münch (eds.). *Psychose und Literatur.* Göttingen: Vandenhoeck und Ruprecht, 2004 (= Forum der psychoanalytischen Psychosentherapie. Vol. 11), 11–22.

Navratil, Leo. "Psychopathologie und Sprache." In: Winfried Kudszus (ed.). *Literatur und Schizophrenie. Theorie und Interpretation eines Grenzgebiets.* Tübingen: Niemeyer, 1977 (= Deutsche Texte. Vol. 45), 113–34.

Seidler, Miriam. *Figurenmodelle des Alters in der deutschsprachigen Gegenwartsliteratur.* Tübingen: Narr, 2010.

Stock, Ulrich. "Vergessen erzählen. Alzheimer bedroht die alternde Gesellschaft. Mehr und mehr wird die Krankheit auch in Film und Literatur Thema. Was macht die Kunst mit der Demenz? " In: *Die Zeit* 10.4.2008.

Warsitz, Rolf-Peter. "Zeichen indirekter Symbolisierung in poetischer Sprache. Variationen der psychoanalytischen Grundregel nach Wilfred R. Bion und Julia Kristeva." In: *Psyche* 68 (2014): 840–65. (Sonderheft: *Suche nach Repräsentanz. Neuere Arbeiten zu seelischen Transformationsprozessen*)

Leonie Süwolto (Paderborn)

„Da mein Vater nicht mehr über die Brücke in meine Welt gelangen kann, muss ich hinüber zu ihm." Zum Verhältnis von Subjektivität und Sprache in Arno Geigers *Der alte König in seinem Exil*

Abstract: The course of dementia goes along with an increasing aphasia. People suffering from dementia lose their possibility to express themselves in the advanced stages of the disease. The speechlessness of patients means a challenge for literary representations of dementia especially from a narratological point of view because an inner perspective cannot be given authentically. That is why subjects suffering from dementia are often represented from the outside. Hence, the narrator serves as a mediator and translator between the patient and the reader and thereby creates a hierarchical order. In my paper I will give a critical perspective on these narratological translations. I will argue in terms of postcolonial theory how those translations may be interpreted as an act of marginalization that represents a threat to subjectivity.

I. Einleitung

Das für den Titel dieses Beitrags gewählte Zitat entstammt Arno Geigers autobiographisch inspirierter, 2011 erschienener Erzählung *Der alte König in seinem Exil*, in der er die Erfahrung der Pflege von und Begegnung mit seinem demenzleidenden Vater August literarisch be- und verarbeitet.[1] Das Zitat zeugt von der Gewissheit einer in Zeiten des fortgeschrittenen Krankheitsverlaufs nurmehr einseitig verlaufenden Kommunikation, einer unerwiderten Ansprache des Sohnes an den Vater. Denn die Krankheit, so lässt der österreichische Autor seine Leserschaft wissen, spannt einen dichotomen Raum auf zwischen den Familienmitgliedern:

---

1 Der folgende Aufsatz enthält Thesen, die ich an anderer Stelle bereits in meiner Dissertation und in einem daran angelehnten Aufsatz entwickelt habe. Vgl. Verf. *Altern in einer alterslosen Gesellschaft. Literarische und filmische Imaginationen*. Paderborn: Fink, 2016, 260–73; 334–59. Siehe auch Verf. "Der Altern(d)e kann sprechen. Sprechen aus dem Exil in Arno Geigers autobiographischer Erzählung *Der alte König in seinem Exil* (2011)." In: *Limbus. Australisches Jahrbuch für germanistische Literatur- und Kulturwissenschaft* 8 (2015): 201–19.

> *Dort drüben*, innerhalb der Grenzen seiner geistigen Verfassung, *jenseits unserer auf Sachlichkeit und Zielstrebigkeit ausgelegten Gesellschaft*, ist er immer noch ein beachtlicher Mensch, und wenn auch nach allgemeinen Maßstäben nicht immer ganz vernünftig, so doch irgendwie brillant. (Geiger. *Der alte König in seinem Exil*, 11; Hervorhebung L.S.)

Die Segregation des dementen Familienoberhauptes, die in der Titelgebung *Der alte König in seinem Exil* bildsprachlich Gestalt annimmt, wird eindeutig begründet durch die normativen Leitbilder der Gesellschaft: Sachlichkeit, Zielstrebigkeit und Vernunft sind die Parameter, die das Exil des Vaters vermessen, denn seine Heimat ist nach Auskunft des Sohnes längst verloren. Nun legt Geiger seiner Erzählung ein sprachbasiertes Verständnis von Heimat zugrunde, das er mit den Worten des römischen Exilanten Ovid beschreibt: Heimat sei dort, wo man jemandes Sprache verstehe. (Vgl. Geiger, *Der alte König in seinem Exil*, 57) Für jemanden, aus dem „die Sprache langsam [...] heraussickert" (Geiger, *Der alte König in seinem Exil*, 12) – und das aufgrund einer im Zuge des Krankheitsverlaufs symptomatisch fortschreitenden Aphasie –, ergibt sich daraus ein existentielles Problem des Heimatverlusts.[2] Seine „ansatzlose[n] [...], unwahrscheinlich[en] [...] und schwebend[en]" Sätze, „wie sie einem manchmal in Träumen kommen", (Geiger, *Der alte König in seinem Exil*, 11) bleiben in einer sich rationalistisch gebarenden Gesellschaft unverstanden. Die betonte Traumlogik der Sprache als Signum des Irrationalen steht dem Paradigma eines rational geleiteten Weltzugangs diametral gegenüber. Die eindeutigen erzählerischen Verflechtungen von Topographie und Sprache weisen den metaphorischen Brückenschlag des titelgebenden Zitats als einen aufgrund der Demenz gescheiterten Dialog zwischen Vater und Sohn aus. Schließlich ergibt sich in fortgeschrittenen Stadien der

---

2 Vgl. „Der quälende Eindruck, nicht zu Hause zu sein, gehört zum Krankheitsbild. Ich erkläre es mir so, dass ein an Demenz erkrankter Mensch aufgrund seiner inneren Zerrüttung das Gefühl der Geborgenheit verloren hat und sich an einen Platz sehnt, an dem er diese Geborgenheit wieder erfährt. Da jedoch das Gefühl der Irritation auch an den vertrautesten Orten nicht vergeht, scheidet selbst das eigene Bett als mögliches Zuhause aus. [...] Weil seine Versuche, Gesprächen zu folgen, immer öfter scheiterten, und auch das Entziffern von Gesichtern immer öfter misslang, fühlte er sich wie im Exil. Die Redenden, selbst seine Geschwister und Kinder, waren ihm fremd, weil das, was sie sagten, Verwirrung stiftete und un-heimlich war." Der kulturhistorische Rekurs auf Freuds Studie zum Unheimlichen zeigt nochmal die existenzielle, das Subjekt bedrohende Dimension des Heimatverlusts, insofern Freuds Phänomene des Unheimlichen wie z.B. der Doppelgänger an Momente der Ich-Spaltung gemahnen. Geigers Text stellt sich unter anderem dar als die Suche nach einem 'Zuhause außerhalb der greifbaren Welt'. (Geiger. *Der alte König in seinem Exil*, 13–14; 57)

Demenz ein manifestes sprachpraktisches Problem,[3] das in seiner literarischen Ausgestaltung zuvörderst – so auch in Geigers Erzählung – als ein erzähltheoretisches Problem der Fokalisierung in Erscheinung tritt, „denn es ist nicht möglich, eine Innensicht fortgeschrittener Demenz zu erzählen",[4] schreibt Heike Hartung in ihrem Aufsatz „Small World? – Narrative Annäherungen an Alzheimer". Das demenzleidende „Subjekt" kann sich nicht selbst bzw. kann nicht sein Selbst erzählen.[5] Seine Darstellung ist auf die Vermittlung durch einen unabhängigen Erzähler, der qua Krankheitsbild keine realistische Innensicht der erkrankten Figur teilen kann, angewiesen, denn „besonders im Erzählen über Krankheit [ist] häufig traditionelles chronologisches Erzählen und ein stabiles Ich erforder[lich]".[6] Der Demenzleidende braucht jemanden, *der für ihn spricht* – einen Vermittler.

Ich werde mich im Folgenden vor dem Hintergrund dieser Problematisierung auf der Grundlage verschiedener Forschungsperspektiven auf jene Geste des Vermittelns, des *für-jemanden-Sprechens*, das in der Literatur über Demenz aufgrund ihrer Symptomatik zu einem zentralen, auch erzähltheoretischen Problem gerinnt, konzentrieren. Die Argumentation folgt dabei der leitenden Überlegung, dass die Erzählliteratur der Gegenwart um das Thema Alzheimer(Demenz) durch die Installation von ‚Übersetzerfiguren', d.h. von Erzählern, die der Leserschaft die von Krankheit gezeichnete Perspektive des Dementen nahebringen, einerseits auf die

---

3 Es werden gewöhnlich drei Stadien des Krankheitsverlaufs unterschieden: die leichtgradige Demenz, die mittelschwere Demenz und die schwere Demenz. Während die kognitive Beeinträchtigung in der ersten Phase zumeist von geringem Ausmaß ist, sodass die Alltagsbewältigung noch weitestgehend möglich ist, sind die Schädigungen im mittelschweren Stadium signifikant und einschneidend: Spätestens im Stadium der mittelschweren Demenz wird die sprachliche Verständigung zum Problem, aus Wortfindungsstörungen werden massive Beeinträchtigungen der verbalen Kommunikation. Vgl. Kurz, Alexander, Freter, Hans-Jürgen, Saxl, Susanna, Nickel, Ellen. *Demenz. Das Wichtigste*. Berlin: Deutsche Alzheimer Gesellschaft e.V., [2]2016, 19–24.

4 Hartung, Heike. "Small World? – Narrative Annäherungen an Alzheimer." In: Cornelia Bogen, Madlen Domaschke, Sabine Pabst (eds.). *Alte Menschen und Medien. Alter im Spannungsfeld zwischen Kultur und Medien*. Frankfurt a.M.: Peter Lang, 2008, 163–78, 165.

5 Die fehlende Möglichkeit der Selbstrepräsentation ist in der literaturkritischen Auseinandersetzung mit Geigers Erzählung mitunter mit Unmut zur Kenntnis genommen worden. Ein besonders eindrückliches Beispiel ist die Kritik von Ulrich Stock in *Die Zeit*. Vgl. Stock, Ulrich. "Material Vater. Der Schriftsteller Arno Geiger schreibt einen Bestseller über den demenzkranken August Geiger, dessen Sohn er ist." In: *Die Zeit* online 18.02.2011. <http://www.zeit.de/2011/08/L-B-Geiger > (letzter Zugriff 20.09.2016).

6 Hartung. "Small World?," 165.

Unvermittelbarkeit einer Innenperspektive des fortgeschrittenen Krankheitsverlaufs reagiert. Andererseits aber wird das Wissen um die tendenziell hierarchisierende Bewegung des Vermittlungsaktes als Voraussetzung der Erzählverhältnisse im Text reflektiert und problematisiert.[7] Geigers Text, so die vertretene These, repräsentiert innerhalb dieser Problemstellung den Versuch eines integrativen Umgangs mit der Krankheit und der von ihr Betroffenen durch die Imagination einer Innenperspektive des Erkrankten – wenn nicht eine Ich-Perspektive, so doch eine nicht eindeutig zuordenbare Erzählstimme, die auf den Dementen verweist. Er leistet damit eine fingierte Teilhabe des Erkrankten am Demenzdiskurs, zeigt dabei zum einen offenkundig das Bestreben, ein Subjekt zu erretten, das im Sinne einer fortschreitenden Aphasie buchstäblich unmündig erscheint, zum anderen illustriert er die damit verbundenen Aporien, ein tendenziell hierarchisierendes Verhältnis des Vermittlungsaktes auch im mimetischen Verfahren nicht überwinden zu können und so wiederum das sprachlose Subjekt neuerlich zum Verschwinden zu bringen.

II. Theoretische Reflexionen zum Verhältnis von (aphasischer) Sprache und Subjektivität

Ich möchte diesem ersten Einblick in Geigers Text nun im Sinne der leitenden Überlegung eine theoretische Reflexion zum Verhältnis von sprachlicher Repräsentation bzw. Erzählen und Subjektivierung folgen lassen, die sich an der zunehmenden Artikulationsunfähigkeit Demenzkranker im literarischen Text ausrichtet.

---

7 Ein weiteres eindrückliches Beispiel aus dem Bereich der Gegenwartsliteratur wäre Ulrike Draesners Erzählung "Ichs Heimweg macht alles alleine," die 2006 in der von Klara Obermüller herausgegebenen Anthologie *Es schneit in meinem Kopf* erschienen ist. Die Erzählung um Hans und seine demenzleidende Ehefrau Sarah zerfällt in zwei Erzählteile. Der erste führt den Leser in die Imagination der Innenperspektive einer Demenzpatientin ein, wird also aus Sarahs Perspektive erzählt, während der zweite Teil aus Hans' Perspektive die Ereignisse des ersten Teils scheinbar sinnverstehend einholt, der nicht zufällig als ‚verkopfter' Naturwissenschaftler den vermeintlichen Gegenpol Sarahs repräsentiert. Tatsächlich wird aber die Diskrepanz der Perspektiven über eine leitmotivische Spiegelmetaphorik zunehmend dekonstruiert und die Binarismen von Gesundheit und Krankheit, Rationalität und Irrationalität lösen sich sukzessive auf. Vgl. Draesner, Ulrike. "Ichs Heimweg macht alles alleine." In: Klara Obermüller (ed.). *Es schneit in meinem Kopf. Erzählungen über Alzheimer und Demenz.* München: Nagel & Kimche, 2006, 59–81.

Die sprachliche Verfasstheit des Subjekts gilt in der Postmoderne längst als Allgemeinplatz: Konstruktivisten, unter ihnen vor allem Judith Butler, begreifen das Subjekt als Ergebnis zitatförmiger Wiederholungen kultureller (Sprach)Normen, durch die sich das Subjekt in der Sprache materialisiert und essentialisiert. Vertreter der Narrativen Psychologie gehen ebenfalls von einer konstitutiven Bedeutung von sinnstiftenden Erzählungen für Subjektivierungsprozesse aus. Narrative Identität versteht sich im Sinne der Narrativen Psychologie als „die Einheit des Lebens einer Person, so wie diese Person sie in den Geschichten erfährt und artikuliert, mit denen sie ihre Erfahrung ausdrückt.“[8] Sowohl die eigene Identität als auch das Verhältnis zur Welt wird in Erzählungen gestaltet, d.h. Narration ist ein „grundlegende[r] Modus der sozialen Konstitution von Wirklichkeit“.[9] Man geht davon aus, dass Subjekte ihre narrativen Selbstentwürfe in Auseinandersetzung mit kulturellen Sinnstrukturen und Ordnungsmustern, s.g. Meta-Erzählungen bzw. gesellschaftlich vermittelten Erzählformen (z.B. Pro- oder Regressionsnarration bis hin zu validen Gattungsmustern wie Tragödie, Komödie, Romanze etc.),[10] entwickeln. Das heißt, die narrative Identität im Sinne eines kohärenten, kausal verbundenen, entwicklungsorientierten, teleologischen Erzählmusters des Selbst bildet sich stets in Interaktion mit dem gesellschaftlichen, kulturellen Umfeld heraus, sie bedarf der Antizipation durch verschiedene handlungstragende Gegenüber, wird also in der kommunikativen Aushandlung immer wieder aufs Neue formiert. Dabei ist die Selbstgeschichte jedoch immer im Plural als Geschichten zu denken. Narrative Identität erweist sich als Konglomerat von Erzählungen, die in Aushandlungsprozessen unter Betonung oder Aussparung je unterschiedlicher Sachverhalte und Erlebnisse stetig reformuliert werden. Als Identitätsentwurf *in actio*, in ihrer Abhängigkeit von Dritten, wird die narrative Identität offen für Erzählungen Anderer, die ebenfalls in den Entwurf einer Lebensgeschichte, eines narrativen Selbst einfließen. Hieraus ergibt sich ein zentraler Ansatzpunkt ethisch interessierter Auseinandersetzungen mit Subjektivität im Kontext von Demenz. Durch die kommunikative Aushandlungssituation, in die Identitätsentwürfe und Lebensgeschichten des Subjekts eingebettet sind, eröffnet sich grundsätzlich die Möglichkeit einer Fortschreibung von Subjektivität im Kontext der Krankheit

8 Widdershoven, G. A. M. “The Story of Life: Hermeneutic Perspectives on the Relationship between Narrative and Life History.” In: R. Josselson, A. Lieblich (eds.). *The Narrative Study of Lives*. Newbury Park: Sage, 1993, 7, zit. n. Kraus, Wolfgang. *Identität als Narration. Die narrative Konstruktion von Identitätsprojekten*. http://web.fu-berlin.de/postmoderne-psych/berichte3/kraus.htm (letzter Zugriff 20.09.2016).

9 Kraus. *Identität als Narration.*

10 Vgl. Kraus. *Identität als Narration.*

durch Erzählungen Dritter.[11] Die Möglichkeit der Forterzählung einer individuellen Lebensgeschichte durch dritte, handlungstragende Akteure aber ist aus einer vornehmlich machtpolitisch fokussierten Perspektive durchaus zu problematisieren. Denn der zunehmende Sprachverlust als Symptom der Demenzerkrankung zeitigt ab einem fortgeschrittenen Krankheitsstadium in erzähltheoretischer Hinsicht den nahezu vollständigen Verzicht auf eine personale Perspektive, sodass die Repräsentation Demenzleidender notwendigerweise einem unabhängigen Erzähler obliegt. Die damit verbundene Geste des *für-jemanden-Sprechens* ist insbesondere durch Vertreter der *Postcolonial Studies* problematisiert worden, die den Zusammenhang von Sprache und vornehmlich politischer Subjektivierung aus einem machtpolitisch geschulten Blickwinkel fokussieren.

An anderer Stelle habe ich bereits in einem Aufsatz versucht,[12] der Validität einer interkulturell interessierten Perspektive auf die Herausforderungen, die das Sujet Demenz an den literarischen Text stellt, in Anlehnung an Gayatri Spivaks wegweisenden Essay „Can the Subaltern Speak?“ mit dem Titel „Der Altern(d) e kann sprechen“ zur Sichtbarkeit zu verhelfen. Es mag in Zweifel stehen, einen Begriff, der maßgeblich durch die postkoloniale Theoriebildung geprägt wurde, in Zusammenhang mit Demenz und Hochaltrigkeit zu bringen. Seine Anwendbarkeit kann im Rahmen dieses Beitrags auch sicherlich nicht umfassend unter Beweis gestellt werden. Eine rudimentäre Skizze der gemeinsamen Interessengebiete von *Age Studies* und *Postcolonial Theory* vermag jedoch ihren Deckungsgrad in Ansätzen zu erhellen. In seinem Aufsatz „‚Ins Graue'. Zur kulturellen Konstruktion von Altern und Alter“ etwa legt Rüdiger Kunow sein Augenmerk auf die Interferenzen der *Gender*, *Postcolonial* und *Age Studies* und vollzieht nicht nur eine Registratur der gemeinsamen Interessengebiete von *Gender* und *Age Studies*,[13]

---

11 Vgl. den Artikel von Martina Schmidhuber "Lebensgeschichte und Personalität bei Demenz" in diesem Band. Schmidhuber stellt unter ethischen Gesichtspunkten das ratio-zentrierte, auf John Locke zurückgehende Verständnis personaler Identität in der klassischen Philosophie einer Perspektive gegenüber, die Personsein und Identität in einer individuellen Lebensgeschichte gründend begreift, die offen ist für Veränderungen und Brüche, dabei leibliche Erfahrungen und Weltzugänge, wie sie mitunter für das Krankheitsbild prägend sind, einschließt. Diese kann in Anlehnung an die grundsätzliche Relationalität narrativer Identität potentiell auch von anderen weitererzählt werden.

12 Vgl. Verf. "Der Altern(d)e kann sprechen. Sprechen aus dem Exil in Arno Geigers autobiographischer Erzählung *Der alte König in seinem Exil*." In: *Limbus. Australisches Jahrbuch für germanistische Literatur- und Kulturwissenschaft* 8 (2015): 201–19.

13 Kunow, Rüdiger. "'Ins Graue'. Zur kulturellen Konstruktion von Altern und Alter." In: Heike Hartung (ed.). *Alter und Geschlecht. Repräsentation, Geschichten und Theorien des Alter(n)s*. Bielefeld: transcript, 2005, 23–43, 34: „[h]ier wie dort geht es um den sozialen

sondern regt ebenfalls eine fruchtbare Betrachtung des Alters aus postkolonialer Perspektive an, die mit den *Gender Studies* und *Age Studies* eine Fokussierung auf Fragen der Identitätspolitik, der Repräsentation, der Machtasymmetrien, der Frage nach dem kulturell Dominanten und Entlegenen, der Marginalisierung, kurzum: „der Beschreibung entmachteter Sozialität" teilt.[14]

Es geht in der vorliegenden Argumentation jedoch nicht bevorzugt um die Profilierung eines theoriebildenden Impulses für die Entwicklung literarischer Altersbetrachtungen,[15] sondern mit der Fokussierung auf Spivaks Studie, die das Verhältnis von Sprache, Repräsentation, Subjektivierung und Macht beleuchtet, wird meines Erachtens das Herzstück von Geigers Text zu Tage befördert: Die Frage nach der Möglichkeit der Selbstrepräsentation, nach einer Erzählung des Selbst im Kontext der Erkrankung und ihren hierarchisierenden Implikationen.

Die Konstitution eines (politischen) Subjekts ist gemäß Spivak genuin gekoppelt an die Möglichkeit der Selbstrepräsentation. Antonio Gramsci prägte in den 30er Jahren des 20. Jahrhunderts mit seinen *Gefängnisheften* den Begriff der Subalternität (z. dt. *von minderem Rang*) für diejenigen, die von dieser Möglichkeit ausgeschlossen sind. Er nahm diesen Begriff seiner Zeit für das Proletariat in Anspruch, während der Begriff in der postkolonialen Theoriebildung der 80er in Gayatri Spivaks Essay „Can the Subaltern Speak?" (1985) auf die indische subalterne Bevölkerung Anwendung findet und insbesondere am Beispiel der indischen Witwenverbrennung auf seine geschlechtsspezifischen Implikationen überprüft wird. Spivaks Kritik gilt dabei – unter anderem ausgehend vom Beispiel indischer Witwen und ihrer doppelten Marginalisierung sowohl durch ein einheimisches Patriarchat als auch durch die Kolonialmacht – Versuchen, Subalterne durch *Experten* und *Übersetzungen*, also durch vermittelnde Instanzen, zum Sprechen zu bringen. Dabei würden Menschen zu Objekten von Wissensproduktion, die jedoch selbst nicht am Diskurs partizipierten. In der Einleitung zur deutschen Ausgabe von Spivaks wegweisendem Aufsatz heißt es bei Hito Steyerl: „Die anderen ‚für sich selbst sprechen' zu lassen, ist also laut Spivak eine uneingestandene Geste der Selbsterhöhung." Sie sei im Gegensatz zu ihrer Intention, das Subjekt zu erretten, einzig die „verdeckte Rehabilitation des Subjekts

und kulturellen Konstruktcharakter scheinbar biologischer Tatsachen, um Fragen der Diskriminierung auf der Basis dieser Konstrukte (sexism bzw. ageism) [...]."

14 Kunow. "'Ins Graue,'" 34.

15 Einen bemerkenswerten Ansatz in dieser Richtung liefert ein *special issue* des *Journal of Aging Studies*. Dyk, Silke van, Küpper, Thomas (eds.). *Postcolonial Perspectives in Aging Studies*. Journal of Aging Studies 2016. <http://www.journals.elsevier.com/journal-of-aging-studies/recent-articles> (letzter Zugriff 20.09.2016).

(der westlichen Mittelklasse)".[16] Der Akt des *für-jemanden-Sprechens* markiere die Fremdheit und Unverständlichkeit des prekären Subjekts, sodass es „nur durch Zerstreutheit und Unfassbarkeit definiert [werde] und [...] letztendlich aus reiner Differenz"[17] bestehe. Hat der Begriff der Subalternität im Laufe seiner Geschichte bereits auf verschiedene Gegenstandsbereiche zwischen der Landbevölkerung Italiens und den indischen Subalternen Anwendung gefunden, so erlaubt die Wortbedeutung „von minderem Rang"[18] die Übertragbarkeit auf verschiedene Formen der Unterprivilegierung, wie sie letztlich auch die Demenzkrankheit als Kontrapunkt der Hegemonie einer ratiozentrierten Gesellschaft darstellt. Die Fruchtbarkeit des Begriffs besteht in einer spezifischen Sensibilisierung für die Machtmechanismen, die den Versuchen, der Krankheit erzählerisch Ausdruck zu verleihen, eingeschrieben sind.

III. Leben mit Demenz erzählen: (Selbst)Repräsentation und Subjektivierung in *Der alte König in seinem Exil*

Schon die Problematik der Gattungszuordnung lässt die Konfliktstellung der Sprechhoheit offen zu Tage treten. Haben wir es im Fall des *alten Königs in seinem Exil* mit einem autobiographischen oder biographischen Text zu tun? Wessen Leben wird erzählt? Die Autobiographie kennzeichnet gemäß dem *Reallexikon der deutschen Literaturwissenschaft* das Folgende:

> Eine Autobiographie ist ein nichtfiktionaler, narrativ organisierter Text im Umfang eines Buches, dessen Gegenstand innere und äußere Erlebnisse sowie selbst vollzogene Handlungen aus der Vergangenheit des Autors sind. Diese werden im Rahmen einer das Ganze überschauenden und zusammenfassenden Schreibsituation sprachlich so artikuliert, daß sich der Autobiograph sprachlich handelnd in ein Verhältnis zu seiner Umwelt setzt.[19]

Demgegenüber steht die Biographie, die ein Leben aus der Außenperspektive erzählt: „Heute meint Biographie fast nur noch die künstlerisch-literarische bzw. wissenschaftliche Darstellung eines fremden Lebenslaufs, wobei meist an eine

---

16 Steyerl, Hito. "Die Gegenwart der Subalternen." In: Gayatri Chakravorty Spivak. *Can the Subaltern Speak? Postkolonialität und subalterne Artikulation*. Wien: Turia + Kant, 2008, 7–16, 11.

17 Steyerl. "Die Gegenwart der Subalternen," 11.

18 Steyerl. "Die Gegenwart der Subalternen," 8.

19 Lehmann, Jürgen. "Autobiographie." In: *Reallexikon der deutschen Literaturwissenschaft: Vol. 1*. Berlin: de Gruyter, 1997, 169–73, 169.

umfassende, das ganze Leben umspannende Darstellung gedacht wird".[20] Selbstverständlich offenbart Arno Geiger im Text *seine* Erfahrungen mit der Pflege seines Vaters. Primär aber geht es um eine *fremde* Lebens- und Leidensgeschichte des Vaters, August Geiger, und zwar weit über die Krankheitserzählung hinaus. Diese Tatsache hat manchen Kritiker dazu bewogen, ein moralisches Verdikt gegen den Autor zu verhängen, der in *Der alte König in seinem Exil* die Geschichte eines Mannes vermittelt, der diese nicht selbst erzählen bzw. autorisieren kann. Ulrich Stock schreibt in einer Rezension mit dem signifikanten Titel „Material Vater" in *Die Zeit*:

> Eine Gattungsbezeichnung fehlt. Sollten wir es einsortieren, wäre es ein Sachbuch, denn es erzählt von den Vorzeichen, dem Ausbruch und dem Verlauf einer Demenz am Fall eines konkret existierenden, noch lebenden Menschen, von dem wir sehr viel erfahren, Name, Wohnort, Ehegeschichten und Peinlichkeiten, die er, wäre er noch bei Verstand, wohl lieber für sich behielte.[21]

Unabhängig von Stocks Qualifikation der Erzählung als Sachbuchliteratur, die in der Forschung durch den Nachweis der ästhetischen Überformung und des Fiktionalisierungsgrades der Figuren zurückgewiesen wurde,[22] richtet der Rezensent mit seinem Vorwurf der Bloßstellung den Fingerzeig auf die Fallstricke

---

20 Scheuer, Helmut. "Biographie." In: *Reallexikon der deutschen Literaturwissenschaft: Vol. 1*. Berlin: de Gruyter, 1997, 233–38, 233.

21 Stock. "Material Vater".

22 Kretzschmar, Dirk. "Alzheimertexte der deutschen Gegenwartsliteratur." In: Ders., Rudolf Freiburg (eds.). *Alter(n) in Literatur und Kultur der Gegenwart*. Würzburg: Königshausen & Neumann, 2012, 117–45, 121: „Die Anwendung von literarischen Verfahren wie der Analepse und des auktorialen Kommentars, die wirkungsvoll verhindern, dass die Beschreibungen des Demenzkranken in die Nähe von Verächtlichmachung oder Verspottung geraten, sind ein deutliches Indiz dafür, dass Geiger sich die Frage, wie er es bei der Darstellung seines Vaters mit der Moral halte, auch selbst gestellt hat. [...] Denn die genannten narrativen Strategeme verweisen eben auch darauf, dass es sich bei Geigers Text um Literatur, also um ein ästhetisch durchkonstruiertes Artefakt handelt. Insofern ist es allzu kurzschlüssig, die reale Person August Geiger mit der gleichnamigen textinternen Figur ‚August Geiger' vollkommen in eins zu setzen und ausschließlich nach der Realitätsadäquatheit und/oder moralischen Rechtfertigung seiner literarischen Gestaltung zu fragen. Die Erzähl- und Fiktionalitätstheorie kennt bekanntlich die Kategorie des pseudo-realen Objekts. Darunter fallen beispielsweise literarische Figuren, die es in der Wirklichkeit gab oder gibt, die aber mit ihrem Eintritt in den Text unhintergehbar literaturspezifischen Formierungen unterzogen werden, sodass ihnen der Status lebensweltlich gedeckter Referenzialisierbarkeit nur noch beschränkt zukommt."

der Repräsentation eines Unmündigen bzw. Sprachlosen. Und tatsächlich erweist sich die Erzählung als Konflikt um die Deutungshoheit einer Lebensgeschichte, die unter anderem erzähltheoretisch ausagiert wird. Denn das titelgebende Exil des Dementen als Metapher seiner Segregation und Isolation entfaltet sich terminologisch ausgerechnet in einer Schreibszene. Zwar wird ein hierarchisch organisierter Raumdualismus zur Darstellung der Krankheit schon zu Anfang des Textes entworfen, der sich zwischen einem „[d]ort drüben, innerhalb der Grenzen seiner geistigen Verfassung" und „unserer auf Sachlichkeit und Zielstrebigkeit ausgelegten Gesellschaft" (Geiger. *Der alte König in seinem Exil*, 11) aufspannt; dennoch findet das Exil erstmals begrifflich Erwähnung, während Arno Geiger an der Erzählung über seinen Vater schreibt: „Da irrt der Vater rat- und rastlos umher *wie ein alter König in seinem Exil.* Dann ist alles, was er sieht, beängstigend, alles schwankend, instabil, davon bedroht, sich im nächsten Moment aufzulösen. Und nichts fühlt sich an wie zu Hause. *Ich sitze seit einiger Zeit in der Küche und tippe Notizen in meinen Laptop.* Im Wohnzimmer läuft der Fernseher […]." (Geiger. *Der alte König in seinem Exil*, 12; Hervorhebung L.S.) Die Verbannung des einstigen Souveräns aus der Heimat, der Machtverlust, der durch die titelgebende Formel impliziert wird, wird in eine assoziative Verbindung mit der Erzählung der Lebens- und Leidensgeschichte gebracht, von der der Vater – in der zitierten Schreibszene dezidiert auch räumlich – ausgeschlossen ist. Der Verlust von Souveränität, der durch das Bild des exilierten Herrschers zum Ausdruck kommt, wird also gestaltet als ein Verlust der erzählerischen Deutungshoheit und Verfügung über die eigene Vita, während der Sohn sich durch „auktorial-sentenziöse[ ] und didaktisierende[ ] Kommentare[ ]",[23] durch seine rationalistische Weltsicht, die den normativen gesellschaftlichen Maßstäben entspricht, zu ihrem Souverän aufschwingt. Zudem wird der Ausschluss vom Erzählen des eigenen Lebens assoziativ mit der Vorstellung des Schwankens, der Instabilität, der Verflüchtigung kurzgeschlossen. Das sich nicht selbst erzählende Ich ist gemäß dem Zitat in Auflösung begriffen.

Die Selbstermächtigung des souveränen erzählenden Ich demgegenüber zeigt sich z.B. in der Repräsentation der Kriegserfahrungen des Vaters. Das Kriegsnarrativ dient hier nicht nur – wie für die Krankheitserzählung kennzeichnend[24] – als

---

23 Kretzschmar. "Alzheimertexte der deutschen Gegenwartsliteratur," 120.

24 Anne Hunsaker Hawkins war Professorin am Institut für Humanwissenschaften am Penn State College of Medicine. Aus Ihren Untersuchungen im Bereich der Narrativen Medizin ist unter anderem die viel beachtete Studie *Reconstructing Illness. Studies in Pathography* hervorgegangen. Am Beispiel von Pathographien, (auto)biographischen Erzählungen physischer Erkrankungen, arbeitet Hunsaker Hawkins verschiedene

Medium der Veranschaulichung einer individuellen Krankheitserfahrung. In Anlehnung an Anne Hunsaker Hawkins schreibt Heike Hartung: „Hawkins ist der Auffassung, dass Pathographien um zugrunde liegende transkulturelle Mythen organisiert sind, wobei häufig die Metaphorik des Kriegs oder Kampfs, der Reise oder Suche, des Todes und der Wiedergeburt wirksam wird.“[25] Die Anreicherung der Krankheitserzählung mit (inter)kulturellen Gemeinplätzen dient dabei nach Hunsaker Hawkins der erzählerischen Verknüpfung von Individual- und Kollektiverleben, sodass ein Erfahrungshorizont für die persönliche Krankheitsgeschichte hergestellt werde. Eine solche, der Krankheit zur Sichtbarkeit verhelfende Metaphorik ist auch in Geigers Erzählung vorhanden: Von einem „Stellungskrieg“, von feindlicher Übernahme (Geiger. *Der alte König in seinem Exil*, 205), von einem „Trümmerfeld“ (Geiger. *Der alte König in seinem Exil*, 205) ist zuweilen die Rede. Doch die Bedeutung der Kriegserzählung geht weit über eine illustrierende Funktion der Leiden hinaus. Zum einen manifestieren sich die Erfahrung von Krieg und Krankheit im existenzbedrohenden Gefühl des Heimatverlusts, der jedoch – in beiden Fällen – durch Sprache aufgehoben wird bzw. werden kann.[26] Krieg und Krankheit berühren sich darüber hinaus – und dieser Aspekt ist hier erkenntnisleitend – in einer Leerstelle, die beide in den Erzählungen des Vaters produzieren. Während die Krankheitssymptomatik bewirkt, „dass die Sprache langsam aus ihm [August Geiger; L.S.] heraussickert“, das symbolische Exil seiner Krankheit also aus der Perspektive des Exilierten unerzählt bleiben muss, ist auch seine Gefangenschaft in einem „Lazarett am Stadtrand von Bratislava“ (Geiger. *Der alte König in seinem Exil*, 43) ein blinder Fleck. Es heißt sinnfällig: „Diese vier Wochen blieben ausgespart, die Erzählungen des Vaters begannen meist erst mit dem Tag, an dem ihn die Sowjets laufenließen, weil [er] nichts mehr wert war.“ (Geiger. *Der alte König in seinem Exil*, 43) Der Kurzschluss von Krieg und Krankheit wird dabei bereits durch ihre räumlich periphere Figuration im Zitat nahegelegt, um beide Erfahrungen hüllt sich überdies Schweigen. Das erzählende Ich vermag die

---

konstitutive Erzählmuster für Krankheitsnarrative heraus, die über die Anwendung hergebrachter Metaphoriken und transkultureller Mythen und Erzählungen eine sinnstiftende Integration von individuellem Krankheitserleben und kollektiver Erfahrung herstellen, die überindividuelle Verstehensangebote offeriert. Vgl. Hunsaker Hawkins, Anne. *Reconstructing Illness. Studies in Pathography*. West Lafayette, Indiana: Purdue University Press, 1999, 18–30.

25 Hartung. “Small World?,” 167.

26 Vgl. Geiger. *Der alte König in seinem Exil*, 45. Nach der Rückkehr aus der sowjetischen Gefangenschaft stellt sich das Gefühl von Heimat mit dem Erkennen der dialektalen Färbung der Region um das österreichische Wolfurt ein. (Ibid., 164)

kriegsbedingte Leerstelle in der Lebensgeschichte des Vaters souverän auszufüllen, ebenso wie er die Krankheit zu beschreiben vermag: „In der Gefangenschaft wurde er zum Verladen von Kriegsbeute vergattert, bis er in der Suppe einen offensichtlich verdorbenen Knochen fand und ihn vor lauter Hunger abnagte. Am Tag darauf hatte er die Ruhr und magerte bis auf vierzig Kilo ab." (Geiger. *Der alte König in seinem Exil*, 43) Nun wird die Deutungshoheit des Sohnes bezüglich der Repräsentation der Kriegsereignisse jedoch jäh durchbrochen, als die Tagebücher des Vaters aufgefunden werden, aus denen – wenngleich indirekt, da durch ein Dokument vermittelt – die Stimme des Vaters hörbar wird:

> Im Gegensatz zu den Tagen waren die Nächte eher kühl, und da uns die russischen Schwestern, die mir in äußerst unangenehmer Erinnerung liegen, nur für je 2 Mann eine Decke erlaubten, fror es mich manchmal. [...] Dieser Zustand dauerte 2 Tage, dann war das Fieber weg. Nicht wunderlich war es, als ich bald darauf wieder Arbeitsdienst machen musste, und zwar musste ich mit, die Toten vergraben. (Geiger. *Der alte König in seinem Exil*, 166)

Die monologische Erzählweise erhält in diesem Moment ein Gegengewicht. Die ‚Sprachermächtigung' des Traumatisierten bezüglich der Kriegserinnerungen präfiguriert die Entwicklung der Krankheitserzählung.

Während in der Erzählung und all den ihren Kapiteln vorangestellten Frage-Antwort-Sequenzen zunächst der Sohn buchstäblich tonangebend ist, indem er das Gespräch durch eine einleitende Frage lenkt, kippt das dadurch entworfene Kräfteverhältnis zwischen dem Erzähler und dem Erkrankten im Verlauf der fortschreitenden Erzählung. Zu Anfang heißt es noch: „‚Wie geht es dir, Papa?' ‚Also, ich muss sagen, es geht mir gut. Allerdings unter Anführungszeichen, denn ich bin nicht imstande, es zu beurteilen.'" (Geiger. *Der alte König in seinem Exil*, 17) Rund einhundert Seiten später dann: „‚Weißt du, ich bin auch schon ein älterer Knabe. Dagegen bist du ein junger Hupfer.' ‚Wo du recht hast, hast du recht.'" (Geiger. *Der alte König in seinem Exil*, 111) Die fast unbemerkt sich in den Text schleichende Ergreifung des Wortes wird unmittelbar eingeleitet durch das metaphorisch zu verstehende Auffinden eines Fotos, das den Vater nach seiner Entlassung aus der Kriegsgefangenschaft zeigt und das, wie auch die heraussickernde Sprache, irreversibel verloren zu sein scheint. Das Foto, so erfährt der Leser, war im Zuge der Krankheitswirren vom Vater unauffindbar verlegt worden:

> Ich bedauerte, dass das Foto gemeinsam mit der Brieftasche meines Vaters verlorengegangen war. Tante Hedwig sagte; ‚Ach, Arno, wir haben eine Kopie. Keine Ahnung, wie die in unseren Besitz gekommen ist. Aber wir haben eine Kopie.' ‚Bist du sicher?' ‚Ja, ich bin sicher. Wenn du willst, suche ich es heraus. Du kannst es morgen holen.' Also holte ich das Foto und machte eine Kopie der Kopie und durfte die Originalkopie behalten; sie ist eines der Dinge, an denen mein Herz hängt. Aus der Kennzeichnung auf der Rückseite

des Fotos geht hervor, dass Emil den Abzug im Jahr 1995 machen ließ, zu einem Zeitpunkt, als er und mein Vater bereits alte Männer waren. 1995 – um diesen Dreh herum hatte das ganze Schlamassel angefangen. (Geiger. *Der alte König in seinem Exil*, 108–9)

Aus dem Zitat lassen sich mannigfache Schlüsse ziehen: Zunächst wird das Foto durch die Datierung unmittelbar mit dem Beginn des Krankheitsverlaufs in Verbindung gebracht, darüber hinaus verbindet es erneut die Motive Krieg und Krankheit. Während das kurz nach der Gefangenschaft aufgenommene Bild Dokument eines durch extreme Auszehrung zu verschwinden drohenden Subjekts ist, leitet die Fotografie ebenfalls das Wiederauftauchen eines durch Krankheit und Aphasie schwindenden Subjekts ein.[27] Allerdings weist das diskutierte Verhältnis von Original und Kopie auf die Tatsache hin, dass wir es mit einer fingierten Sprachermächtigung zu tun bekommen. Der Fund des Fotos erfüllt die Funktion eines Kippmoments in der Erzählung: Die vorausgehenden Interviewsequenzen verändern ihre Vorzeichen und im unmittelbar folgenden Erzähltext beginnt sich der fortschreitende Sprachverlust indes druckgraphisch zu materialisieren. Sichtbar zerfasert nun das Textgefüge, eine sukzessive Reduktion der Erzählteile bei gleichzeitiger Zunahme der typographischen Lücken im Text ist zu beobachten und scheint der Bewegung des Schwindens und *Heraussickerns*, die durch das Krankheitsbild vorgegeben wird, poetologisch Rechnung zu tragen. Dabei ist die Bewegung des Schwindens als Inszenierung der Krankheitssymptomatik paradox, sie nähert sich zwar druckgraphisch dem Verschwinden und verhilft dabei doch der Perspektive des Erkrankten zur Sichtbarkeit. Auf die erste Wortergreifung des Vaters in den Frage-Antwort-Passagen folgt im Erzähltext die Antizipation der eigenen Sprachlosigkeit. Zitat: „‚Ich bin einer, der nichts zu melden hat. Da ist nichts mehr zu machen.' Es waren Sätze wie dieser, die auch ein Held von Franz Kafka oder Thomas Bernhard gesagt haben könnte, ich dachte mir, *da haben sich zwei gefunden, ein an Alzheimer erkrankter Mann und ein Schriftsteller.*" (Geiger.

27 Ursprünglich soll das Bild als Identitätsnachweis während der Heimkehr aus der sowjetischen Gefangenschaft dienen. (Geiger. *Der alte König in seinem Exil*, 44) Der Verlust des Bildes wird erzählerisch mit den krankheitsinduzierten Verlusten kurzgeschlossen, im übertragenen Sinn geht es also um den drohenden Identitätsverlust: „Die Anfänge der Krankheit waren eine schreckliche Zeit, ein vollkommener Fehlschlag. Außerdem waren sie die Zeit der großen Verluste. Das betrifft sowohl das biographische Gedächtnis des Vaters als auch das konkrete Verschwinden von Dingen, die im Leben des Vaters wichtig gewesen waren. […] Das Brustbild, unmittelbar nach dem Krieg aufgenommen, ein Jugendlicher mit nur wenig mehr als vierzig Kilogramm – verloren. Mein Vater hatte das Foto fast sechzig Jahre lang in seiner Geldtasche mit sich herumgetragen, gemeinsam mit einem Foto seiner Mutter. Dinge, an denen sein Herz gehangen hatte." (Ibid., 26)

Der alte König in seinem Exil, 114; Hervorhebung L.S.) Just in dem Moment, da das Subjekt zu verschwinden droht – der Vater sagt ‚Ich bin nichts mehr.' –, inszeniert Geiger die rettende Begegnung zwischen Schriftsteller und Patienten als Begegnung zweier Erzähler, die flankiert wird von Exponenten der Sprachexperimente der literarischen Moderne wie Franz Kafka und James Joyce, die fortan zur poetologischen Bezugsgrößen des Erzählverlaufs werden. Die aphasische Sprache des Vaters erinnert den Erzähler dabei frappierend an die Sprachvirtuosität der literarischen Moderne:

> Diese Ausdrucksweise beeindruckte mich, ich fühlte mich in Berührung mit dem magischen Potential der Wörter. James Joyce hat von sich gesagt, er habe keine Phantasie, überlasse sich aber einfach den Offerten der Sprache. So kam es mir auch beim Vater vor. Aus zukünftig machte er kuhzünftig, das Ende des Lateins, das ich bekundete, konterte er, er selber befinde sich nicht am Ende des Lateins, sondern am Ende des Daseins. Dabei betonte er die Wörter so, dass die lautliche Verwandtschaft unüberhörbar war. Er verwendete Wörter wie pressant, pressiert, dawei und bistra. (Geiger. *Der alte König in seinem Exil*, 101)

Im Analogieschluss eröffnen die krankheitsinduzierten semantischen Fehlleistungen vielversprechendes poetisches Potential, das schlussendlich eine Begegnung von Erzähler und Erkranktem auf Augenhöhe erlaubt, die zu Beginn der Erzählung durch den Schreibprozess noch deutlich separiert erschienen: Es ist eine Allianz, die in der Assimilation des kreativen poetologischen Potentials der Krankheit realisiert wird.[28] Das Kräftemessen um die Erzählhoheit im Text, das zunächst zu Ungunsten des Vaters ausging, steht durch das poetische Potential der Krankheitssymptomatik neuerlich zu Disposition. Es wird wiederum entschieden in einer erneut metaphorisch zu lesenden Begegnung von Vater und Sohn. Das erzählerische Kräftemessen wird dabei substituiert und präfiguriert durch ein physisches: „Bei einem meiner Besuche in dieser Woche überredete ich den Vater nochmals zum Armdrücken. Zunächst drückte er in die falsche Richtung, ich erklärte ihm, wie wir es machen müssen, er begriff es, dann ließ ich ihn zweimal gewinnen." (Geiger. *Der alte König in seinem Exil*, 127) Diese zunächst unbedeutend erscheinende Anekdote aus dem Leben mit der Krankheit läutet den finalen und symbolischen ‚Triumphzug' des Demenzleidenden ein, der sich schlussendlich sowohl formalästhetisch zeigt als auch über die Erzählverhältnisse Gestalt annimmt. Das Narrativ tritt im schließenden Kapitel typographisch

---

28 Zum poetologischen Potential der Erkrankung bzw. zum Vergleich von Ausprägungen der Aphasie und der Poetik der Literatur der Moderne vgl. Stanzel, Franz K. "Gerontologisches in Literatur und Poetik." In: *Arbeiten aus Anglistik und Amerikanistik* 29 (2004): 3–21, 11.

nun vollends als ein Konglomerat von Versatzstücken in Erscheinung. Damit wird schon in visueller Hinsicht ein Übergewicht jener durch die Krankheit hervorgebrachten *ansatzlosen, unwahrscheinlichen* und *schwebenden* Sätze geschaffen, die anfänglich noch durch ihre vom Erzähler behauptete Traumlogik den Gegensatz zur Rationalität der Gesellschaft und des Sohnes begründeten, die in einem geschlossenen, kohärenten, linearen und auf Logizität zielenden Narrativ ihre Entsprechung fand. Zudem wird das Erzählte, das im Fortgang des Kapitels dem *Heraussickern der Sprache* Form verleiht, von einem eindeutig zu identifizierenden Erzähler-Ich abgekoppelt. Sätze wie jener: „In der Zeitung steht, schwarze Schafe werden wegen der Erderwärmung seltener", (Geiger. *Der alte König in seinem Exil*, 188) erinnern jedoch frappant an solche, die zu Beginn der Erzählung noch zur Illustration des korrumpierten Verstandes des Vaters gelten konnten. Doch sie haben im Verlauf der Erzählung ihre Vorzeichen deutlich verändert. Sind sie zu Beginn noch unübersehbar durch das erzählende Ich vermittelt, stehen sie am Ende für sich selbst; die Erzählstimme mischt sich nicht mehr sichtbar in die Aussagen des Dementen ein, sondern tritt ihnen nebengeordnet an die Seite. Während zu Beginn die Erzählerstimme deutlich vernehmbar ist, [vgl. „Eine Katze streift durch den Garten. *Der Vater sagt*: ‚Früher hatte ich auch Katzen, nicht gerade für mich allein, aber als Teilhaber.' *Und einmal als ich ihn frage, wie es ihm gehe, antwortet er*: ‚Es geschehen keine Wunder, aber Zeichen.'" (Geiger. *Der alte König in seinem Exil*, 11; Hervorhebung L.S.) tritt der Ich-Erzähler am Ende in den Hintergrund. Und erst nach einer typographischen Lücke im Text tritt das erzählende Ich wieder aus dem Schatten in die Erzählung ein: „Meine Befürchtungen, dass der gute Teil vorbei sei, hatten sich oft genug als ungerechtfertigt erwiesen, meine Vorhersagen waren selten eingetroffen." (Geiger. *Der alte König in seinem Exil*, 188) Während die Vermittlung durch den Sohn zu Anfang explizit in der Rede des Vaters hervortritt, wird diese Form der Einmischung gen Ende aufgegeben. Durch die Nebenordnung von erzählendem Ich und den von einer klar markierten Erzählinstanz losgelösten Versatzstücken entsteht der Eindruck einer Polyphonie,[29] welche die monologische Deutungshoheit des Sohnes durchbricht. Scheinbar wird gen Ende der Erzählung eine „mimetische Darstellungsweise [eingenommen], die sich der besonderen Herausforderung (an das Schreiben) stellt,

29 Ursprünglich bezeichnet der Begriff diverse Arten der Mehrstimmigkeit in der Musik. 1929 wird er von Michail Bachtin zur Beschreibung des mehrstimmigen Erzählverfahrens von Fjodor Dostojewski für die Literaturbetrachtung adaptiert. Vgl. Bachtin, Michail. *Probleme der Poetik Dostoevskijs*. Aus dem Russischen von Adelheid Schramm. München: Hanser, 1971. Als tendenziell anti-hierarchische Stimmenvielfalt haben polyphone Erzählverfahren auch das Interesse der *Postcolonial Studies* geweckt.

die Innensicht einer dementen Person zu imaginieren".[30] Die sprachbasierte, auf Ovid zurückgehende Definition von Heimat als Ort, wo man jemandes Sprache verstehe, ebnet den Weg für diese sinnbildliche Raumergreifung, gleichwohl der Textraum natürlich lediglich eine imaginäre Heimat für den Exilierten zur Verfügung stellt. Denn die Tatsache, dass hier die zu Anfang klar als ‚Sinnfreiheiten' markierten Äußerungen des Vaters unkommentiert für sich selbst stehen, zeugt von der Gewissheit, dass sie – ohne Übersetzung und Vermittlung – auf Verständnis stoßen. Dergestalt wird ihnen das Stigma des Unverständlichen und Fremdartigen genommen, die Synthese des sich zwischen Rationalität und Irrationalität aufspannenden Raumbinarismus wird durch eine schließende Bezugnahme zum Titel bekräftigt: „Es heißt: Wer lange genug wartet, kann König werden", (Geiger. *Der alte König in seinem Exil*, 189) lautet es dort nicht ohne Pathos. Sein Exil wird aufgehoben, indem die Deutungshoheit gewissermaßen zurückerlangt wird. Zeitgleich jedoch ist die letzte Sentenz mehrdeutig in ihrer Verweisstruktur. Verweist sie durch die sprachbildliche Bezugnahme zur Titelgebung scheinbar eindeutig auf die Figur des dementen Vaters, so rekurriert das lange Warten tendenziell auf die Beharrlichkeit des Sohnes, der während der Entstehung der Erzählung den sprichwörtlichen ‚langen Atem' aufbringt:

> Ich wollte mir mit diesem Buch Zeit lassen, ich habe sechs Jahre darauf gespart. Gleichzeitig hatte ich gehofft, es schreiben zu können, bevor der Vater stirbt. Ich wollte nicht nach seinem Tod von ihm erzählen. Ich wollte über einen Lebenden schreiben, ich fand, dass der Vater, wie jeder Mensch, ein Schicksal verdient, das offenbleibt. (Geiger. *Der alte König in seinem Exil*, 188–89)

Damit reüssiert am Ende vor allem der Erzähler, dem hier tatsächlich in seiner künstlerischen Schaffenskraft erneut die Deutungshoheit über das väterliche Leben zukommt, dem er hier ein offenes Ende offeriert. Es bleibt also der fade Beigeschmack eines allenfalls zugestandenen Triumphes, der sich mit der gönnerhaften Geste des Sohnes, der seinem Vater im eben zitierten Duell im Armdrücken den Sieg ‚selbstlos' schenkt, bereits einschleicht. So wie diese Episode metaphorisch den ‚Triumphzug' des Vaters durch das ‚Auftauchen' seiner Stimme im Text präfiguriert, so überschattet sie ihn gleichzeitig, denn sie unterwirft seine Wortergreifung einer „uneingestandenen Geste der Selbsterhöhung", wie sie für Spivak für das *jemanden-für-sich-sprechen-lassen* kennzeichnend ist, obschon das

30 Hartung, Heike. "Fremde im Spiegel. Körperwahrnehmung und Demenz." In: Sabine Mehlmann, Sigrid Ruby (eds.). *'Für dein Alter siehst du gut aus!' Von der Unsichtbarkeit des alternden Körpers im Horizont des demographischen Wandels. Multidisziplinäre Perspektiven*. Bielefeld: transcript, 2010, 123–38, 126.

erzählende Ich sich von seiner Position als sichtbarer Vermittler oder Übersetzer zunehmend zurückzieht. Natürlich ist diese Form der Selbsterhöhung nicht im Kontext (inter)kultureller Hegemonien und Machtverhältnisse zu lesen, wie sie Spivak und die Vertreter postkolonialer Theorie interessieren. Doch auch hier festigen sich einige für die Wahrnehmung des Demenzleidenden folgenschwere Binarismen mit deutlichen machtpolitischen Implikationen zwischen Gesundheit und Krankheit, Rationalität und Irrationalität, die seine Stimme überlagern. Hier wird durch den Vermittlerstatus ein Subjekt bestätigt, das sich durch seine „allgemeinen Maßstäben" Genüge leistende „Sachlichkeit und Zielstrebigkeit" (Geiger. *Der alte König in seinem Exil*, 11) autorisiert. Immer wieder reflektiert der Text die damit verbundenen Gesten der Souveränität und Machtergreifung, z.B. im spielerischen Duell im Armdrücken, auch explizit, die Frage nach Herrschaft und Macht gehört schließlich gemäß der Titelgebung zu seiner Programmatik.

Gleichzeitig problematisiert das Erscheinungsbild der fingierten erzählerischen Selbstpräsentationen die Anforderungen an subjektivitätsstiftende Selbstnarrationen wie Kohärenz, Linearität und Kausalität[31] und regt einerseits dazu an, einen hergebrachten Subjektbegriff zu hinterfragen, andererseits selbstverständlich auch dazu, sich die Grundlagen der Segregation Erkrankter vor dem Hintergrund etablierter kultureller Muster bewusst zu machen.

Bibliographie

Bachtin, Michail. *Probleme der Poetik Dostoevskijs*. Aus dem Russischen von Adelheid Schramm. München: Hanser, 1971.

Draesner, Ulrike. "Ichs Heimweg macht alles alleine." In: Klara Obermüller (ed.). *Es schneit in meinem Kopf. Erzählungen über Alzheimer und Demenz*. München: Nagel & Kimche, 2006, 59–81.

Dyk, Silke van, Küpper, Thomas (eds.). *Postcolonial Perspectives in Aging Studies*. Journal of Aging Studies 2016. <http://www.journals.elsevier.com/journal-of-aging-studies/recent-articles> (letzter Zugriff 20.09.2016)

Geiger, Arno. *Der alte König in seinem Exil*. München: dtv 2011.

Hartung, Heike. "Fremde im Spiegel. Körperwahrnehmung und Demenz." In: Sabine Mehlmann, Sigrid Ruby (eds.). *'Für dein Alter siehst du gut aus!' Von der Unsichtbarkeit des alternden Körpers im Horizont des demographischen Wandels. Multidisziplinäre Perspektiven*. Bielefeld: transcript, 2010, 123–38.

Hartung, Heike. "Small World? – Narrative Annäherungen an Alzheimer." In: Cornelia Bogen, Madlen Domaschke, Sabine Pabst (eds.). *Alte Menschen und*

31 Kraus. *Identität als Narration*.

Medien. Alter im Spannungsfeld zwischen Kultur und Medien. Frankfurt a.M.: Peter Lang, 2008, 163–78.

Hunsaker Hawkins, Anne. *Reconstructing Illness. Studies in Pathography*. West Lafayette, Indiana: Purdue University Press, 1999, 18–30.

Kraus, Wolfgang. *Identität als Narration. Die narrative Konstruktion von Identitätsprojekten*. <http://web.fu-berlin.de/postmoderne-psych/berichte3/kraus.htm> (letzter Zugriff 20.09.2016).

Kretzschmar, Dirk. "Alzheimertexte der deutschen Gegenwartsliteratur." In: Ders., Rudolf Freiburg (eds.). *Alter(n) in Literatur und Kultur der Gegenwart*. Würzburg: Königshausen & Neumann, 2012, 117–45.

Kunow, Rüdiger. "'Ins Graue'. Zur kulturellen Konstruktion von Altern und Alter." In: Heike Hartung (ed.). *Alter und Geschlecht. Repräsentation, Geschichten und Theorien des Alter(n)s*. Bielefeld: transcript, 2005, 23–43.

Kurz, Alexander, Freter, Hans-Jürgen, Saxl, Susanna, Nickel, Ellen (eds.). *Demenz. Das Wichtigste*. Berlin: Deutsche Alzheimer Gesellschaft e.V., [2]2016.

Lehmann, Jürgen. "Autobiographie." In: *Reallexikon der deutschen Literaturwissenschaft: Vol. 1*. Berlin: de Gruyter, 1997, 169–73.

Scheuer, Helmut. "Biographie." In: *Reallexikon der deutschen Literaturwissenschaft: Vol. 1*. Berlin: de Gruyter, 1997, 233–38.

Stanzel, Franz K. "Gerontologisches in Literatur und Poetik." In: *Arbeiten aus Anglistik und Amerikanistik* 29 (2004): 3–21.

Steyerl, Hito. "Die Gegenwart der Subalternen." In: Gayatri Chakravorty Spivak. *Can the Subaltern Speak? Postkolonialität und subalterne Artikulation*. Wien: Turia + Kant, 2008, 7–16.

Stock, Ulrich. "Material Vater. Der Schrifsteller Arno Geiger schreibt einen Bestseller über den demenzkranken August Geiger, dessen Sohn er ist." *Die Zeit* online 18.02.2011. <http://www.zeit.de/2011/08/L-B-Geiger > (letzter Zugriff 20.09.2016).

Süwolto, Leonie. *Altern in einer alterslosen Gesellschaft. Literarische und filmische Imaginationen*. Paderborn: Fink, 2016.

Süwolto, Leonie. "Der Altern(d)e kann sprechen. Sprechen aus dem Exil in Arno Geigers autobiographischer Erzählung *Der alte König in seinem Exil* (2011)." In: *Limbus. Australisches Jahrbuch für germanistische Literatur- und Kulturwissenschaft* 8 (2015): 201–19.

Widdershoven, G. A. M. "The Story of Life: Hermeneutic Perspectives on the Relationship between Narrative and Life History." In: R. Josselson, A. Lieblich (eds.). *The Narrative Study of Lives*. Newbury Park: Sage, 1993.

Sara Strauss (Paderborn)

Narrative Ethics and Dementia in Alice LaPlante's *Turn of Mind*

Abstract: Within the field of narrative ethics this article is interested in the way in which the narrative voice and structure of a fictional dementia narrative can convey moral values and stimulate the reader to ethical reflections. By analysing Alice LaPlante's novel *Turn of Mind* (2011) the article examines the potential of second person and present tense narration to create narrative empathy with the fictional characters.

As a result of the high prevalence of dementia and Alzheimer's disease in contemporary society, there is a growing public interest in getting an insight into the consciousness of dementia patients. Numerous literary texts and films show this increasing public awareness of the disease and move the subjective experience of dementia patients into the centre of attention. Due to this focus on the patients' subjectivity, narrative fiction can contribute another perspective to the present discourse on dementia than the predominant medical view. By representing individual experience, fictional narratives also address ethical challenges that arise with dementia and Alzheimer's disease. With reference to Martha Nussbaum, who differentiates literature's approaches to ethics from the abstractions of analytic philosophy, James Phelan states that "novels explore the concrete particularity of ethical dilemmas faced by fully realized characters, and those explorations harness the cognitive power of the emotions".[1] In consequence of engaging the reader's emotions, literature is able to stimulate the reader to ethical reflections, and thereby it contributes to public discourses on dementia and the ethical dilemmas the disease poses to contemporary society. With regard to dementia narratives, Irmela Krüger-Fürhoff points out that

> these stories are significant from an ethical point of view because they offer first-person-based or imaginary insights into the experience of people with dementia, which no other discourse (e.g., that of the medical community or of caregivers) can provide.[2]

---

1 Phelan, James. "Narrative Ethics." In: Peter Hühn, John Pier, Wolf Schmid, Jörg Schönert (eds.). *Handbook of Narratology: Vol. 2*. Berlin/Boston: De Gruyter, 2014, 531–46, 541.

2 Krüger-Fürhoff, Irmela Marei. "Narrating the Limits of Narration – Alzheimer's Disease in Contemporary Literary Texts." In: Mark Schweda, Aagje Swinnen (eds.). *Popularizing Dementia: Public Expressions and Representations of Forgetfulness*. Bielefeld: Transcript, 2015, 89–108, 91.

Yet, the symptoms of the disease, which causes a severe loss of the patients' cognitive and linguistic faculties, pose fundamental challenges to narrative representation. As Krüger-Fürhoff notes, "[t]he neurodegenerative breakdown of memory and language will continue to demand new narrative approaches".[3] Authors of narrative fiction meet this challenge of representing the situation of mentally confused, disoriented characters with the help of different, sometimes experimental, narrative modes and techniques. As regards the inexpressibility of dementia patients' first-hand experience in consequence of their memory loss and aphasia, narrative fiction thus attempts to "narrat[e] the unnarratable".[4]

This article analyses the use of innovative narrative devices, such as second person and present tense narration as well as a fragmentation of the narrative voice, as means of conveying a fictional inside perspective of the reality of dementia patients. By analysing Alice LaPlante's novel *Turn of Mind*, published in 2011, the paper examines the high potential of these techniques to imitate the disoriented mind of a dementia patient, to create narrative empathy with the fictional character and thereby inspire the reader to ethical reflections on dementia and its implications for contemporary society. With reference to narrative ethics, the paper focuses on "the ethics of the told", i.e. the plot and the characters' actions, and principally on "the ethics of the telling", which James Phelan describes as "the ethical dimensions of the narrative's techniques".[5]

I. Immersion into the Consciousness of a Fictional Dementia Patient

Told from the perspective of the protagonist, Alice LaPlante's murder-mystery story *Turn of Mind* blends genre conventions of crime fiction with the narrative of a fictional dementia patient.[6] It employs what Brian Richardson terms "multipersoned narration"[7] and combines traditional first person and figural narrative

---

3 Krüger-Fürhoff. "Narrating the Limits of Narration," 105.

4 Rimmon-Kenan, Shlomith. "What Can Narrative Theory Learn from Illness Narratives?" In: *Literature and Medicine* 25,2 (2006): 241–54, 241.

5 Phelan, James. "Narrative Ethics," 531.

6 For a detailed analysis of the way in which *Turn of Mind* challenges the genre conventions of detective fiction and thereby interrogates dominant discourses on dementia see Sako, Katsura. "Dementia and Detection in *Elizabeth is Missing* and *Turn of Mind*." In: *Contemporary Women's Writing* 10,3 (2016): 315–33.

7 Richardson, Brian. "I Etcetera: On the Poetics and Ideology of Multipersoned Narratives." In: *Style* 28,3 (1994): 312–28, 312.

situations with second person narrative. The protagonist and homodiegetic narrator, 64-year-old Jennifer White, suffers from late-stage dementia. Already in the opening lines of the novel the first person narrator reveals her confused state of mind and describes this confusion as a condition rather normal to her:

> Something has happened. You can always tell. [...] This time, I am in a room, sitting on a cold metal folding chair. The room is not familiar, but I am used to that. I look for clues. (LaPlante. *Turn of Mind*, 3)

The first person narrator's admission that she is used to not being familiar with her surroundings makes the reader anticipate a peculiar mental condition of the protagonist. At the same time the protagonist reacts rationally and reasons logically how to resolve her disorientation. Being used to states of bewilderment, she has found strategies of coping with strange situations; strategies such as immediately looking for clues to make sense of her whereabouts. In this rational behaviour the protagonist does not differ from other, healthy persons since her actions seem to be led by intuition and logical conclusions and thereby she exhibits faculties exceedingly cherished in contemporary society. By use of the pronoun "you" the narrator generalises her act of drawing conclusions and trusting her intuition in the same way as other people do: "You can always tell." (LaPlante. *Turn of Mind*, 3) Before describing the protagonist's personal experience with the pronoun "I", the narrative starts with the more general, yet not impersonal pronoun "you". This generic "you" also includes the reader, whereby, from the beginning of the novel onwards, the narrative voice encourages him or her to identify with the protagonist's point of view.

Due to the homodiegetic narrative situation the reader's comprehension of the plot is for long parts of the novel limited to the character's subjective point of view. After some fragmented paragraphs, which fully confirm the fictional character's state of mental confusion, both, the protagonist and the reader, are presented with the main facts when the protagonist reads a sign "taped to the kitchen wall" (LaPlante. *Turn of Mind*, 4):

> My name is Dr. Jennifer White. I am sixty-four years old. I have dementia. My son, Mark, is twenty-nine. My daughter, Fiona, twenty-four. A caregiver, Magdalena, lives with me. (LaPlante. *Turn of Mind*, 4)

With the help of this sign Jennifer is at times able to remember some facets of her identity. Mostly, however, she forgets about her recent past and neither recognizes her children nor her carer. As typical of Alzheimer's disease this feeling of estrangement causes anxiety in the patient. Only seconds after reading the sign Jennifer forgets its message:

> It is all clear. So who are all these other people in my house? People, strangers, everywhere. A blond woman I don't recognize in my kitchen drinking tea. A glimpse of movement from the den. Then I turn the corner into the living room and find yet another face. I ask, So who are you? Who are all the others? (LaPlante. *Turn of Mind*, 4–5)

Although Jennifer and her carer Magdalena are alone in the house, her own reflection in the window and Magdalena's movement from one room to another perturb Jennifer so much that she believes to be surrounded by several strangers in her own house.

As characteristic of the symptoms of dementia, the protagonist's memory lapses and her recuperations of memory occur randomly and are unpredictable. Her mental state differs from day to day and often even changes from one moment to the next. The narrative situation reflects this state of living in the present without a memory of the recent past or plans for the future. In contrast to "the traditional role of past tense as the 'unmarked' or default tense of fiction and of narration generally",[8] Alice LaPlante's novel is told in the present tense with extensive interior monologues. "[O]pting […] for a 'poetics of immediacy'"[9] the peculiar decision for the present tense enables the narrator to represent the character's feeling of embodiment in time and space in the way the dementia patient might experience it. The present tense thereby fulfils the function described by Monika Fludernik "to foreground the time of the narrated experience […] and therefore concentrate on the psychology of the protagonist".[10] For LaPlante's protagonist the past frequently merges into the present. She does not remember that she is a 64-year-old widow with dementia retired from her profession but recalls being a doctor and a mother of two. Thus she acts accordingly:

> I wake early, hoping to get some work done before the children start clamoring for their breakfast, but someone is up even earlier. That blond woman [i.e. her carer Magdalena, S.St.]. Damn. Only this time she's not alone. Another woman is with her, drinking coffee out of my favorite cup. (LaPlante. *Turn of Mind*, 55)

The homodiegetic narrative situation and internal focalization through the protagonist give an insight into Jennifer's inner thought processes. They explain her actions to be caused by her temporal disorientation in consequence of which she inhabits a time span in the past and confuses it with her present reality. The

8 Fleischman, Suzanne. "Tense in Narrative." In: Paul Schellinger (ed.). *Encyclopedia of the Novel: Vol. 2*. Chicago/London: Fitzroy Dearborn, 1998, 1320–21, 1320.

9 Fleischman. "Tense in Narrative," 1320.

10 Fludernik, Monika. "Chronology, Time, Tense and Experientiality." In: *Language and Literature* 12,2 (2003): 117–34, 124–25.

narrator's use of first person narrative situation, internal focalization and the present tense together with prolepses and analepses as well as a fragmentation of the narrative mimics Jennifer's confused state of mind.

In this way the narrator also succeeds in presenting Jennifer's fragmented and abruptly changing lines of thought when her present reality is governed by her former profession as a doctor. As an orthopaedic surgeon Jennifer specialised on hand surgery, a profession that earned her high respect. The memories and hallucinations of operating on patients that Jennifer frequently has show her complete dedication to her profession:

> I am performing a complex brachial plexus procedure where the total plexus lesions have permeated all the nerve roots. The patient is under general anaesthesia. His (her?) face is covered. Things are not going well. [...] I miscalculate and hit the subclavian vein. Horrifying quantities of blood. [...]
> Then the room undergoes a sort of seismic shift and I am no longer in the OR. No patient anesthetized on a table. Instead I am gazing down at a bed with rumpled floral sheets. [...] I want the OR back, the soothing green walls, the steel instruments reflected large in the steel cabinetry. Everything placed just so. But this. This richly furnished, unsterile environment. It makes me uncomfortable. (LaPlante. *Turn of Mind*, 114–15)

It is these moments when she mentally returns to the job which strongly shaped her identity that Jennifer feels at one with herself. The present tense of the protagonist's thoughts strongly expresses the immediacy of her conviction that she is conducting surgery on a patient and it reveals her actions to stem from this hallucination. As Jennifer's identity has chiefly been formed through her profession as a surgeon and her considerable success in it, she is unable to identify with her new role as a private person and even less as a patient. Instead, the sterile order of an imagined OR gives structure to her environment and it provides her existence with a purpose.

The dementia patient's confusion of past and present and her hallucinations lead her to perform actions that appear to be unreasonable to the outside observer, for example leaning over a bed and moving her hands as if operating on a patient. The internal focalization and interior monologue though reveal the motivation behind the dementia patient's actions and serve as examples of those narrative techniques which Suzanne Keen considers to convey narrative empathy, i.e. "the sharing of feeling and perspective-taking induced by reading, viewing, hearing, or imagining narratives of another's situation and condition".[11] In addition to these

11 Keen, Suzanne. "Narrative Empathy." In: Peter Hühn et al. (eds.), *Handbook of Narratology: Vol. 2*. Berlin/Boston: De Gruyter, 2014, 521–30, 521.

techniques, "high levels of imagery [as in the scene depicted above] invit[e] mental simulation and immersion"[12] on the part of the reader. Taking the perspective of the fictional character Jennifer White and immersing into her world can thus contribute to a change in the readers' perceptions of dementia in general. As a consequence of "catch[ing] the emotions and sensations of a representation"[13] and feeling narrative empathy with this fictional representation, readers might assess the medical condition and the process of identity transformation, the suitable surroundings and individual needs of real dementia patients differently.

II. Processes of Identification and Fragmentation

As regards the identity of the fictional character in *Turn of Mind*, the climax of the third part of the novel, which is told in second person narrative, evokes how strongly Jennifer White's identity is still shaped by her former profession as a physician. Having escaped from her care home, Jennifer returns to the hospital where she did voluntary work before her Alzheimer's diagnosis:

> You [i.e. Jennifer, S.St.] are awakened by a crack of thunder [...]. You see that you are already dressed, shoes even. You must have been on call. [...] You catch sight of the clock still ticking above the sink. Eight forty-five. The clinic opened at 8 AM. You are late. (LaPlante. *Turn of Mind*, 267)

Here, in part III of her novel, Alice LaPlante chooses what Richardson terms "standard second-person narration [...], in which the protagonist, focalizer, and governing consciousness of the text is a single figure designated by the second-person pronoun".[14] In LaPlante's novel this second person narrative is introduced at a stage in the development of the woman with dementia which is strongly marked by the severe progress of the disease and therefore by an increasing fragmentation of the patient's identity. The current situation that she has just had to relocate from her own house into a care home causes even further anxiety in the fictional character. The quotation above represents Jennifer's logical reasoning when she finds herself in bed but fully dressed. Due to the description of events in second person narrative, the reader can follow the protagonist's line of thought and realises that he or she might draw similar conclusions if he or she were a doctor accustomed to being on call.

---

12 Keen. "Narrative Empathy," 522.

13 Keen. "Narrative Empathy," 522.

14 Richardson. "I Etcetera: On the Poetics and Ideology of Multipersoned Narratives," 316.

> You run through the rain to the front door [of the clinic, S.St.]. The waiting room is full of people. [...] You walk into the back area and are surprised at all the strange faces. A medium-sized dark-skinned man stops you. *I'm sorry,* he says, *staff only here.* His name tag says Dr. Aziz. It's okay, you tell him. I'm Dr. Jennifer White. [...] You go to the wardrobe, take a white coat, button it over your dress. What do you have for me? you ask. The other doctor hesitates, then shrugs. *Room three, a rash, could be shingles, could be poison oak,* he says. *The chart is on the door.* (LaPlante. *Turn of Mind*, 268–69. LaPlante's italics)

Jennifer acts as she used to act thousands of times before. Her professionalism and routine actions dispel the other doctor's doubts, who then leaves her in charge of diagnosing and treating a patient's symptoms. As in parts I and II of the novel, Alice LaPlante uses internal focalization and represents the action exclusively from the protagonist's perspective. The second person narrative, however, generalizes the experience and includes the reader while, at the same time, removing the strong closeness to the focalizer typical of a first person narrative situation. Monika Fludernik highlights the playfulness of this multifunctionality of second person narrative:

> Second-person fiction (typically) plays with the multifunctionality of the second-person pronoun (*you* as address, as generic 'one', or *you* as self-address, etc.) and with the reader's attempt at constructing a situation for the discourse, at naturalizing the disparities within the text.[15]

In her analysis of authentic patient narratives, Jarmila Mildorf shows that patients use second person pronouns for specific purposes when narrating their experiences, for example in doctor-patient interlocution. Mildorf describes "several discursive functions" of the you-narrative:

> it generalizes the experience as generic 'you' would do (everyone can experience this); at the same time it addresses the interlocutor and implies him/her in the experience as though he or she could potentially experience the same (this can happen to you, too); [...] finally, 'you' is also related to the speaker herself since she talks about her own personal experience. In this last context, 'you' seems to have a distancing effect because the patient chooses precisely not to use the first-person pronoun.[16]

---

15 Fludernik, Monika. "Second-Person Narrative as a Test Case for Narratology: The Limits of Realism." In: *Style* 28,3 (1994): 445–79, 455 (Fludernik's italics).

16 Mildorf, Jarmila. "Unreliability in Patient Narratives: From Clinical Assessment to Narrative Practice." In: Vera Nünning (ed.). *Unreliable Narration and Trustworthiness: Intermedial and Interdisciplinary Perspectives.* Berlin/Boston: De Gruyter, 2015, 395–413, 409.

When implementing a second person narrative at the climax of her novel, Alice LaPlante chooses a narrative situation that is an experimental and still a rather infrequent device in narrative fiction. In the context of LaPlante's fictional work, the second person narrative fulfils similar functions as those described by Mildorf: it generalizes the experience of dementia, implying that it could potentially be experienced by everyone, including the reader. Apart from the severe mental confusion caused by dementia, the second person narrative also relates events that could be experienced by any person, who does not necessarily have to suffer from dementia. The scene depicted above when Jennifer is abruptly awakened and thinks she is late for work is a situation which most readers can identify with. Finally, when the narrator refers to Jennifer herself with the second person pronoun instead of the first person pronoun, this has a distancing, defamiliarising effect. As Richardson concludes about multipersoned narration "[p]assages like these effectively dramatize the intersubjective constitution of 'the' self, the instability of the classical ego, and pose interesting questions about gender, speech, and subjectivity [...]".[17] In its narrative structure, *Turn of Mind* thus subverts the predominant public discourse about dementia as the complete loss of a patient's identity and instead draws attention to the fact that a person's individual sense of self is founded upon a variety of intersubjective aspects and that identity formation involves processes of personal development and transformation. In *Turn of Mind*, second person narrative represents the dementia patient's fragmented self and foregrounds certain aspects of Jennifer's identity, for example her dedication to her profession, whereas, in the course of Alzheimer's disease, it likewise shows her growing detachment from other social roles that co-constituted her former identity, such as her role as a wife and mother.

III. Maintaining a Sense of Self despite Dependence

In the ensuing, final part of the novel the ambiguous effect of creating identification and achieving a distancing effect on the part of the reader is further increased by figural narrative situation and fragments of unmediated dialogue and thought representation. Just as Jennifer only spontaneously remembers separate facets of her former identity, she is now unable to differentiate the hallucinations she has of her dead mother from the real persons surrounding her, for example carers, doctors and visitors (see LaPlante. *Turn of Mind*, 296). As a matter of fact, the dementia patient does no longer recognize her children:

17 Richardson. "I Etcetera: On the Poetics and Ideology of Multipersoned Narratives," 314.

> She does not know this person. Is it male or female? She cannot tell anymore. Whoever it is, they are speaking.
> *Mom?*
> She doesn't answer. She thinks something has happened, something important, but she can't remember what.
> *Mom? Do you know who I am?*
> No, not really, she says. (LaPlante. *Turn of Mind*, 297. LaPlante's italics)

Due to the figural narrative situation, the complete focalization through Jennifer and the unmediated dialogue, the reader is as ignorant of the visitor's identity as the demented protagonist herself. As Katsura Sako points out, "the hermeneutic experience of the text also helps the reader to grasp what it may mean to live with dementia and with the unknown".[18] Although the words spoken by the visitor make it easy to conclude that he or she is one of Jennifer's children, the narrative does not specify if it is the protagonist's daughter or her son. Instead, the narrative voice represents an unmediated version of Jennifer's thoughts in free direct style. This technique conveys the patient's abrupt changes of thought from being aware of the present situation, though not making complete sense of it, to extreme confusion: "She's still not sure who this young person is, but she cannot stay here too long. There are a rabbit and a cat to feed and a donkey to ride." (LaPlante. *Turn of Mind*, 298) Although free direct style closely resembles the character's line of thoughts, in comparison to the first- and second person narrative earlier, the use of third person pronouns and the absurdity of Jennifer's conclusions distance the reader from the patient's point of view.

Apart from the severe progress of the disease, Jennifer's condition also deteriorates due to the appalling standards of care since she has been transposed from her former luxurious private care home, "[t]he Ritz for the mentally infirm", to a state hospital (LaPlante. *Turn of Mind*, 154). Here six patients share a room while the low staff-to-patient ratio does not allow the nurses to provide care that responds even to the basic human needs of the patients. Jennifer feels deeply humiliated by the disregard for her personal desires and by the fact that she is dependent on another person to tend to her physical needs and urges:

> She is not hungry. So why do they keep placing food in front of her? Tough meat, applesauce. A cup of apple juice, as though she is a baby. She hates the sticky sweet smell, but she is thirsty, so she drinks. She wants to brush her teeth afterward, but they say, *Not now, we'll do that later.* Then, much later, the sloppy hard scrubbing, the rasp of bristles against her tongue, the cup of water brought to her lips and then taken away too soon. *Rinse. Spit.* The bulky diaper, the shame. Take me to the bathroom.

---

18 Sako. "Dementia and Detection in *Elizabeth is Missing* and *Turn of Mind*," 326.

> *No, I can't, we don't have the staff today, everyone's on sixteen-hour shifts. Someone will change you later.* (LaPlante. *Turn of Mind*, 295. LaPlante's italics)

Far from allowing the patients autonomous decisions about what they prefer to drink and to opt for eating when they are hungry, the strict hospital routine and the time pressure do not permit the carers to respond even to the patients' most urgent requests. In consequence of this disrespect to her personal preferences, the indispensable reliance on others and the paternalism involved, Jennifer has the impression of being degraded to the social status of an infant. She is embarrassed of her natural human urges, the lack of privacy and the ultimate loss of her dignity. In addition to the physical harm that may be caused by bedsores, malnutrition, dehydration, insufficient dental hygiene and missing physical exercise, the poor conditions of care thus also cause emotional pain to the patient. Jennifer's situation in *Turn of Mind* vividly illustrates the way in which deficient care worsens the effects of advanced Alzheimer's disease and, beyond the existing cognitive impairment, severely affects the physical and psychosocial well-being of the patient. "Accordingly, the novel not only seeks to represent Jennifer's self but also explores the ethical questions that dementia raises about subjective positions in the care relationship."[19] As regards the mental and emotional turmoil Jennifer endures, she considers her existence to be ultimately reduced to states of physical well-being that relieve her from the horrors and pains she experiences otherwise:

> But when all is done, when the end is near, what is left? What is one left with? Physical sensation. The pleasure that comes from relieving one's bowels under hygienic conditions. From laying one's head on a soft pillow. The release of the straps after a long hard night of pulling and pushing. To awaken from nightmares and find that they were, comparatively, the sweetest of dreams. (LaPlante. *Turn of Mind*, 297)

IV. Ethical Implications in *Turn of Mind*

Beyond the mimetic imitation of the dementia patient's gradual change of personality, the identification and later distancing effect on the reader also gains high semantic and ethical relevance. Against the background of the crime fiction genre of the novel, *Turn of Mind* addresses manifold ethical dilemmas with regard to dementia, patients' autonomy, their advance healthcare directives, the legal responsibility and social stigmatisation of dementia patients. In consequence of Jennifer White's own advance directive, her children hold the medical and financial powers of attorney. At some stage in the progress of dementia the authorized

19 Sako. "Dementia and Detection in *Elizabeth is Missing* and *Turn of Mind*," 325.

person is usually confronted with the moral dilemma of deciding on the binding force of a patient's advance directive.[20] The authorized person has to determine to respect the patient's interests expressed in the advance directive or else adhere to the donor's "experiential interests"[21] and declaration of intent in his or her current confused state of mind, which might contradict prior instructions. Against Jennifer's present resolve for maintaining her independence, her son, for example, urges his mother to consent to his efforts of declaring her mentally incompetent in order to pre-empt legal charges against her. In view of Jennifer's cognitive impairment and reluctance to adhere to his advice, her son decides that "it's time for [him] to exercise the medical power of attorney" (LaPlante. *Turn of Mind*, 70).

Turn of Mind likewise exposes difficulties as regards the binding force of advance directives from the patient's perspective. With the events filtered through the protagonist's consciousness the reader realizes that both, son and daughter, at times try to manipulate their confused mother. It is contestable whether the children execute their powers of attorney for the patient's or for their own benefit. The fragmentation of the narrative and the unreliable narration make it impossible to decide whom to trust, especially since the brother and sister discredit each other in private communications with their mother as well as in their letters and entries into her diary (see LaPlante. *Turn of Mind*, 8–9, 20–24, 70–72). The reader's reception of the homodiegetic narrative situation, due to which the reader cannot rely on the accuracy and credibility of the narrator's presentation of events and characters, thus mimics the situation of the demented woman, who has difficulties to rely on her trust in her children and carers as much as on the trustworthiness of her own mental capacity.[22] *Turn of Mind* thereby raises questions of autonomy, dependence, trust and reliability in family and care relationships.

---

20 For the philosophical discussion of the binding force of advance directives see the article by Oliver Hallich in this volume as well as the controversy discussed in Dworkin, Ronald. *Life's Dominion. An Argument about Abortion, Euthanasia, and Individual Freedom.* New York: Vintage, 1994, 218–42; and Dresser, Rebecca. "Dworkin on Dementia: Elegant Theory, Questionable Policy." In: James Lindemann Nelson, Hilde Lindemann Nelson (eds.). *Meaning and Medicine: A Reader in the Philosophy of Health Care.* London/New York: Routledge, 1999, 47–56.

21 Ronald Dworkin distinguishes persons' "critical interests" in the way people wish to lead their lives and the ideals to pursue thereby as expressed in advance directives from their "experiential interests" fulfilled in the pleasure of desirable experiences of the moment. Dworkin. *Life's Dominion*, 201–04. See also the article by Daniela Ringkamp in this volume.

22 For an analysis of the way in which the "thriller narrative [...] dramatize[s] tensions between Jennifer and those who are in the position of caring for her" see Sako. "Dementia and Detection in *Elizabeth is Missing* and *Turn of Mind*," 325–26.

In the context of the murder-mystery plot, the novel accentuates the relevance of decisions about the diminished or legal responsibility of mentally incapacitated people. Thus, after the death of Jennifer's friend Amanda, the police hold Jennifer as a murder suspect although evidence for her involvement in the crime is wanting and she is unable to remember even the fact that her friend died. Not only the professional surgical dissection of the victim's fingers but moreover Jennifer's confused state of mind and the aggression that is a typical symptom of many Alzheimer's patients are considered to be clues for her likely involvement in the crime. The police, the press and the neighbourhood hence eagerly stigmatise the dementia sufferer as insane and as capable of committing murder. Accordingly, the police repetitively question Jennifer even though, as a result of her memory loss, the contradictory testimonies do not assist the police in their inquiries, yet the interviews provoke great distress in the woman with dementia (see LaPlante. *Turn of Mind*, 39–43). They repeatedly confront the suspect with the information that her best friend was murdered, a fact that she keeps forgetting. Learning anew about Amanda's death in each police interview causes deep shock, anxiety and grief in the dementia sufferer. With the help of internal focalization Alice LaPlante is able to represent the extreme sorrow, emotional suffering and suicide tendencies the friend's death produces in the protagonist (see LaPlante. *Turn of Mind*, 7–8). LaPlante here points to several jurisprudential and ethical issues which are related to a defendant's fitness to stand trial: Does it require the defendant's recollection of committing the offense in order to convict a criminal? Do the means of solving a crime for the sake of a just punishment of the perpetrator justify causing mental harm to a witness or suspect with a fatal disease like dementia?[23]

It is questions like these that LaPlante's novel poses through the "ethics of the told" and "the ethics of the telling".[24] As a result of the diverse techniques that create narrative empathy, the reader is able to identify with the subjective perspective of the protagonist and through large parts of the novel understands the protagonist to be innocent. Yet, when the narrative voice turns to the less personal second person- and figural narrative situation in parts III and IV and thereby achieves a distancing effect from the protagonist, the reader calls Jennifer's complete innocence into question. When, during the dissolution of the plot, the protagonist's daughter Fiona conveys how she herself killed the victim and that her mother became an involuntary witness and an accomplice in the removal of the evidence,

23 For a philosophical discussion of similar ethical and jurisprudential concerns see the article by Annette Dufner in the present volume.

24 Phelan. "Narrative Ethics," 531.

it becomes apparent that the dementia patient is found guilty of a crime that she did not commit. Free indirect style reveals that Jennifer mistakes her memory of finding Fiona over Amanda's bleeding body and her own surgical removal of the evidence from the victim's hand for her usual routine of conducting an operation in hospital:

> [Fiona:] *How are things today? I'm sorry I'm late. Work's been insane.*
> Yes, she knows how insane work can be. One patient after another, bones bursting out of skin, how fragile the human body is, how easily penetrated and broken, how difficult to put together again. But the work doesn't need to be so sloppy. Who made this mess? She cannot believe it. She cannot believe her eyes. Who would do such a careless job. [sic]
> You didn't clean up the OR, she says.
> *It's Fiona, Mom, your daughter. Here to say hello.* (LaPlante. *Turn of Mind*, 298. LaPlante's italics)

Jennifer's confusion of the crime scene with an operating room and of her daughter with one of her medical students conveys that the convict does not recollect the scene as a criminal act. Yet, since the narrative sets in after Amanda's murder and the circumstances of her death are revealed retrospectively through the confused witness's consciousness, *Turn of Mind* remains indefinite about the protagonist's mental capacity at the moment of dissecting the dead Amanda's hand and therefore as regards her legal and moral responsibility at that time. The narrative effect of reader identification and distancing, and the resultant ambiguity of belief and doubts in the protagonist's innocence or legal culpability, consequently put the endeavour of accomplishing a completely rational assessment of a dementia patient's situation to question.

Apart from the wider, societal and legal relevance, LaPlante's novel exposes an ethical dilemma most families with a late-stage dementia patient have to face in everyday life: Should they inform dementia patients who forgot their spouses', parents' or relatives' death about their bereavement and thereby cause emotional harm to the patient? Or should they keep the patients in ignorance and make them live under the false assumption that their beloved one is still with them? *Turn of Mind* here addresses the double bind of, on the one hand, ensuring the emotional welfare of a person with Alzheimer's while, on the other hand, not patronising them by preventing them from making their own decisions. As Rita Charon and Martha Montello conclude about illness narratives in general, the choices patients and their relatives are confronted with in the presence of fatal diseases transcend mere questions of health care but predominantly concern "*the ethics of life*":

> Perhaps another result of narrative ethics' emergence will be the realization that, for patients and their families, the ethics under question are not located primarily in the

> technical questions of providing or withholding health care, allocating scarce resources, or preserving autonomy in the face of death. Those are ethicists' ethical considerations. In large part, the ethics in question are the ethics of ordinary life: how to fulfill life goals, to honor obligations, and to make sense of events in ways that make it possible to go on. These ethical issues have not only to do with *bioethics*; they are also the *ethics of life*.[25]

V. Conclusion

The fragmented narrative structure of LaPlante's novel with its use of three different narrative situations, i.e. first person-, second person- and figural narrative situation, as well as present tense narration, unmediated dialogue, interior monologue and free direct style, mimetically imitates the fragmentation of a fictional dementia patient's sense of self. In the course of the disease and with increasing memory loss Jennifer's personality changes but, at the same time, the protagonist's strong identification with her former profession contests the dominant discourse about dementia patients' complete loss of identity. When experimenting with the combination of diverse introspective narrative techniques, LaPlante's novel succeeds in transposing this transformation of the fictional character to the reader's experience of the story. Whereas the reader is encouraged to identify with the fictional character in the beginning, the degree of close reader identification gradually decreases in the following parts of the novel. It is by means of these narrative techniques as well as the plot, which depicts the protagonist's cognitive and physical deterioration, her false conviction for murder and the discrepancies in different care situations she experiences, that *Turn of Mind* addresses ethical implications arising with memory loss and cognitive impairment. It exposes problems involved in care ethics and advance directives and reveals moral dilemmas families are confronted with as regards maintaining the patient's well-being and questions of trust, paternalism and a patient's autonomy.

Of course, LaPlante's use of multipersoned narrative does not propose that people with dementia necessarily refer to themselves by second- and third person pronouns, but second person narrative here fulfils the function described by Monika Fludernik "to undermine realist narrative parameters and frames".[26] Just as the symptoms of dementia make the representation of a first-hand experience

---

25 Charon, Rita, Montello, Martha. "Introduction: Memory and Anticipation: The Practice of Narrative Ethics." In: Rita Charon, Martha Montello (eds.). *Stories Matter: The Role of Narrative in Medical Ethics*. New York/London: Routledge, 2002, ix-xii, xi (Charon's and Montello's italics).

26 Fludernik. "Second-Person Narrative as a Test Case for Narratology: The Limits of Realism," 445.

of the disease inexpressible through language, second person- and multipersoned narration reach out to "[t]he [l]imits of [r]ealism"[27] in order to "narrat[e] the unnarratable".[28]

References

Charon, Rita, Montello, Martha. "Introduction: Memory and Anticipation: The Practice of Narrative Ethics." In: Rita Charon, Martha Montello (eds.). *Stories Matter: The Role of Narrative in Medical Ethics*. New York/London: Routledge, 2002, ix-xii.

Dresser, Rebecca. "Dworkin on Dementia: Elegant Theory, Questionable Policy." In: James Lindemann Nelson, Hilde Lindemann Nelson (eds.). *Meaning and Medicine: A Reader in the Philosophy of Health Care*. London/New York: Routledge, 1999, 47–56.

Dworkin, Ronald. *Life's Dominion. An Argument about Abortion, Euthanasia, and Individual Freedom*. New York: Vintage, 1994.

Fleischman, Suzanne. "Tense in Narrative." In: Paul Schellinger (ed.). *Encyclopedia of the Novel: Vol. 2*. Chicago/London: Fitzroy Dearborn, 1998, 1320–21.

Fludernik, Monika. "Chronology, Time, Tense and Experientiality." In: *Language and Literature* 12,2 (2003): 117–34.

Fludernik, Monika. "Second-Person Narrative as a Test Case for Narratology: The Limits of Realism." In: *Style* 28,3 (1994): 445–79.

Hühn, Peter, Pier, John, Schmid, Wolf, Schönert, Jörg (eds.). *Handbook of Narratology: Vol. 2*. Berlin/Boston: De Gruyter, 2014.

Keen, Suzanne. "Narrative Empathy." In: Peter Hühn, John Pier, Wolf Schmid, Jörg Schönert (eds.), *Handbook of Narratology: Vol. 2*. Berlin/Boston: De Gruyter, 2014, 521–30.

Krüger-Fürhoff, Irmela Marei. "Narrating the Limits of Narration – Alzheimer's Disease in Contemporary Literary Texts." In: Mark Schweda, Aagje Swinnen (eds.). *Popularizing Dementia: Public Expressions and Representations of Forgetfulness*. Bielefeld: transcript, 2015, 89–108.

LaPlante, Alice. *Turn of Mind*. London: Vintage, 2012.

Mildorf, Jarmila. "Unreliability in Patient Narratives: From Clinical Assessment to Narrative Practice." In: Vera Nünning (ed.). *Unreliable Narration and*

27 Fludernik. "Second-Person Narrative as a Test Case for Narratology: The Limits of Realism," 445.

28 Rimmon-Kenan. "What Can Narrative Theory Learn from Illness Narratives?," 241.

Trustworthiness: Intermedial and Interdisciplinary Perspectives. Berlin/Boston: De Gruyter, 2015, 395–413.

Phelan, James. "Narrative Ethics." In: Peter Hühn, John Pier, Wolf Schmid, Jörg Schönert (eds.). *Handbook of Narratology*: *Vol. 2*. Berlin/Boston: De Gruyter, 2014, 531–46.

Richardson, Brian. "I Etcetera: On the Poetics and Ideology of Multipersoned Narratives." In: *Style* 28,3 (1994): 312–28.

Rimmon-Kenan, Shlomith. "What Can Narrative Theory Learn from Illness Narratives?" In: *Literature and Medicine* 25,2 (2006): 241–54.

Sako, Katsura. "Dementia and Detection in *Elizabeth is Missing* and *Turn of Mind*." In: *Contemporary Women's Writing* 10,3 (2016): 315–33.

Elaine Lux (New York)

Narrativity in Dementia, through Fiction: Alice Munro's "The Bear Came over the Mountain", Elie Wiesel's *The Forgotten*, and Lisa Genova's *Still Alice*

Abstract: In Alice Munro's "The Bear Came over the Mountain", Elie Wiesel's *The Forgotten*, and Lisa Genova's *Still Alice*, the authors create compelling fictional evocations of memory loss in complex, vibrant, and beloved human beings. Lux examines how Munro, Wiesel, and Genova use poesis – especially point of view, dialogue, cultural context, and limited disclosure – to convey a humanity that endures even despite dementia's destruction of ongoing narrative identity.

I. Introduction

According to Michael White, "the narrative metaphor proposes that persons live their lives by stories [...] – and that these stories provide the structure of life."[1] A key ingredient in a person's having an ongoing narrative identity is memory. Molly Andrews calls memory "a cornerstone of identity." Andrews observes that "[w]ithout recollection, it is difficult to have a sense of who we are in the present, much less to configure a past for ourselves."[2] Especially because dementia impairs the narrative function, literary treatments may be a key part of making a "bind[ing] together" experience relevant and meaningful to readers.[3] The loss of narrative identity that results when memory, that "cornerstone of identity", is less and less accessible to an individual is devastating and grievous – both to the person who senses the fog coming in and to those who love that person. Thus, to tell the story of a person experiencing dementia or Alzheimer's disease is difficult, as that person progressively loses his or her ability to articulate the experience or his or her resultant sense of self.

1 See Freedman, Jill, Combs, Gene. *Narrative Therapy: The Social Construction of Preferred Realities*. New York: Norton, 1996, 77.
2 Andrews Molly. *Narrative Imagination and Everyday Life*. New York: Oxford, 2014, 3.
3 Hawkins, Anne Hunsaker. *Reconstructing Illness: Studies in Pathography*. West Lafayette. Purdue University Press, 1993, 3.

Fiction has shown itself to be one effective way that the incapacitating loss of memory, through progressive disease, can be enstoried and made real to someone not undergoing that experience. Perhaps the art provides some sort of catharsis for our fears, as well, by suggesting there is a story, even if we no longer can tell it. The primary challenges to the author are to make the dementia or Alzheimer's real while, at the same time, making the fictional narrative cohesive enough to grasp, and compelling, relevant, and aesthetically pleasing. Anne Hunsaker Hawkins says that the most important "task" of the author of any pathography is "to restore to reality its lost coherence and to discover, or create, a meaning that can bind it together again".[4] In Alice Munro's short story "The Bear Came over the Mountain," Elie Wiesel's novel *The Forgotten*, and Lisa Genova's novel *Still Alice*, the artistic challenges are met effectively.

In his reflections on hindsight's importance, Mark Freeman suggests that there is a parallel between hindsight and *poesis*, calling both hindsight and artistic renderings of experience "potential vehicles of what might be termed *recuperative disclosure*; they are agents of insight and rescue, recollection and recovery, serving to counteract the forces of oblivion".[5] We will examine here how Munro, Wiesel, and Genova use *poesis* – especially point of view, dialogue, cultural context, and limited disclosure – to create narratives that capture what the characters themselves become unable to put into story and to thus "counteract the forces of oblivion."

II. Alice Munro's "The Bear Came over the Mountain"

In Alice Munro's "The Bear Came over the Mountain", the person with dementia, a woman named Fiona, is sketched with a light but deft stroke. The story is filtered through her husband Grant's perspective, with third person limited viewpoint. The very spare story is divided into many brief sections, separated from one another by asterisks, and it seems to flow through time in a narrative that is a bit disjointed, picking up pieces of the past as it flows through the present. Fiona's name is the first word of the story, placing the focus on her. Yet what she is thinking and feeling is rarely disclosed to us, except through another's mind. The first sentence links Grant to her: "Fiona lived in her parents' house, in the town where she and Grant

4 Hawkins. *Reconstructing Illness*, 2–3.

5 Freeman, Mark. *Hindsight: The Promise and Peril of Looking Backward.* New York: Oxford University Press, 2010, 43–44.

went to university" (Munro. "The Bear," 1).[6] And the first section ends with a hint this may be a love story:

> 'Do you think it would be fun' – Fiona shouted. 'Do you think it would be fun if we got married?' He took her up on it, he shouted yes. He wanted never to be away from her. She had the spark of life. (Munro. "The Bear," 2)

This enigmatic "spark of life" regarding Fiona's magnetism is the underlying thread of the story. Despite the vicissitudes of their relationship, including years of infidelity by Grant with students, and perhaps even with colleagues' wives, Grant never has wanted to leave Fiona.

The story provides only limited disclosure about Fiona's problem and the years of onset. About a year before the real time of the story, we are told "Grant had started noticing so many little yellow notes stuck up all over the house" (Munro, "The Bear," 3). Fiona had always left some notes around, but "[t]he new notes were different. Taped onto the kitchen drawers – Cutlery, Dishtowels, Knives" (Munro. "The Bear," 4). She began getting lost when she drove out somewhere or went for walks. Very poignantly, in the house, "[s]he would stand in doorways trying to figure out where she was going. She forgot to turn on the burner under the vegetables or put water in the coffeemaker. She asked Grant when they'd moved to the house. 'Was it last year or the year before?' He said that it was twelve years ago. She said, 'That is shocking'" (Munro. "The Bear," 5).

We do not get a lot of Fiona's inside thinking, even in the beginning when she would have been capable of articulating her feelings, but we learn early on that it was Fiona who first suggested Grant would need to put her in a care facility: "'You know what you're going to have to do with me, don't you? You're going to have to put me in that place. Shallowlake?'" (Munro. "The Bear," 7). The narrative slides from Grant's saying they are not "at that stage yet" to the next section, in which Fiona is getting admitted. The reader then understands that the leaving the house, even in the second section of the story, was for the nursing home.

The story does not disclose in detail the process of deterioration in Fiona's memory, but she emerges in the story as having an inherent dignity and individuality as we meet her through Grant's impressions, memories, and reconstructions of their life together and of his life in the midst of their life together. Thus, memories of Grant's life and foibles are interspersed with his eager visits to Meadowlake home (the proper name of the facility) to visit Fiona. It is clear that he misses

---

6 Munro's original title for the story is used in this paper, for literary purposes. The title of the film based on the story is substituted as "Away from Her," in the collection *Away from Her: Stories by Alice Munro.* New York: Penguin, 2007, 1–65.

her, although it is also clear that their marriage has had its challenges because of his infidelities. After the first thirty days of her stay at Meadowlake, a period in which Grant is not allowed to visit Fiona, she does not seem to know him. She has taken up a relationship with a wheelchair-bound man named Aubrey, and she treats Grant like some unknown new patient, greeting him politely but not familiarly, and Grant cannot tell if this is an act or not. Grant feels unable to talk to her because she is always with Aubrey and because of the invisible barrier she seems to place between Grant and herself.

This seeming romance with Aubrey forms part of what Nuria Casado-Gual refers to as an "unexpected turn in lifelong sentimental journeys."[7] Casado-Gual sees a feminist subtext in the late life romance of Fiona and Grant through Fiona's seeming ability to "'perform' remembrance and oblivion at her own convenience" in much of the story and, thus, "to re-construct her own self-esteem by finally responding to Grant's undeclared unfaithfulness."[8] Casado-Gual sees self-assertive significance in Fiona's pre-Meadowlake story about following fences when she became lost on her usual walk and had to follow "the fence line – a very long way round." Through her telling Grant "she'd counted on fences always taking you somewhere" (Munro. "The Bear," 4), Fiona at last may have been alluding to Grant's extramarital affairs. For, according to Casado-Gual, the fences "can be read in an ironic light if Grant's past affairs are interpreted as the fences that had kept Fiona isolated in their marriage and which, eventually, led them to the physical and social isolation of her family's farm."[9] Later on, at Meadowlake, observing Fiona's relationship with Aubrey, Grant is amazed to observe her possibly intentional reversal of the earlier pattern of their marriage in which Grant was the "philanderer" (Munro. "The Bear," 15).[10]

Then, after a time, almost mysteriously, Fiona's awareness of her connection to Grant re-emerges: she

> lifted her arms to put them around him. Her skin or her breath gave off a faint new smell, a smell that seemed to him like that of the stems of cut flowers left too long in their water. 'I'm happy to see you,' she said, and pulled his earlobes. 'You could have just driven away,' she said. 'Just driven away without a care in the world and forsook me. Forsooken me. Forsaken.' He kept his face against her white hair, her pink scalp, her sweetly shaped skull. He said, 'Not a chance.' (Munro. "The Bear," 65).

---

7 Casado-Gual, Nuria. "Unexpected Turns in Lifelong Sentimental Journeys: Redefining Love, Memory and Old Age through Alice Munro's 'The Bear Came Over the Mountain" and its Film Adaptation, *Away from Her*." In: *Ageing & Society* 35 (2015): 389–404, 389.

8 Casado-Gual. "Unexpected Turns," 395.

9 Casado-Gual. "Unexpected Turns," 395.

10 Casado-Gual. "Unexpected Turns," 395.

Although late life romance has more texture and ambiguity than we might have imagined, the shared words between Fiona and Grant evoke a sense in us that love can linger beyond the loss of narrative identity, that the "spark of life" in an individual and in a relationship is more important even than the ability to tell about ourselves.

Especially because the ending suggests that Fiona has been offering her husband the chance to leave her for good, Fiona is lent dignity and character, even in her dementia/Alzheimer's. The story's limited disclosure and its medically non-technical and narratively non-linear telling keep readers from finding a refuge in our minds to intellectualize Fiona's condition. We have no technical diagnosis of Fiona's condition. Nor do we have a revelation of the struggles with sadness and fear Fiona may have experienced. The sorrow of it all is implied but not stated. We as readers imagine it, but are not forced to enter into it, as we remain with Grant's perspective primarily. However, as Casado-Gual observes, "the interconnection of memory, old age and love in [Munro's narrative, E.L.] enables an alternative discourse of ageing where old age and dementia are deprived of their alleged meaninglessness and become, instead, part of a new quest for meaning" – a quest in which "small moments of (mutual and self-) discovery are still possible in desolate scenarios."[11]

Through limiting disclosure to things Grant sees and thinks, Munro has managed to affirm the person beneath the dementia. Munro does not describe what "the spark of life" in Fiona is, nor does she demonstrate it. Yet in her story we believe in it and in the living spark that enables one individual to love another. Thus, Munro counters the forces of oblivion by bringing to life in us the story of a woman whose own narrative capacity is gone but whose "spark of life" somehow remains.

III. Elie Wiesel's *The Forgotten*

In contrast to Munro's story, Eli Wiesel's powerful novel *The Forgotten* takes us into the whirlpool of terror that the somewhat elderly holocaust survivor Elhanan Rosenbaum experiences as he loses his memory and his narrative capability, even though, in this narrative too, we are given no diagnosis, no name to hang Elhanan's condition on. This is explained as being Elhanan's refusal to name the disease, and this refusal is respected by his son Malkiel Rosenbaum, to whom Elhanan's story is transmitted and through whom much of the third person limited viewpoint

11 Casado-Gual. "Unexpected Turns," 401.

of the novel is filtered. *The Forgotten*'s narrative is comprised of a complex intertwining of the cultural and individual memory of the father and the son, of their stories and of how the charge of containing his father's story as well as his own impacts Malkiel. Elhanan's story of memory loss is essential not just because of his individuality but because of his experience as a Jewish person during the years of the holocaust. Whereas the culture of free love in the 1960s was relevant to the unfolding of Grant's relationship with Fiona, showing the personal vicissitudes of individuals and couples as they live through their time, Elhanan's story is presented not just as a personal or a family struggle, but as an essential part of the history and survival of a people.

The physical text begins with an epigraph from *The Talmud*: "Respect the old man who has forgotten what he learned. For broken Tablets have a place in the Ark beside the Tablets of the Law" (Wiesel. *Forgotten*, 7). Thus, the metaphor that each living soul, however broken, is a living tablet of importance reinforces the spiritual tone that is set by reference to *The Talmud*. Then, the first introductory section of Wiesel's novel is entitled "Elhanan's Prayer." It is in Elhanan's own voice, and its content places memory in the foreground of human identity. Elhanan's prayer begins:

> God of Abraham, Isaac and Jacob, forget not their son who calls upon them now. You well know, You, source of all memory, that to forget is to abandon, to forget is to repudiate. Do not abandon me, God of my fathers, for I have never repudiated You. (Wiesel. *Forgotten*, 9)

The prayer ends

> Know, God, that I do not wish to forget You. I do not wish to forget anything. Not the living and not the dead. Not the voices and not the silences. I do not wish to forget the moments of abundance that enriched my life, nor the hours of anguish that drove me to despair. Even if you forget me, O Lord, I refuse to forget You. (Wiesel. *Forgotten*, 10)

Can Elhanan succeed in keeping his word and not forgetting God? The novel suggests that his word may need to be fulfilled through what he has transmitted to his son. Elhanan's prayer is followed by an introductory section entitled "Malkiel's Words," and it expresses the son's fear that what is happening to his father could also happen to him, that he could lose his memory, too. He is very aware that his memory has a double burden now, as it "harbors my father's memories, too, since his mind has become a sieve" (Wiesel. *Forgotten*, 11).

Once into the novel itself, we as readers move through the intertwined stories of father and son, mostly in the third person limited viewpoint, with no advance-orientation as to which character's viewpoint is coming up or where the character is in time and space. Through the inner thoughts that are interspersed with the outward action, Wiesel's novel conveys the individual and communal importance of shared memory. David Patterson speaks of memory as "the defining theme" of *The Forgotten,* saying that, for Wiesel, "the task of remembrance is the task of creating a dwelling place for God in a world where He has been uprooted through the uprooting of humanity." And storytelling is sacred for Wiesel, Patterson explains: "Because creation is made of a tale, [humans, including writers, E.L.] do not impose meaning upon the world [...]. The storyteller is not a maker of meaning [...] but a messenger of meaning." He notes, too, the significance in Wiesel's naming of his characters, pointing out that "many of Wiesel's characters bear the names of 'angels' or *malakhim,*" as is seen in Malkiel's name in *The Forgotten.*[12]

The narrative itself begins in a graveyard, through the experience of Elhanan's son. Malkiel is in Communist Romania, at his grandfather's grave, crying out on behalf of his father. He has been sent there by his father so as to remember his father's memories, even by going to the place of his father's childhood. The grave is both a literal burial place and a metaphor for Elhanan's mind. The respect Malkiel and his father hold for the dead will soon need to include respect for Elhanan, who will outlive his mind.

Even with its patriarchal religious emphasis on the father and son story, Wiesel's *The Forgotten,* like Munro's "The Bear Came over the Mountain," is a quest-for-meaning tale tempered by a love story motif, with each of the two romances featuring a strong-female element. Elhanan's decision not to remarry after the death of his wife Talia, but to nurture her memory for the rest of his life, makes their romance one that lasts beyond youth into old age, indeed beyond the grave, only that Elhanan is losing his memory. This romance is, as it were, passed down to Malkiel and Tamar to both treasure and to live. The women that father and son have chosen are very political and active in the world around them: Talia was a Zionist fighting in the underground for the establishment of Israel as a Jewish state, and Tamar is a reporter for the *New York Times*, sometimes writing pieces on dangerous topics and exploring her news coverage fearlessly. Both women are self-actualizing, and both desire to love and to create a family even in the face of danger in the world around them. The love stories of Elhanan and Talia and Malkiel and Tamar are integral to the fraught story of Elhanan's loss of memory and are essential to the subtle affirmation of life in the novel.

---

12 Patterson, David. "Wiesel's Aggadic Outcry." In: Steven T. Katz, Alan Rosen (eds.). *Elie Wiesel: Jewish, Literary, and Moral Perspectives.* Bloomington: Indiana University Press, 2013, 190–200, 196, 191.

The first chapter weaves between Malkiel's own thoughts and Elhanan's mental despair over losing his memory. In his own life, Malkiel is not only dealing with the weight of carrying his father's memories, but with his own reluctance to marry and to have children. He says he is unwilling to bring children into this world of suffering. By the end of the novel, Malkiel seems to have been transformed inwardly by what he has discovered from the past. As he prepares to return from Romania, he stands at the grave of his paternal grandfather, who carries his same name: Malkiel. He speaks within his heart to Tamar, the woman he loves:

> 'We are going to be married, Tamar. [...] Let's take whatever comes along – the good and the less good alike – simply and in harmony. Despite pain and sorrow, we'll put our trust in what exalts us – my father's relentless sufferings – and in what thwarts us, too – the ambiguities of life, most of all Jewish life in the diaspora. We'll forge new links from which new sparks will rise. Spoken words will become signs, words unspoken will serve as warnings. And we'll invent the rest. And my father's memory will sing and weep in mine. And yours will blossom in our children's. You win: we'll have many children, Tamar. And one day, Grandfather, they'll tell the story of your son, in their turn, Elahanan son of Malkiel. Malkiel son of Elhanan.' (Wiesel. *Forgotten,* 310)

Despite the suffering in the Jewish past and the contemporary sufferings of other peoples all around the globe, despite the increasing erosion of his father's ability to remember, Malkiel discovers within himself courage and even eagerness to say yes to life. This shift in Malkiel is an important part of the novel's affirmation of life, even if memories cannot be held onto fully by those who carry them or by those who try to carry others' memories. However, the novel does not end on Malkiel's hope for the future. It concludes with a chapter called "Farewell." This chapter consists of Elhanan's first person musings. He is talking to his son, but as the musings unfold, we see that his son is not physically present as he speaks to him, for Malkiel still has not returned from the journey to Romania. Elhanan experiences awareness that his "reason" is "near death" (Wiesel. *Forgotten,* 312). He suffers with inward blame for having failed "to pass on" something "vital" but has forgotten what it was (Wiesel. *Forgotten,* 314). His grief over his loss of identity via his loss of the past is great. He tries to keep faith in the benevolence of a creator, yet he sees his mental "dissolution" (Wiesel, *Forgotten,* 313) as a punishment. The novel ends with Elhanan's struggle to affirm meaning, but his final thoughts end mid-sentence: "God cannot be so cruel as to erase everything forever. If He were, He would not be our father, and nothing would make sense. And I who speak to you cannot say more, for" (Wiesel. *Forgotten,* 316). Thus, the novel suggests a somewhat hopeful but highly nuanced ambiguity.

As readers, we need to construct part of the novel's story line because of the poetic way in which time and point of view move in the novel. Perhaps our involvement in making sense of the novel increases our involvement in Elhanan's and Malkiel's lives. We get few quotidian details of their lives, to ground us, yet we are deeply moved by the suffering of Elhanan. We can relate to Malkiel's questions about the wisdom of bringing new life into this world. We rejoice in Malkiel's breakthrough near the end, yet we retain a sense of the sorrow and unpredictability of life, too, through Elhanan's fading and incomplete last sentence.

IV. Lisa Genova's *Still Alice*

Lisa Genova's *Still Alice* focuses primarily on the experience of the person who undergoes deterioration from early onset Alzheimer's disease. The novel, told in the third person, is mostly limited to what Alice sees, feels, and knows. However, as Alice's mind deteriorates, the narrator-author supplements Alice's increasingly limited ability to place her thoughts into words with clues to the reader. The impact of Alice's early onset Alzheimer's on her husband and family is interwoven into the narration, but the central experience we enter into is that of the Alzheimer's sufferer. According to Genova, "stories are what move us as human beings and connect us to each other, whether [we're] talking about physics or biology or a woman who has early onset Alzheimer's."[13] Naturally, the emotional import of the novel is increased by the author's choosing to make her protagonist an exceedingly bright person. Alice Howland's rapid deterioration highlights the relentless progress of Alzheimer's. When the novel opens, in September 2003, we meet her as a high-powered Harvard professor of linguistics, publishing books in her field, serving as expert speaker at conferences, teaching and mentoring bright students through their doctoral process. She is married to a high-powered scientific researcher and is comfortable in an elitist and high-pressure academic culture. In this first chapter, we catch her at the vulnerable moment of detecting that something is going terribly wrong. Suddenly and significantly, as she jogs a familiar route near her home, one she has taken every day for years, she is unnerved and struck with terror; she cannot figure out whether to go right or left to get home. She is lost, blocks from home.

Poignantly, less than two years later, in a chapter dated Summer 2005, Alice finds a book that looks familiar. She says to someone she perceives as "the man":

---

13 Birge, Sarah. "Brainhood, Selfhood, or 'Meat with a Point of View': The Value of Fiction for Neuroscientific Research and Neurological Medicine." In: Melissa M. Littlefield, Jenell M. Johnson (eds.). *The Neuroscientific Turn: Transdisciplinarity in the Age of the Brain*. Ann Arbor, MI: University of Michigan Press, 2012. 98.

> 'I think I've read this book before'[…]. The man looked over at the book she held and then at her. 'You've done more than that. You wrote it. You and I wrote that book together.' Hesitant to take him at his word, she closed the book and read the shiny blue cover. *From Molecules to Mind* by John Howland, Ph.D. and Alice Howland, Ph.D. She looked up at the man in the chair. *He's John.* (Genova. *Still Alice,* 284)

Here, we see Genova's skill in communicating the inside feelings while revealing the outside behaviors. The person beneath the Alzheimer's suddenly, inexplicably, fleetingly surfaces. She recognizes her husband and herself. Alice reads to herself these words from the book: "'An infinite possibility of expression, learned yet instinctive, semanticity, syntax, case grammar, irregular verbs, effortless and automatic, universal.' The words she read seemed to push past the choking weeds and sludge in her mind to a place that was pristine and still intact, hanging on" (Genova. *Still Alice,* 284). The image of weeds and sludge in the mind makes Alice's experience real to us. The irony that Alice no longer has any of these universal language-making gifts is not lost on readers. But the narrative helps us to feel the loss from Alice's viewpoint:

> 'John,' she said.
> 'Yes.' […]
> 'I wrote this book with you,' she said.
> 'Yes.'
> 'I remember. I remember you. I remember I used to be very smart.'
> 'Yes, you were, you were the smartest person I've ever known.'
> […]
> She wanted to tell him everything she remembered and thought, but she couldn't send all those memories and thoughts, composed of so many words, phrases, and sentences, past the choking weeds and sludge into audible sound. She boiled it all down and put all her effort into what was most essential. The rest would have to remain in the pristine place, hanging on.
> 'I miss myself.'
> 'I miss you, too, Ali, so much.'
> 'I never planned to get like this.'
> 'I know.' (Genova. *Still Alice,* 285)

Though the novel is highly informative about such medical aspects of Alzheimer's as the possible drugs that can be used for treatment, the diagnostic procedures, the symptoms of onset and decline, the testing for genetically inherited early-onset genes, and the scarcity of group support resources for the Alzheimer's sufferer, the characters in this novel are individualized, and Genova manages to convey the human experience of a person afflicted with Alzheimer's from the inside out, even while providing readers with an education about the disease. Alice is very real to us, as we find out about her background, her marriage, her children, and they all are given personalities and stories, too. The strong patterning of the novel helps us to note and to feel Alice's deterioration. Throughout, readers are moved along, as is Alice, in a tide of unyielding calendar time. Almost every chapter, with the exception of a brief epigram and the concluding Epilogue, is marked by a date: usually a month and year. Skillfully, as Alice's mind deteriorates, Genova renders Alice's perceptions in a narrative we can understand, but which we know she cannot form for herself. The first chapter is dated September 2003. The novel's final chapter is undated and simply called "Epilogue." It shows us Alice's life as she lives it, dateless and always in the present, encircled by her daughters, in a family setting. Specifics are gone for Alice, even her grasp of names and her relationship to the others. We as readers can glean that the disease has continued to progress, as the twins that were born in March 2005 are still babies, but Genova does not give us a date. This is the end of the novel, but, of course, not of Alice's deterioration. Genova chooses not to take us to the end of Alice's life, perhaps so as to leave us with a sense of hope for the precious in-between days, which yet can be pleasurable to an Alzheimer's sufferer who is living with massive cognitive impairment but surrounded by love.

The speed of the deterioration has been astonishing: two years. This woman who wrote books on linguistics barely has individual names for those closest to her, or a sense of their relationship to her. The romance element of the novel, centering around the closeness between two like-minded people who are still attracted to and supportive of one another, has dissipated. Alice's journey of transformation has led her to increasingly shift her inner values in the direction of simple human caring over intellectual accomplishment and status, but her request that her husband take a leave from work to spend time with her while she is still somewhat like herself goes unheeded. He is unwilling and emotionally unable to stay with her full-time. Instead he takes a position in New York City, a position with wonderful research opportunities. John would have taken Alice with him, but she and her daughters are not willing for her to relocate away from her home and family in Boston. This is one of Alice's last opportunities for self-determination, and she takes it. Like Fiona, of "The Bear Came over the Mountain," and Talia and Tamar of *The Forgotten,* Alice has been a strong-minded, independent partner in the marriage. Even in her Alzheimer's, like Fiona, she participated fully in the early decisions about her condition, but, by the end of the novel, the self-determination elements dissipate, too, like the romance in the marriage. In effect, the romance between the couple transitions into a family romance, with much of Alice's support coming from her daughters, in particular. As Mike Bender observes: "the book ends with Lydia, coming East to study, and Anna, now with newborn twins, helping their mother. John, as expected, can only give limited support, given the demands of his new post. Tom plays little part in helping his mother, being involved in his medical studies. Men cannot be expected to stop giving their careers priority, even when Alice has manifestly only a few months left to live."[14] Alice's strongly feminist personality is modified by a basic need to give and receive nurturing love. The vulnerability of such simplicity helps enrich the power of the narrative to evoke empathy in the reader. As Bender aptly observes, *Still Alice* is "a disquieting book," even regarding the health care system's coldness to Alzheimer's sufferers.[15]

However, it is also an encouraging book. At her worst moments, Alice still has love. Alice's daughter Lydia, whom Alice perceives as "the actress," has acted out a monologue for Alice and, treating Alice with respect, asks her how the monologue affects her:

> 'When I'm done, tell me how I made you feel, okay?' […] The actress stopped and came back into herself. She looked at Alice and waited. 'Okay, what do you feel?' 'I feel love. It's about love.' The actress squealed, rushed over to Alice, kissed her on the cheek, and smiled, every crease of her face delighted. 'Did I get it right?' asked Alice. 'You did, Mom. You got it exactly right.' (Genova. *Still Alice,* 292)

These words end the novel.

V. Closing Reflections

Severe dementia is a physical affliction that cannot be overcome by effort or will power, and this progressive brain deterioration eventually erases the person's awareness of his or her narrative identity. This inability to overcome the mind's relentless descent into forgetfulness appears in the works of literature discussed here, and, of course, in life. Reading these fictional accounts of dementia and Alzheimer's is humbling, for it reminds us of the importance of the body to our human identity. As Rita Charon puts it: "The self depends on the body for its presence, its location. Without the body, the self cannot be uttered."[16]

Through the artistry of Munro, Wiesel, and Genova, however, the haunting quality of the loss of identity in the characters suffering from rapidly advancing dementia is made somewhat less bleak by the presence of others who remember

14 Bender, Mike. "A Disquieting Look at Dementia." In: *Psychologist* 28,3 (2015): 222–23, 223.

15 Bender. "A Disquieting Look," 223.

16 Charon, Rita. *Narrative Medicine: Honoring the Stories of Illness.* New York: Oxford University Press, 2006, 87.

who the dementia/Alzheimer's suffers were and cherish them even in the now. Interestingly, each of the authors has chosen to enhance the positive ambience for the dementia sufferers, as well, by removing financial problems from the picture. Good facilities and support people are readily available because all three dementia sufferers are wealthy. The artistic choice to use educated and affluent families and protagonists allows for a more palatable care situation for both characters and readers, but it also makes more salient the stark truth that no amount of intelligence, funds, or knowledge and no number of medical or scientific resources can make a difference in the condition of the dementia/Alzheimer's character's situation at this time. The helplessness of characters in each work to fix the problem helps readers to sense our own vulnerability more – and perhaps to become more sensitive to the gift of order in the quotidian life we lead – to thus become awakened from a numbness, at least for a time, that Hawkins describes this way: "And indeed most of us, at some time or another, have recognized that the apparent orderliness and coherence of our lives is something of an accident, or a gift, or a miracle that renews itself day after day. Yet most of us behave as though this miracle were quite natural."[17] In addition, Munro, Wiesel, and Genova all choose to end their stories before the characters suffering dementia become totally unrecognizable. Thus, their artistic choices of when and how to close the work soften the heartbreaking reality of the worst case scenarios that often occur in real life, especially in cases of early onset Alzheimer's.

Through *poesis*, using what Freeman has called "recuperative disclosure," Munro, Wiesel, and Genova have been "agents of insight and rescue, recollection and recovery, serving to counteract the forces of oblivion" in their characters' – and perhaps their readers' – lives.[18] Although the characters themselves, by the end of the works, cannot any longer know or tell their own story, through artistic disclosure, the authors have done so for the characters, and each author has entrusted, within the fictional world of the narrative, a metaphorical holding womb in another character, a space that can enfold the story of the one unable to formulate who he or she is. In each of these fictional worlds, others have treasured the narrative self for the memory-deprived person, and have continued to love that person even in this altered mental state approaching oblivion of self. The degree of comfort for a reader in the possibility of such a virtual holding will vary by individual, of course, but each of these fictional works has affirmed hope experientially, through the artistic telling of a seemingly untellable story.

---

17 Hawkins. *Reconstructing Illness,* 2.

18 Freeman. *Hindsight,* 43–44.

In addition, there is a subtle suggestion in "The Bear Came over the Mountain," *The Forgotten*, and *Still Alice* that there may be an essential worth of being that transcends narrative. This suggestion, implied though unarticulated in the works themselves, takes us away from historical time into what narrative theorist Mark Freeman describes as an "overriding ontological commitment made in the context of mythical time – namely, that life, rather than having meaning imposed upon it, actually bears meaning within it."[19]

These powerful works, individually and taken together, allow us to experience what is termed *katabasis* in classical heroic journeys, a descent to the underworld, into the darkness. In myth, the protagonist who takes such a journey is enriched. I suggest that we, too, are enriched in reading "The Bear Came over the Mountain," *The Forgotten*, and *Still Alice*. The stories they tell help us to listen to what Arthur Frank calls "voices bespeak[ing] conditions of embodiment that most of us would rather forget our own vulnerability to" and thus to perform what Frank calls "a fundamental moral act," for "in listening to the other, we listen for ourselves."[20] By their artistically conveyed depictions of love's ability to survive even a loved one's loss of narrative identity, Munro, Wiesel, and Genova succeed in fulfilling the primary task Hawkins says belongs to an author of a pathography: "discover[ing], or creat[ing], a meaning that can bind [reality, E.L.] together again".[21] These works help us to face our own fear of the unknowns in our life, our own human vulnerability. They enrich and stretch us and give us, at least vicariously, the ability to have empathy for those who suffer severe memory loss. Above all, they challenge our sense that our identity and worth are contained in our ability to have a narrative self.

References

Andrews, Molly. *Narrative Imagination and Everyday Life*. New York: Oxford University Press, 2014.

Bender, Mike. "A Disquieting Look at Dementia." In: *Psychologist* 28,3 (2015): 222–23.

Birge, Sarah. "Brainhood, Selfhood, or 'Meat with a Point of View': The Value of Fiction for Neuroscientific Research and Neurological Medicine." In: Melissa

19 Freeman. "Mythical Time, Historical Time, and the Narrative Fabric of the Self." In: *Narrative Inquiry* 8,1 (1998): 27–50, 39.

20 Frank, Arthur. *The Wounded Storyteller: Body, Illness, and Ethics*. Chicago: University of Chicago Press, 1997, 25.

21 Hawkins. *Reconstructing Illness*, 2–3.

M. Littlefield, Jenell M. Johnson (eds.). *The Neuroscientific Turn: Transdisciplinarity in the Age of the Brain.* Ann Arbor, MI: University of Michigan Press, 2012, 89–104.

Casado-Gual, Nuria. "Unexpected Turns in Lifelong Sentimental Journeys: Redefining Love, Memory and Old Age through Alice Munro's 'The Bear Came Over the Mountain' and Its Film Adaptation *Away from Her*." In: *Ageing and Society* 35 (2015): 380–404.

Charon, Rita. *Narrative Medicine: Honoring the Stories of Illness.* New York: Oxford University Press, 2006.

Frank, Arthur. *The Wounded Storyteller: Body, Illness, and Ethics.* Chicago: University of Chicago Press, 1997.

Freedman, Jill, Combs, Gene. *Narrative Therapy: The Social Construction of Preferred Realities.* New York: Norton, 1996.

Freeman, Mark. *Hindsight: The Promise and Peril of Looking Backward.* New York: Oxford University Press, 2010.

Freeman, Mark. "Mythical Time, Historical Time, and the Narrative Fabric of the Self." In: *Narrative Inquiry* 8,1 (1998): 27–50.

Genova, Lisa. *Still Alice.* New York: Gallery, 2009.

Hawkins, Anne Hunsaker. *Reconstructing Illness: Studies in Pathography.* West Lafayette, Purdue University Press, 1993.

Munro, Alice. "The Bear Came over the Mountain," renamed as "Away from Her" in this edition. In: *Away From Her: Stories by Alice Munro.* New York: Penguin, 2007, 1–65.

Patterson, David. "Wiesel's Aggadic Outcry." In: Steven T. Katz, Alan Rosen (eds.). *Elie Wiesel: Jewish, Literary, and Moral Perspectives.* Indiana: Indiana University Press, 2013, 190–200.

Wiesel, Elie. *The Forgotten.* Trans. Stephen Becker. New York: Schocken, 1992.

Alexander Schwieren (Köln)

Lebendige Tote: Zum Status der Dementen in der Gegenwartsliteratur

Abstract: What are we talking about when we talk about dementia? This article analyzes the current figuration of dementia patients in the light of contemporary German-speaking literature. Its main aim is to discuss how dementia patients are related to the premodern staging of the dead and which meaning is attributed to dementia due to this relation. Both topics lead to the question in which way dementia could help us reflect on the notion of life in the twenty-first century.

I. Einleitung

Vor dem Hintergrund des ‚demographischen Wandels' stehen Auseinandersetzungen mit der Demenz in Konjunktur: Nicht nur in der Pflegewissenschaft und in ökonomischen Diskursen (‚Pflegeversicherung', ‚Renten') stellt die prozentuale Zunahme von Demenzerkrankungen eine Herausforderung dar, auch in sozial- und kulturwissenschaftlichen Zusammenhängen sind die Demenz und die an ihr Erkrankten zu einem symptomatischen Phänomen geworden, dessen Zusammenhang mit der ‚Kultur des Vergessens' frag- und forschungswürdig erscheint. Wie schwierig es ist, dieses Phänomen zur Sprache zu bringen, macht nicht zuletzt der Soziologe Gronemeyer deutlich, wenn er die Demenzerkrankten als „Flüchtlinge aus unserer Gesellschaft" bezeichnet.[1] Die Metapher vom Flüchtling ist unglücklich, vor allem weil ein Flüchtling oftmals eine Alternative zu seiner Flucht besitzt, auch wenn diese häufig bedeutet, in der Gefahr des Todes zu leben. Anders als die Flucht ist die Demenz, wenn sie denn eintritt, ohne Alternative, mit der Medizin gesprochen: progredient. Während das Ziel eines Flüchtlings in der Regel der Frieden ist, erwartet den Demenzerkrankten letztendlich der Tod.

Dennoch ist Gronemeyers Formulierung nicht belanglos, sondern vielmehr als Versuch zu respektieren, ein weitgehend sprachloses Phänomen zur Sprache zu bringen. Eine ähnliche Konstellation hat Thomas Macho in seiner Monographie über die *Todesmetaphern* interessiert: „*Worüber sprechen wir, wenn wir*

---

1 So Reimer Gronemeyers Formulierung auf dem 3. Demenzkongress in St. Gallen (2016). Vgl. zu Gronemeyers Perspektive insgesamt seine Monographie *Das 4. Lebensalter. Demenz ist keine Krankheit*. München: Pattloch, 2013.

vom Tod sprechen?"[2] Da sich die Erfahrung des Todes nicht einholen lässt, kann unser unentwegtes Reden vom Tod nur metaphorisch sein: Wie genau – das war Machos Interesse – sehen diese Metaphern aber aus und worüber geben sie Aufschluss, wenn nicht über den Tod? Die Demenz ist keine Todesart, sie teilt mit dem Tod aber die Uneinholbarkeit ihrer Erfahrung. Insofern erscheint es nicht unangebracht, Machos Frage neu zu stellen: *Wovon sprechen wir, wenn wir von der Demenz sprechen?* Im Angesicht des Grabens, der die Dementen von den Nicht-Dementen zweifellos und – zumindest in späteren Krankheitsstadien – fundamental trennt, scheint es interessant, einen Diskurs zu verfolgen, „dem die Unversöhnlichkeit der Differenz zwischen unseren Reden" und dem Diskurs der Dementen „eingebrannt" ist, einen Diskurs, „der die Erfahrung solcher Differenz nicht immanent verleugnen" muss, „ein[en] Diskurs ohne den therapeutischen Eros jeglicher *ars moriendi.*"[3] Eine Figur, die in diesem Zusammenhang wesentlicher sein könnte als die des Flüchtlings, ist die Figur des Todes selbst.

Diese Untersuchungsperspektive verdankt sich mehreren Anlässen. Zunächst findet sich die Nähe zum Tod und mehr noch, die Rede von einem Dasein „zwischen Leben und Tod" immer wieder in gegenwärtigen Auseinandersetzungen mit der Demenz.[4] Die Figur des Todes ist aber darüber hinaus auch im Versuch, das Alter – im Zuge der demographischen Untergangsszenarien zu Beginn des einundzwanzigsten Jahrhunderts – kulturhistorisch zu verorten, ins Spiel gebracht worden: Das Alter, so etwa Ulrike Vedder in einem Beitrag für die *Zeitschrift für Germanistik*, sei an die ‚Stelle des Todes' getreten.[5] Demnach haben ‚die Alten' in der Gegenwart den Status der Toten in der Vormoderne eingenommen. Doch was genau soll dieser Auftritt des Alters an der Stelle des Todes beinhalten: Ist mit diesem Auftritt eine kulturtheoretische Metapher formuliert, die das Alter als Begriff oder präziser als Figur der Gegenwart zu beschreiben und reflektieren erlaubt? Oder ist das Alter kulturhistorisch in den Fluchtpunkt einer Energie

---

2 Macho, Thomas. *Todesmetaphern. Zur Logik der Grenzerfahrung*. Frankfurt/M.: Suhrkamp Verlag, 1987, 23.

3 Die zitierten, hier auf die Demenz übertragenen Passagen finden sich bei Macho. *Todesmetaphern*, 22. Versuche, sich in einen Demenzerkrankten hineinzuversetzen und aus dessen Perspektive zu sprechen, sind nicht Teil des hier angedeuteten Diskurses und werden im Folgenden aus diesem Grund vernachlässigt.

4 Vgl. etwa Gronemeyer. *Das 4. Lebensalter*, 185–94, oder Jens, Inge. *Langsames Entschwinden*. Reinbek bei Hamburg: Rowohlt Verlag, 2016.

5 Vgl. Vedder, Ulrike. "Gegenwart und Wiederkehr der Toten. Sterben, Erben, Musealisieren vor und nach der Moderne." In: *Zeitschrift für Germanistik* Neue Folge XVII,2 (2007): 389–97, 392.

geraten, die in der Vormoderne dem Tod und den Toten zuteil wurde und die im Zuge der Moderne ihren Fluchtpunkt verloren hat? Wie auch immer diese Fragen beantwortet werden – die Toten der Vormoderne versprechen offenbar, als Vorgeschichte, die Gegenwart des Alters zu erhellen. Sie verheißen – im Jenseits physiologischer, psychologischer, soziologischer und ökonomischer Begriffe – Aufschluss über die Figuration des Alters.

Ich möchte versuchen, dieses Versprechen für die Frage nach einem über die medizinischen Konzepte hinausgehenden Begriff der Demenz anschlussfähig zu machen und werde die genannte These dazu etwas enger fassen: *Sprechen wir, wenn wir von der Demenz sprechen, vom Tod?* Oder besser: *Ist der Tod eine Metapher der Demenz?* Wenn das Alter im zwanzigsten Jahrhundert an die Stelle des Todes getreten ist, dann sollte das an der Schwelle zum einundzwanzigsten Jahrhundert in besonderem Maße auch für die Demenz Geltung haben.[6] Welche Beziehung besteht also zwischen dem kulturellen Status der Dementen und demjenigen der Toten in der Vormoderne? Welche Ähnlichkeiten zwischen Demenz und Tod, zwischen Dementen und Toten finden sich auf dem Schauplatz der Literatur?[7] Und: Was heißt das dann für die Demenz und die an ihr Erkrankten?

Diesen Fragen soll mit einer Lektüre begegnet werden, die zeitgenössische Literatur als Schauplatz liest: In der Literatur werden nicht nur die Figuren in Szene gesetzt, die uns im Angesicht eines letztlich nicht vermittelbaren und insofern sprachlosen Phänomens – metaphorisch – zur Hilfe kommen. Diese Figuren werden auch reflektiert und erlauben deshalb eine Lesart, die ihre Reichweite zu hinterfragen sucht.[8] Zuvor bedarf es allerdings einer Klärung, oder genauer, einer

---

6 Eine andere Perspektive verfolgt der Beitrag von Nicolai Glasenapp, der zwar gleichfalls den Konnex von Demenz und Tod in der Gegenwartsliteratur untersucht, dabei aber nicht an einer kulturgeschichtlichen Perspektive interessiert ist, vgl. Glasenapp, Nicolai. "Lebt man in Vergessenheit? Zum Konnex von Sterben, Tod und Demenz in der deutschsprachigen Gegenwartsliteratur." In: *Limbus* 8 (2015): 147–66.

7 Von Interesse ist hier also weniger, inwiefern die Literatur der Demenz einen fragwürdigen Sinn zuschreibt, um Erkrankte „nicht bloß als lebende Tote darzustellen", vgl. dazu Vedder, Ulrike. "Erzählen vom Zerfall. Demenz und Alzheimer in der Gegenwartsliteratur." In: *Zeitschrift für Germanistik* Neue Folge XXII,2 (2012): 290–305, 289. Es geht vielmehr darum, die Reichweite und vor allem die Figuration dieser ‚lebenden Toten' zu fokussieren.

8 Vgl. zu diesem Lektüreverfahren Weigel, Sigrid. *Literaturgeschichte als Voraussetzung der Kulturgeschichte. Schauplätze von Shakespeare bis Benjamin*. München: Wilhelm Fink Verlag, 2004. Die Verbindung von Literatur und Demenz diskutieren in diesem Sinne auch Neufeld, Anna Katharina und Vedder, Ulrike: "An der Grenze: Sterben und

Annäherung an die vermeintliche Vorgeschichte: Was ist vorzustellen unter dem Status der Toten in der Vormoderne?

II. Das Vorbild des Todes

In seiner epochemachenden Studie über die Kulturgeschichte des Todes bezeichnet Philippe Ariès den ‚gezähmten Tod' als grundlegende Konfiguration in der Geschichte des Todes: Der Tod, der schon in der Antike als Einbruch der wilden Natur in die Kultur des Menschen inszeniert worden ist, erscheint demnach vom fünften bis ins achtzehnte Jahrhundert vor allem als Prüfung der Gemeinschaft, die am Fortbestehen der Gattung interessiert ist.[9] Der Tod, der trotz aller mit dem Christentum verbundenen Umbrüche immer mit dem Bösen in Verbindung steht, wird „nicht sich selbst und seiner Maßlosigkeit überlassen", sondern „in Zeremonien eingefangen" und damit zumindest in seiner dramatischen Wirkung gebändigt.[10] Die Abschieds- und die Trauerszenen verknüpfen den Toten mit der Vergangenheit und der Zukunft der Gattung und verdrängen damit die Unruhe, die die Nähe des Todes bei den Trauernden hervorruft: Der Sterbende blickt zurück auf sein Leben, er versammelt die Nachkommen um sein Bett, gibt letzte Anweisungen, nimmt Abschied und empfiehlt Gott seine Seele.[11] Er fügt sich damit in ein vertrautes Schicksal und stirbt einen ‚einfachen Tod'. Zu diesem Tod gehört ganz wesentlich seine Öffentlichkeit: „Der Sterbende muss den Mittelpunkt einer Versammlung bilden."[12] Diese Versammlung ist durch eine starke Ritualisierung geprägt: Handlungs- und Sprechweisen, Gesten des Abschiednehmens und der Trauer, Anordnungen des Raumes und der anwesenden Menschen, Regelungen der Gebete, des Redens und des Schweigens gelten der Ehrung und der Zeugenschaft, die die bedrohliche Natur des Todes zu bannen sucht. Robert Harrison hat derartige Praktiken als „Werk der Trennung" bezeichnet, das den Tod des Verstorbenen „in mir" zu begleiten hat, soll dessen Sterben distanziert und nicht geteilt werden – „oder ich sterbe mit dem Toten".[13] Von Homer bis in

Tod in der Gegenwartsliteratur. Einleitung." In: *Zeitschrift für Germanistik* Neue Folge XXV,3 (2015): 495–98, 497.

9 Anzumerken ist an dieser Stelle, dass Ariès' Geschichte auf die *westliche* Moderne zuläuft – eine Einschränkung, die auch die folgenden Ausführungen teilen.

10 Ariès, Philippe. *Geschichte des Todes*. München: DTV, [9]1999, 776.

11 Vgl. Ariès. *Geschichte des Todes*, 25–28.

12 Ariès. *Geschichte des Todes*, 30.

13 Harrison, Richard. *Die Herrschaft des Todes*. München/Wien: Carl Hanser Verlag, 2006, 95.

die Gegenwart entdeckt Harrison in diesem Sinn eine Kultur, die die Bedrohung, die der Tod eines anderen Menschen hervorruft – die „Bedrohung durch die psychische Katastrophe" –, zu bannen sucht, in dem sie eine Grenze zwischen Toten und Lebenden zieht.[14]

Diese Grenze ist nach Ariès immer stabiler geworden: Das Nachleben der Toten, das in der Vormoderne als „Warten (et excepto)" vorgestellt wurde,[15] verliert in der Moderne an Bedeutung. Der Tod und die Toten werden aus dem Leben der Lebenden ausgeschlossen –Tod und Leben erscheinen als fundamentale Gegensätze.[16] Die Furcht vor den Toten, die Sorge der Antike, die Toten könnten wiederkehren und die Lebenden stören, wird in diesem Sinn aber schon mit dem Christentum immer schwächer. Die Toten werden als friedlich Ruhende vorgestellt: Im Mittelalter zeigt die häufigste Ikonographie die Toten im Schoß Abrahams, wo sie – wie die Kinder in der Wiege – geborgen sind. Trotz dieses beruhigenden Bildes werden aber auch Praktiken bedeutsam, die das eigene Nachleben betreffen: Messen werden bestellt, Stiftungen ins Leben gerufen, Testamente werden verfasst. Die Liebe der Lebenden soll erhalten bleiben, zugleich gilt es aber auch, in den Himmel zu investieren – ein Kalkül, das Historiker als ‚Jenseitsökonomie' beschrieben haben.[17] Die Toten führen ein Nachleben, das im Idealfall einen schlafähnlichen Zustand – im Himmel – mit einem anhaltenden, ehrenvollen Einfluss auf die Nachwelt – die Lebenden – verbindet.

Die *Natur des Todes* hingegen wird weiter distanziert, nicht zuletzt durch das zuvor noch unverhüllte, nun zunehmend verborgene Gesicht. Ariès schreibt, dass das Gesicht „von Leichentuch, Sarg und Katafalk oder *représentation* verlarvt" wird: „Die Hülle des Toten wird, spätestens seit dem vierzehnten Jahrhundert, zum theatralischen Monument",[18] das die Distanzierung des ‚nackten Todes' mit der Repräsentation eines individuellen Nachlebens zu verbinden hat.

---

14 Harrison. *Herrschaft des Todes*, 90–112, 95.

15 Ariès. *Geschichte des Todes*, 776.

16 Das Sterben erscheint mit anderen Worten nicht mehr als „Jenseits-Passage", sondern als „absolute [...] Grenze", vgl. Solhdju, Katrin, Vedder, Ulrike. "Das Leben vom Tode her. Zur Einleitung." In: Dies. (eds.). *Das Leben vom Tode her. Zur Kulturgeschichte einer Grenzziehung*. München: Wilhelm Fink Verlag, 2015, 7–15, 11.

17 Vgl. dazu Willer, Stefan, Weigel, Sigrid, Jussen, Bernhard (eds.). *Erbe. Übertragungskonzepte zwischen Natur und Kultur*. Berlin: Suhrkamp Verlag, 2013, besonders den Beitrag von Kressin, Urban. "Geistliches Erbe. Theologie von Abstammung und Besitz im Frühmittelalter." In: Willer et al. *Erbe*, 65–84.

18 Ariès. *Geschichte des Todes*, 780.

Eine entscheidende Veränderung in dieser Kultur des Todes verzeichnet Ariès vor allem im neunzehnten Jahrhundert, wenn sowohl die eher abstrakte Bedeutung der Gattung als auch der Horizont des eigenen, individuellen Todes hinter die Sorge und Trauer um nahestehende Verwandte und Freunde zurücktritt, „von denen getrennt zu werden man nicht mehr erträgt: die Trennung löst eine dramatische", von Ariès bekanntlich als der „Tod des Anderen" bezeichnete „Krise aus".[19] Im Wesentlichen tritt die Kernfamilie damit an die Stelle von Gattung und Individuum. Die ursprünglich ritualisierte Trauer, die sich noch ganz wesentlich auf die Sorge um die Zukunft der Gemeinschaft bezogen hatte und eine dementsprechend kollektive Begleitung des Sterbenden erforderlich machte, ist nach Ariès einer individualisierten, romantischen Anteilnahme (am Schicksal einiger weniger) gewichen, die den eigenen Tod verdrängt und gleichzeitig den *Tod des Anderen* als Inbegriff höchster Schönheit verklärt. Das Jenseits „wird vor allem zum Ort der Wiedervereinigung derer, die durch den Tod getrennt worden sind und diese Trennung" nicht akzeptieren können.[20]

Neben dieser Konzentration der Todesvorstellung auf den *Tod des Anderen* hat Ariès die Scham vor dem Tod als wesentlichen Grund für die Einstellung zum Tod in der zweiten Hälfte des zwanzigsten Jahrhunderts ausgemacht: Nachdem die Aufklärung die Hoffnung genährt hat, alles Böse auszumerzen, erscheint der Tod, dessen Kontingenz trotz aller Distanzierungsversuche immer mit dem Bösen in Verbindung gestanden hatte, als Skandal, den es zu verschweigen gilt. Der Tod wird so weit wie möglich verdeckt: durch Krankenhaus- und Hospizwände, durch das Verbergen des nahenden Todes gegenüber dem Sterbenden – „weder das Individuum noch die Gesellschaft sind stark und stabil genug, den Tod anzuerkennen".[21] Der individuelle Tod unterbricht das alltägliche, gesellschaftliche Leben nicht mehr.

Thomas Macho hat diese These verschoben und insbesondere dem zwanzigsten Jahrhundert eine Verschmelzung von Schweige- und Todessehnsucht attestiert: Dem Wunsch, die nach Ausschwitz, Hiroshima und anderen unfassbaren Todeserfahrungen einzig legitime Position, die Position eines Toten einzunehmen und sich damit auf die Seite der Opfer zu stellen, korrespondiert der Wunsch zu schweigen und damit nicht zuletzt das unmögliche Gespräch mit den Toten *in deren Sprache* fortzusetzen. Allein im Schweigen, so ließen sich Ariès' und Machos Arbeiten vielleicht verknüpfen, vermag das zwanzigste Jahrhundert dem Tod zu

19 Ariès. *Geschichte des Todes*, 783.
20 Ariès. *Geschichte des Todes*, 785.
21 Ariès. *Geschichte des Todes*, 788.

begegnen: Das Schweigen bezeichnet sowohl die Strategien, mit dem *Tod des Anderen* umzugehen, als auch den Fluchtpunkt jener Anstrengungen, die den Katastrophen des zwanzigsten Jahrhunderts Rechnung zu tragen suchen. Das Schweigen markiert eine Verdrängung des Todes und zugleich eine Seinsweise, die sich mit den Toten gemein zu machen sucht. In beiden Fällen wird der Tod distanziert, denn auch die Todessehnsucht als Wunsch, das „ausgelebte Unheil im Moment des Verschwindens aller Subjektivität endlich vergessen zu dürfen",[22] räumt dem Tod keinen Raum unter den Lebenden ein. Im Gegenteil: Der Wunsch nach dem Tod entspricht vielmehr einer Distanz zum ‚falschen' Leben (Adorno) als einer Annäherung an die Präsenz und Kontingenz des Todes. Wie das Verdrängen eines nahenden Todes hinter einer verschwiegenen Diagnose und den Wänden eines Hospizes ist der Wunsch, tot zu sein, alles andere als ein Versuch, dem Tod im Leben *wieder* einen Platz einzuräumen, einen Platz, wie etwa denjenigen des ‚gezähmten Todes'.

Ist das Alter, ist die Demenz tatsächlich, oder vielmehr: metaphorisch mit der damit allein vormodernen Annäherung an die Natur des Todes verbunden? Wird der Demenz auf ähnliche Weise begegnet wie dem Tod, bevor seine natürliche Brutalität romantisiert und schließlich fast vollständig verdrängt wurde? *Sprechen wir, wenn wir von der Demenz sprechen, vom vormodernen Tod?*

Konkret gefragt heißt das: Wird die Erfahrung der Demenz ritualisiert, wird ihr in ähnlichen Pathosformeln begegnet wie ehedem der Präsenz eines Toten? Kommt die Demenz als Abschied zur Sprache und wenn ja, inwiefern ist dieser Abschied mit dem Tod zu vergleichen? Wie wird die Präsenz eines Dementen in der Literatur organisiert? Inwiefern erinnert diese Präsenz an das Nachleben der Toten in der Vormoderne?

III. Korrespondenzen zwischen Tod und Demenz auf dem Schauplatz der Literatur

Ritualisierung. Denken wir an die Ehrung der Toten und die Bezeugung des Todes in der Vormoderne, dessen natürliche Gewalt eben durch die ritualisierten Sprechakte, Gesten, Haltungen und Handlungen distanziert werden sollte, so ist die Korrespondenz zur Demenz zunächst kaum mehr als oberflächlich zu nennen. Die Literatur liefert allerdings eine ganze Reihe von Szenen, die Ehrerbietung und Zeugenschaft auf eine spezifische Art und Weise in Verbindung setzen und damit eine fragwürdige Distanzierung zur Sprache bringen. Die Besuchsszenen,

22 Macho. *Todesmetaphern*, 16.

besonders in Betreuungseinrichtungen, bieten dafür einen reichen Fundus: „Dienstags um kurz vor halb fünf warten Professor Sander und Frau von Kanter neben der Drehtür von Haus Ulmen, ein kleines hilfloses Empfangskomitee." (Pehnt. *Schildkröten*, 9) Gleich dieser erste Satz von Annette Pehnts Roman *Das Haus der Schildkröten* (2006) setzt eine ausgeprägte Regelhaftigkeit in der Begegnung von Dementen und Angehörigen in Szene. Der Besuch der Eltern durch die beiden erwachsenen Kinder, die im Mittelpunkt von Pehnts Roman stehen, findet nicht nur immer zur gleichen Zeit statt. Auch die Handlungen und Gespräche ähneln sich stark – genauso, wie die Versuche, die Erinnerung an die Besuche möglichst mit dem Verlassen des Heims zu verdrängen.[23] Interessanter als diese oberflächlichen Parallelen ist die Beschreibung der Besuche als Tauchgänge: Beim Eintritt in das Heim „zögern" die Kinder noch, „in die andere Zeit einzutauchen, eine kinderlose, appetitlose, schlaflose, trockene Zeit" (Pehnt. *Schildkröten*, 51). Diese andere Zeit ist so grundsätzlich von der eigenen unterschieden, dass sich ihr Sinn in keiner Weise feststellen lässt – und darin korrespondiert sie dem Tod: Als Professor Sander seine unentwegt fortgesetzten Aufzeichnungen mit seinem nicht als Sohn erkannten Besucher diskutieren möchte, kann dieser nur „winzige Bleistiftkrakel [...], Seite um Seite gefüllt mit zarten Linien und Strichen" (Pehnt. *Schildkröten*, 55) erkennen – die Demenz hat ihre eigene Schrift, die sich sehen, aber nicht lesen lässt. Die regelmäßigen Versuche, die Nähe eines Dementen „großzügig" (Pehnt. *Schildkröten*, 53) auszuhalten, scheitern, weil alle Zeichen der Demenz verstören und in keinem Sinn aufzugehen scheinen: Diese Gleichzeitigkeit einer Ungleichzeitigkeit, die mit dem Eintauchen in eine andere Zeit ins Bild gesetzt wird, bringt eine fundamentale Distanz zur Sprache. Und doch wird diese Distanz ausgehalten. Der uneinholbare Sinn der Demenz, die zunehmend unverständliche Sprache (und Schrift) der Dementen, werden ausgehalten, auch wenn die Erkrankten selbst diese Beharrlichkeit oftmals nicht zu würdigen wissen, ja, meist nicht einmal bemerken. Auch wenn die in der Literatur inszenierten Rituale im Umgang mit der Demenz weit vom Formalisierungsgrad des vormodernen Todes entfernt sind – mit dem krampfhaften Festhalten an gesellschaftlichen Kommunikationskonventionen wird die Verstörung, die die Demenz mit sich bringt, nicht verschwiegen, sondern begrenzt, und zwar auf ähnliche Art und Weise, wie zuvor die Verstörung des Lebens durch den Tod. Auch hier wird dem Einbruch einer mehr oder weniger natürlichen Gewalt, die in diesem Fall nicht direkt den Tod, aber eben doch eine Zäsur der

23 In Ergänzung zu dieser Ritualisierung der Handlungen konstatiert Ulrike Vedder, dass auch „die räumliche Ordnung [...] ganz auf Ausweglosigkeit ausgerichtet" ist. Vedder. *Erzählen vom Zerfall*, 280.

menschlichen Kultur bezeichnet, mit Strategien begegnet, die Wiederholung, Nähe und Distanz zu verbinden suchen.

Katharina Hacker hat in ihrem Roman *Die Erdbeeren von Antons Mutter* (2010) eine sehr bodenständige Metapher für derartige Versuche in Szene gesetzt: die Kultivierung von Erdbeeren zur Unzeit. Anton, die zentrale Figur des Romans, versucht mit allen Mitteln die Anzeichen der Demenz seiner Mutter – vor allem: das Vergessen der rechtzeitigen Anpflanzung von Erdbeeren – unsichtbar zu machen. Er holt die Anpflanzung heimlich nach und scheitert trotz aller Anstrengung an einer Schneckeninvasion, die sich gleichsam als Metapher des Todes und des neurophysiologischen Demenzbegriffs lesen lässt:

> Wie sie aus dem Wald und sogar aus den umliegenden Gärten sich näherten, die nackten, roten Körper, schleimig glänzend, sie zogen sich und streckten sich rhythmisch und ohne Unterlaß, der Duft war es, der sie anlockte, auch von fern her, sie fraßen systematisch die Früchte an, eine nach der anderen. (Hacker. *Erdbeeren*, 151–52)

Der Kampf gegen diese Invasion bringt alle Abwehrversuche, die in Hackers Roman der Demenz entgegengebracht werden, ins Bild: Da sind zunächst die hoffnungslosen Versuche der Mutter selbst, die mit ihrem Küchenmesser ganze zwei Schnecken zerlegt (vgl. Hacker. *Erdbeeren*, 146). Hinzu kommen die Anstrengungen des ehemaligen Geliebten, der die Gefahr verbergen will und die Schnecken vom Erdbeerfeld in einen Eimer sammelt und abdeckt, als ließe sich der Einbruch der Natur, „ein ekelhaftes Gewimmel, das in ihm Grauen weckte [...], es hatte etwas Unzüchtiges und Verzweifeltes", nachträglich isolieren (Hacker. *Erdbeeren*, 154) – eine Hoffnung, die ein unbedachter Fußtritt gegen den Eimer begräbt. Eine dritte Form der Abwehr wird mit der Naivität der Kinder ins Bild gesetzt, die die Gefahr für die Erdbeeren schlichtweg verdrängen. Zuletzt versucht auch noch ein Fremder zu helfen, aber auch er kommt zu spät, er verliert den Halt, den er geben wollte – „seine dicken Schuhsohlen hatten auf den glitschigen Körpern keinen Halt" (Hacker. *Erdbeeren*, 166). Am Ende aller Hoffnungen auf eine Rettung sitzen die Schnecken „zwischen den Blättern und auf den Erdbeeren, umschl[i]ngen die Früchte, überall [sind] ihre Schleimspuren" (Hacker. *Erdbeeren*, 166). Die Erdbeeren werden faulen. Obwohl eine Vielzahl von Menschen, genauer, eine Vielzahl von Männern mit unterschiedlicher Expertise (der Gärtner, der schulmedizinisch ausgebildete Sohn und nicht zuletzt ein bei der Fremdenlegion ausgebildeter Fremder) der Demenzerkrankten die Konfrontation mit ihrer Krankheit ersparen wollen, bahnt sich die Natur unerbittlich ihren Weg.

Das Beharren auf der Regelmäßigkeit, die Vermeidung von Veränderungen, die zumindest in der Literatur an vielen Stellen als zentrale Verhaltensweise im Umgang mit der Demenz, insbesondere auch durch professionelle Hilfskräfte, inszeniert wird, verfolgt wie die Ritualisierung des Todes das Ziel, die Demenz in ihren Extremen zu distanzieren, zu begrenzen, ihre Natur zu verbergen. Selbstredend sind die Strategien im Umgang mit der Demenz anders begründet, oftmals in (pflege)wissenschaftlichen und nicht in religiösen Diskursen; und nicht zuletzt durch diese unterschiedliche Herkunft sind sie von dem, was wir als Rituale bezeichnen würden, ein gutes Stück entfernt. Im engeren Sinne lassen sich Rituale, wie sie den Toten einst zugekommen sind, im Umgang mit Demenzerkrankten kaum beobachten und ganz sicher entspricht der Öffentlichkeit vormoderner Todesszenen kein vergleichbares Publikum auf den Schauplätzen der Demenz. Die Gefährdungen, die vom Tod in der Vormoderne wie von der Demenz in der Gegenwartsliteratur ausgehen, betreffen aber auf ähnliche Weise den Kern dessen, was jeweils als Leben verstanden wird. Das lässt sich einerseits im Hinblick auf ihre zeitliche Organisation (1) und andererseits im Verhältnis von An- und Abwesenheit (2) deutlich machen.

(1) Abschiede. Selbstredend ist die Demenz eine ‚Krankheit zum Tode', sie ist irreversibel – nach ihr kommt allein der Tod. Und doch markiert die Diagnose Demenz in der Regel – im Gegensatz etwa zu bestimmten Krebsdiagnosen – nicht den Anfang des Sterbens. Mit Demenz lässt sich leben. Und dennoch kommt sie in der Literatur meist als Zulauf auf den Tod zur Sprache. Das wird schon in einer älteren Erzählung Irene Disches, *Der Doktor braucht ein Heim* (1990), deutlich, die im Hinblick auf die zeitliche und grammatische Organisation der Demenz durchaus zeitgemäß erscheint: Für den an Demenz erkrankten Erzähler ist die „Anwendung des Futurs" nicht nur ungewöhnlich, sie ist – wie sonst nur vor dem Tod – „praktisch verboten" (Dische. *Der Doktor*, 23–24). Dieses Verbot geht offenbar nicht von den Erkrankten aus, die mitunter ihren Widerstand planen: „Trotzdem werde ich es [das Futur, A.S.] demnächst verwenden." (Dische. *Der Doktor*, 24) Die Imagination einer Zukunft wird in der Literatur vielmehr von denen durchgestrichen, die die Demenz eines Anderen (eines Geliebten, einer Angehörigen, eines Patienten etc.) erleben. In Urs Faes' Erzählung *Er ist nicht mehr da, wenn er da ist* (2006) resümiert die erzählende Ehefrau eines an Demenz Erkrankten dementsprechend: „Seit sieben Jahren nehme ich Abschied, langsam, langsam […] und dennoch unaufhaltsam." (Faes. *Er ist nicht mehr da*, 24) Oder bei Katharina Hacker: „[S]o also entfernte sich jemand endgültig." (Hacker. *Erdbeeren*, 22) Die Demenz erscheint als – mitunter gewaltsame – Sterbeszene in *Slow Motion*, „Abschiede in Zeitlupe, unumkehrbar": „Alles wird erstickt" (Faes. *Er ist nicht mehr da*, 35, 33). Ähnlich auch in Arno Geigers *Der alte König in seinem Exil* (2011): „Es ist, als würde ich dem Vater in Zeitlupe beim Verbluten zusehen. Das Leben sickert Tropfen für Tropfen aus ihm heraus." (Geiger. *Exil*, 12) Deutlich

wird auch das Exemplarische der Demenz: Die als linear beschriebene Erfahrung der Krankheit des Anderen erscheint als Beispiel, wenn nicht als Inbegriff der Vergänglichkeit: „[I]ch habe gelernt, was vergehen heißt." (Faes. *Er ist nicht mehr da*, 45)[24] Die in der Literatur als Beispiel der ‚Vergänglichkeit' inszenierte Demenz unterscheidet sich dabei vom Prozess des Alterns, der vor dem Hintergrund einer Demenzerkrankung eher als schnell wahrgenommen wird, etwa in Michael Ignatieffs Roman *Die Lichter auf der Brücke eines sinkenden Schiffs* (1993), in dem der Sohn seine an Alzheimer erkrankte Mutter beschreibt: „Sie altert entsetzlich schnell [...]. Alles ist beschleunigt" (Ignatieff. *Lichter*, 62). Während sich das Altern beschleunigt, verlangsamt sich der Moment des Abschieds. Derartige Abschiede werden zwar einerseits als Zäsur, als „Riss durch das Wir" (Faes. *Er ist nicht mehr da*, 35), beschrieben. Sie führen aber dennoch nicht zwangsläufig zu einer Distanzierung, im Gegenteil: In der Reflexion der Abschiedsszenen wird die Nähe zum Kranken vielmehr emphatisch als Bewältigung einer existentiellen Erfahrung beschrieben: „Ich weiß, dass ich noch immer dahin gehöre, zu ihm, diesem Mann, bei allen Abschieden, trotz der Sprachlosigkeit, die sich aufgetan hat." (Faes. *Er ist nicht mehr da*, 46) Obwohl der Erkrankte aus der Außenperspektive immer weiter *verschwindet* – „Was die Erinnerung nicht bewahrt, ist nicht mehr da." (Faes. *Er ist nicht mehr da*, 38) –, obwohl der erkrankte Mensch den Schauplatz seines eigenen Abtritts verlässt, gilt es offenbar, seine Nähe auszuhalten. Wie die Sterbeszene erscheint die Demenzerkrankung als Abschiednehmen und als Prüfung derjenigen, die dem Kranken nahestehen bzw. nahegestanden haben. Sie können mit der Bewältigung dieser Aufgabe wachsen. Die Demenz des Anderen zu meistern, heißt hier, sie auszuhalten – auch dann, wenn der Andere die eigene Nähe nicht wünscht.[25]

(2) Präsenz und Abwesenheit. Dem Abschiednehmen entspricht eine bedenkenswerte Konfiguration von An- und Abwesenheit der Dementen. Arno Geiger hat diese Konfiguration als Exil bezeichnet, in dem der Betroffene „rat- und rastlos" umherirrt, seine Sinneseindrücke werden „schwankend, instabil, davon bedroht, sich im nächsten Moment aufzulösen" (Geiger. *Exil*, 12). In seinem Text erzählt das Gesicht des Kranken von dessen „tiefer Heimatlosigkeit": Dem „König im Exil" ist „die ganze Welt fremd geworden". Diese Bedrohung fällt in der Außenperspektive

---

24 Eine Ausnahme zu dieser Irreversibilität stellt Martin Suters Roman *Small World* dar, in dem eine Heilung der Demenz antizipiert wird. Es ist die Frage, ob sich Suters Roman aufgrund dieser Ausnahmestellung heute noch schreiben ließe.

25 Diese Unerwünschtheit wird in vielen Texten ausführlich inszeniert, beispielsweise in Thorup, Kirsten. *Niemandsland*. Aus dem Dänischen von Angelika Gundlach. Frankfurt/Main: Suhrkamp Verlag, 2007.

auf den Erkrankten zurück: Mit seinen immer disparateren Wahrnehmungen droht auch er sich aufzulösen. Geigers Text ist sicherlich eine Ausnahme, weil er diese Bedrohung nicht Realität werden lässt, sondern, im Gegenteil, den Kranken dem Verlust seiner Identität entkommen lässt: „Er hatte seine Erinnerungen in Charakter umgemünzt, und der Charakter war ihm geblieben.“ (Geiger. *Exil*, 73) Als paradigmatisch für die Inszenierungen des – langen – Abschieds mag eher schon der zitierte Roman von Ignatieff gelten:

> Jeden Morgen erwacht sie ein wenig weiter weg von uns. Aber noch gelingt es ihr, wenn auch nur mit einem Blick, etwas von der Welt, in die sie eingeht, zu vermitteln. Es gibt hier, scheint sie zu sagen, jenseits von Angst und Verlust, am dunklen Rand, wo alles zerbröckelt, verfällt und undeutlich wird, es gibt hier eine Art von Leben. (Ignatieff. *Lichter*, 63)

Die Demenzkranke erscheint auf dem Schauplatz der Literatur als Grenzgängerin, wobei die Grenze ihre eigene Existenz durchzieht: Einerseits ein schwindender Lebenszusammenhang, verblassende Erinnerungen, abreißende Beziehungen, andererseits eine Dunkelheit, die sich allen Worten entzieht. Die Kranke führt in dieser Dunkelheit „eine Art von Leben“, das sich „uns“ allein in Form eines „Blicks“ zu erkennen gibt. Die Augen sind das einzige, letzte Medium zwischen Dunkelheit und Licht[26] – aber auch dieses Medium ist flüchtig, mit dem Fortgang der Krankheit schwindet jede Verbindung. Die Kranken, die vollständig auf die ‚*andere* Seite‘ übergetreten sind, erscheinen auf *dieser* Seite abwesend, sie sitzen, schreibt Urs Faes, „alle da und warten. [...] Warten immerzu.“ (Faes. *Er ist nicht mehr da*, 39) Sie sind „nur noch da [...]. Nur da. Zeitlos“ (Faes. *Er ist nicht mehr da*, 40).

Mit wenigen Ausnahmen[27] gilt das Interesse, das in der Literatur den Dementen entgegengebracht wird, den Grenzgängen der Dementen. Ein Teil ihrer Existenz ist in der Sprache nicht einzuholen. Was eher oberflächlich als Selbstverlust beschrieben wird, kommt deshalb in der Literatur verstärkt als ein besonderer Rhythmus von Präsenz und Absenz zur Sprache, der auch über das Verhältnis von Subjektivität und Passivität nicht präzise beschrieben werden kann. Der „leere[] Blick“ der Kranken, heißt es bei Ignatieff, scheint „darauf zu warten, daß die Zeit verg[eht], daß das Gefühl aufhört[e]“ (Ignatieff. *Lichter*, 123). Der leere Blick, das

---

26 Der Titel *Die Lichter auf der Brücke eines sinkenden Schiffs* lässt sich somit auch als ‚Augenlicht einer Dementen‘, als ‚letztes Zeichen‘ also, dechiffrieren.

27 Zu nennen wäre etwa der ‚Demenz-Klassiker‘ *Small World* von Martin Suter, der zuallererst als Kriminal- und Familiengeschichte zu lesen ist, oder Tilman Jens' Buch über seinen Vater Walter Jens, das in erster Linie eine Auseinandersetzung mit der moralischen Integrität des Vaters darstellt. In beiden Fällen ist die Demenz kaum mehr als ein Mittel zum Zweck.

ist aber nicht zuletzt der Blick einer Maske. In Kirsten Thorups Roman *Niemandsland* (2007) wird das noch deutlicher: „Die Augen waren klein, sein Blick war unklar. Das Gesicht war erstarrt. Die feinen Muskeln und Nervenbahnen streikten. Er hatte keine Falten. Die Haut war geglättet wie in einer Art Vor-Tod." (Thorup. *Niemandsland*, 88) Eine Maske repräsentiert eine Individualität, deren Präsenz sie niemals einholen kann. Anders gesagt: Die individuelle Maske verweist auf die Präsenz einer Individualität, die abwesend ist.[28] Ariès hat beschrieben, wie die Totenmaske im späten Mittelalter Teil der Abschiedsszenen zwischen Tod und Begräbnis geworden ist: „der Leichnam, ehedem vertrauter und bildlicher Ausdruck des Schlafes, verfügt fortan über eine solche bannende Macht, daß sein Anblick unerträglich wird."[29] Der Leichnam wird folgerichtig verhüllt, er wird aber nicht anonymisiert, sondern – zumindest im besten Fall, in dem Geld keine Rolle spielt – durch eine Figur ersetzt: die *„représentation"*, bei der die Bildhauer „genaueste Ähnlichkeit zu erzielen" suchten. „Es ist unschicklich geworden, das Antlitz der Toten allzu lange den Blicken preiszugeben, und doch ist ihre Präsenz noch immer vonnöten, weil sie es sich in ihren Testamenten so ausbedungen haben, weil sie zur Bekehrung der Lebenden unverzichtbar sind."[30] Die Maske der ‚représentation' erlaubt es in der Vormoderne, die Verdrängung des Leichnams und damit des natürlichen, fleischlichen Todes mit dem Nachleben der Toten zu verbinden. In Korrespondenz zu dieser Geschichte des Todes ließe sich formulieren: Indem die Literatur die Dementen maskiert, lässt sie deren Abwesenheit präsent werden. Die Dementen betreten die Bühne, die sie zugleich verlassen. Mit anderen Worten: Die Literatur inszeniert weniger die Anwesenheit von Menschen, die geistig abwesend sind, sondern vielmehr die Abwesenheit dieser Menschen selbst, die nur über Masken *re*präsentiert werden.[31]

Die Dementen sind abwesend, ‚fast' tot. Ihre Handlungen erscheinen mechanisch, sie könnten – so konstatiert Ignatieffs Erzähler – „von einer Maschine stammen" (Ignatieff. *Lichter*, 181). Die Unterbrechung zwischen der verminderten, aber eben doch fortgesetzt vorhandenen Handlungsfähigkeit und dem Ich, das diese Handlungen motiviert, bewirkt eine gespenstische Gegenwart. Die Dementen sind an- und abwesend zugleich. Sie handeln und handeln – im engeren Sinne

---

28 Vgl. dazu Belting, Hans. *Faces. Eine Geschichte des Gesichts*. München: C.H. Beck, 2013, 120.

29 Ariès. *Geschichte des Todes*, 216.

30 Ariès. *Geschichte des Todes*, 218–19 und 222.

31 Als weitere Maske ließe sich die Stimme diskutieren, die angesichts der Regression der Sprache auf Worthülsen, Redewendungen etc. auf ähnliche Weise Präsenz und Absenz ins Verhältnis setzt.

eines autonomen Subjekts – nicht. Als Grenzfall dieser Ambiguität gilt nicht nur in Ignatieffs Roman das Erkennen der eigenen Familie: „Wenn sie einen nicht mehr erkannte, hörte man auf zu existieren. Man war nicht mehr der Sohn, man war niemand mehr. Bestätige meine Existenz. Bestätige deinen Sohn." (Ignatieff. *Lichter*, 193)

IV. Schluss: Wessen Demenz?

Der Grenzfall der Krankheit, mit dem die ‚letzte Stufe' erreicht, die letzten Verbindungen zum einstigen Leben gekappt werden, provoziert nicht nur die Frage nach dem Status dieser letzten Stufe. Er stellt auch die Legitimität der Nachkommen in Frage. Wenn in der Literatur mit der Demenz die Fundamente einer Person in Frage gestellt werden, dann gerät nicht allein die demente Person an dieser Stelle ins Wanken. Der „Anhauch des Todes" (Ariès), der Abgrund, der sich im Leben mit dem Tod eines Anderen auftut, wird mit der Demenz sicht- und spürbar. Die Literatur beschäftigen also nicht allein die Fragen, welche Schwierigkeiten die Pflege/der Umgang mit der Demenz beinhaltet, welche Zäsuren in den Beziehungen von Kranken und Gesunden mit der Demenz verbunden sind oder wie die Demenz aus der Perspektive eines Kranken vielleicht erlebt wird. Die Literatur setzt die Demenz auch als Auftritt einer Jenseitigkeit in Szene, die die Grundlage des Lebens, die eigene Herkunft, infrage stellen kann. In diesem Sinn korrespondiert die Demenz dem vormodernen Tod: Ihre Inszenierung im Diskurs der Literatur greift auf eine Vielzahl von Bildern zurück, die – bewusst oder nicht – mit dem Tod in der Vormoderne in Verbindung stehen.

Wenn es stimmt, dass die Dementen an die Stelle der Toten getreten sind, dann vor allem in dem Sinn, dass sie den Einbruch der Natur vor Augen führen: einer Natur, die unseren Vorstellungen von Autonomie, Individualität und Normalität jeden Boden entziehen kann.

Die zu Beginn formulierte Frage nach dem Status dieser Kulturgeschichtsschreibung lässt sich aber auch jetzt noch nicht abschließend beantworten: *Als Metapher* führt der Tod in der Vormoderne zwar zu einem veränderten Blick auf literarische Inszenierungen der Demenz. Sie macht vor allem deutlich, dass diejenigen, die die Erkrankung erleben, ohne selbst erkrankt zu sein, in der Literatur viel tun, um den ‚Anhauch der Demenz' zu distanzieren. Die Nähe, die es in der ‚Demenzliteratur' der letzten zwei bis drei Jahrzehnte oftmals zu ertragen gilt, ist sicher weniger die Nähe eines Menschen, sondern vielmehr die Nähe von dessen Abwesenheit – die Nähe seines Todes (unabhängig davon, wie viele Jahre er noch leben wird). Das erklärt vielleicht auch, warum diese als extrem lange, ‚langsam' beschriebene Krankheit in der Literatur stellenweise in brutalen Figuren zur

Sprache kommt. Der Tod als Metapher der Demenz ist, das lassen diese Lektüren plausibel werden, keine Metapher für die Inszenierungen der Demenz in der Gegenwartsliteratur, sondern eine Metapher der Gegenwartsliteratur für die Demenz.

Ob sich aber über diese metaphorische Bedeutung eine tiefere kulturhistorische Verbindung zwischen dem Tod und der Demenz beschreiben lässt, das bleibt an dieser Stelle ungeklärt – vielleicht könnte eine Studie, die die späten Spuren des Todes in der Vormoderne mit den frühen Spuren der Demenz, etwa in den Diskursen der Aufklärung, zueinander in Beziehung zu setzen versuchte, darüber entscheiden.

Bibliographie

Ariès, Philippe. *Geschichte des Todes*. München: DTV, ^{9}1999.

Belting, Hans. *Faces. Eine Geschichte des Gesichts*. München: C.H. Beck, 2013.

Dische, Irene. *Der Doktor braucht ein Heim. Erzählung*. Aus dem Amerikanischen von Rainer Kaiser. Frankfurt/M.: Suhrkamp Verlag, 1990.

Geiger, Arno. *Der alte König in seinem Exil*. München: Carl Hanser Verlag, 2011.

Glasenapp, Nicolai. "Lebt man in Vergessenheit? Zum Konnex von Sterben, Tod und Demenz in der deutschsprachigen Gegenwartsliteratur." In: *Limbus* 8 (2015): 147–66.

Gronemeyer, Reimer. *Das 4. Lebensalter. Demenz ist keine Krankheit*. München: Pattloch, 2013.

Faes, Urs. "Er ist nicht mehr da, wenn er da ist." In: Klara Obermüller (ed.): *Es schneit in meinem Kopf. Erzählungen über Alzheimer und Demenz*. München/Wien: Nagel & Kimche, 2006, 23–46.

Hacker, Katharina. *Die Erdbeeren von Antons Mutter*. Frankfurt/M.: S. Fischer Verlag, 2012.

Harrison, Richard. *Die Herrschaft des Todes*. München/Wien: Carl Hanser Verlag, 2006.

Ignatieff, Michael. *Die Lichter auf der Brücke eines sinkenden Schiffs*. Frankfurt/M.: Suhrkamp Verlag, 1998.

Jens, Inge. *Langsames Entschwinden*. Reinbek bei Hamburg: Rowohlt Verlag, 2016.

Jens, Tilman. *Demenz. Abschied von meinem Vater*. Gütersloh: Gütersloher Verlagshaus, 2009.

Kressin, Urban. "Geistliches Erbe. Theologie von Abstammung und Besitz im Frühmittelalter." In: Willer, Stefan, Sigrid Weigel, Bernhard Jussen (eds.). *Erbe. Übertragungskonzepte zwischen Natur und Kultur*. Berlin: Suhrkamp, 2013, 65–84.

Macho, Thomas. *Todesmetaphern. Zur Logik der Grenzerfahrung*. Frankfurt/M.: Suhrkamp Verlag, 1987.

Neufeld, Anna Katharina und Ulrike Vedder. "An der Grenze: Sterben und Tod in der Gegenwartsliteratur. Einleitung." In: *Zeitschrift für Germanistik* Neue Folge XXV,3 (2015): 495–98.

Pehnt, Annette. *Haus der Schildkröten*. München: Piper Verlag, 2006.

Solhdju, Katrin, Vedder, Ulrike. "Das Leben vom Tode her. Zur Einleitung." In: Dies. (eds.). *Das Leben vom Tode her. Zur Kulturgeschichte einer Grenzziehung*. München: Wilhelm Fink Verlag, 2015, 7–15.

Suter, Martin. *Small World*. Zürich: Diogenes Verlag, 1997.

Thorup, Kirsten. *Niemandsland*. Aus dem Dänischen von Angelika Gundlach. Frankfurt/M.: Suhrkamp Verlag, 2007.

Vedder, Ulrike. "Gegenwart und Wiederkehr der Toten: Sterben, Erben, Musealisieren vor und nach der Moderne." In: *Zeitschrift für Germanistik* Neue Folge XVII,2 (2007): 389–97.

Vedder, Ulrike. "Erzählen vom Zerfall. Demenz und Alzheimer in der Gegenwartsliteratur." In: *Zeitschrift für Germanistik* Neue Folge XXII,2 (2012): 290–305.

Weigel, Sigrid. *Literatur als Voraussetzung der Kulturgeschichte. Schauplätze von Shakespeare bis Benjamin*. München: Wilhelm Fink Verlag, 2004.

Willer, Stefan, Sigrid Weigel, Bernhard Jussen (eds.). *Erbe. Übertragungskonzepte zwischen Natur und Kultur*. Berlin: Suhrkamp Verlag, 2013.

Letizia Malottke (Freiburg)

Lücken, Listen, Lexikonausschnitte. Die literarische Demenz-Darstellung in Max Frischs *Der Mensch erscheint im Holozän*

Abstract: One early example for the literary treatment of dementia is Max Frisch's narration *Man in the Holocene* from 1976. The novella can be read as an aesthetic proceeding to cope with mental illness and speechlessness. While the collage full of quotations and original dictionary-documents is related to postmodern forms of intertextuality, the narrative situation stands in the tradition of Georg Büchner's *Lenz*.

I. Wie lässt sich Vergessen, wie Sprachverlust erzählen?

Das literarische und auch literaturwissenschaftliche Interesse an deutschsprachigen Demenz-Narrativen hat seit Mitte der 1990er Jahren stetig zugenommen.[1] Ein Blick auf die Literaturgeschichte zeigt, dass eine solche gesteigerte Auseinandersetzung mit einer bestimmten Krankheit nicht ungewöhnlich ist: Hatten zuvor literarische Darstellungen von Tuberkulose, Neurasthenie oder beispielsweise Krebs eine Phase der Hochkonjunktur erfahren,[2] kommt in gegenwärtigen Texten insbesondere Demenz-Erkrankungen Aufmerksamkeit zu. Dieses Interesse mag zum einen in der fortwährend steigenden Zahl von Demenz-Diagnosen begründet liegen. Darüber hinaus scheint die literarische Auseinandersetzung aber um die Auflösung eines Paradoxons bemüht: Schließlich stellen sie den Versuch dar, Phänomene des Schwindens und der Sprachlosigkeit schriftlich zu fixieren und an der Textoberfläche sichtbar zu machen. Am Beispiel einer frühen Demenz-Darstellung aus dem Jahr 1974 – Max Frischs *Der Mensch erscheint im Holozän* – soll

1 Vgl. z.B. Vedder, Ulrike. "Erzählen vom Verfall. Demenz und Alzheimer in der Gegenwartsliteratur." In: *Zeitschrift für Germanistik* 22,2 (2012): 274–89. Oder: Helbig, Holger. s.v. "Alzheimer-Krankheit." In: Bettina v. Jagow, Florian Steger (eds.). *Literatur und Medizin: Ein Lexikon.* Göttingen: Vandenhoeck & Ruprecht, 2005, 46–50.

2 Die verstärkte literarische Hinwendung zu Krankheiten wie Tuberkulose, Krebs oder Aids hat u.a. Susan Sontag in ihrem prominenten Essay "Krankheit als Metapher" analysiert. Vgl. Sontag, Susan. *Krankheit als Metapher.* Frankfurt a.M.: Fischer Taschenbuchverlag, 1981. Zu Neurasthenie-Narrativen vgl. Bergengruen, Maximilian, Müller-Wille, Klaus, Pross, Caroline (eds.). *Neurasthenie. Die Krankheit der Moderne und die moderne Literatur.* Freiburg i.Br./Berlin/Wien: Rombach Verlag, 2010.

im Folgenden herausgearbeitet werden, welche literarischen Schreibweisen entwickelt und herangezogen werden, um ein disparates Phänomen wie Demenz zu erzählen.

Dieser Text wurde zum Zeitpunkt seines Erscheinens eher zurückhaltend aufgenommen. Zwar mehrten sich schon in den frühen 1980er Jahren Stimmen, die *Der Mensch erscheint im Holozän* als herausragendes Spätwerk des Autors einordneten.[3] Im Vergleich zu vorherigen Arbeiten Frischs kam der Erzählung jedoch verhältnismäßig wenig Aufmerksamkeit zu. Erst in den vergangenen fünfzehn Jahren ist der Text verstärkt in den Fokus der Forschung geraten. Unter anderem wurden Deutungen aus raum-zeitlicher Perspektive oder unter geologischen Gesichtspunkten angestellt,[4] die einhellig die hohe Elaboriertheit von Frischs Text herausstellen. Diese Ansätze erfassen zentrale Aspekte, lassen hingegen die Krankheitsdarstellung außer Acht. Im Jahr 2015 sind jedoch drei Beiträge im australischen Jahrbuch *Limbus* erschienen, die die Erzählung als Demenz- und Altersdarstellung werten. Diese Analysen generieren wertvolle Erkenntnisse, indem sie den Text unter den Aspekten der Bedeutsamkeit und Endlichkeit beleuchten oder die Archivierungs- und Erosionsprozesse innerhalb der Erzählung herausarbeiten.[5] Im Rahmen dieses Aufsatzes wird jedoch untersucht, welches

---

3 Die Sekundärliteratur konstatiert bis heute, die Erzählung sei stets abwertend beurteilt worden. Vgl. z.B. Charbon, Rémy. "Zeit und Raum, Zeit-Raum in Max Frischs Erzählung *Der Mensch erscheint im Holozän*." In: Dariusz Komorowski (ed.). *Jenseits von Frisch und Dürrenmatt. Raumgestaltung in der gegenwärtigen Deutschschweizer Literatur*. Würzburg: Königshausen & Neumann, 2009, 15–24, 15. Dass es sich hierbei um eine bloße Behauptung handelt, beweisen frühe und viel rezipierte Aufsätze, die bereits zu Beginn der 1980er Jahre die literarische Qualität des Texts betonten. Vgl. Butler, Michael. "Die Dämonen an die Wand malen. Zu Max Frischs Spätwerk: *Triptychon* und *Der Mensch erscheint im Holozän*." In: *Text und Kritik* 47/48 (1983): 88–107. Bauer Pickar, Gertrude. "'Es wird nie eine Pagode': Frisch's *Der Mensch erscheint im Holozän*." In: *Seminar. A Journal of Germanic Studies* 19,1 (1983): 33–56. Rossbach, Karlheinz. "Lesevorgänge. Zu Max Frischs Erzählung *Der Mensch erscheint im Holozän*." In: Paul Lützeler (ed.). *Zeitgenossenschaft. Zur deutschsprachigen Literatur im 20. Jahrhundert*. Frankfurt a.M.: Athenäum Verlag, 1987, 252–65.

4 Zur raum-zeitlichen Perspektive vgl. Charbon. "Zeit und Raum", 15–24; Zur geologischen Dimension des Werks vgl. Braungart, Georg. "'Katastrophen kennt allein der Mensch, sofern er sie überlebt'. Max Frisch, Peter Handke und die Geologie." In: Carsten Dutt, Roman Luckscheiter (eds.). *Figurationen der literarischen Moderne*. Heidelberg: Universitätsverlag Winter, 2007, 23–41.

5 Hajduk, Stefan. "Montauk erscheint im Holozän. Literarisches Schreiben und Altern bei Max Frisch." In: *Limbus. Australisches Jahrbuch für germanistische Literatur- und Kulturwissenschaft* 8 (2015): 67–84. Röthinger, Julia. "'Erosion ist ein langsamer Vorgang'.

narrative Repertoire innerhalb der Erzählung aufgerufen oder entwickelt wird, um Vergessen, Sprachlosigkeit und die Unkenntnis über die Demenz zu literarisieren. Auch soll herausgearbeitet werden, auf welche narrativen Traditionen der Text referiert und wie er diese modifiziert. Dabei werden insbesondere die deutlich markierten intertextuellen Referenzen auf Georg Büchners *Lenz* beleuchtet.

II. Der lange Weg ins *Holozän*: Ein Überblick über Textgenese und Inhalt

Zwölf verschiedene Fassungen, wechselnde Titel, unterschiedliche Erzählperspektiven: Insgesamt sieben Jahre rang Max Frisch mit seiner Erzählung *Der Mensch erscheint im Holozän.*[6] Dieser langwierige Entstehungshintergrund scheint insbesondere aufgrund der inhaltlichen Parallelen zu früheren Prosatexten verwunderlich, schließlich waren alternde Männer, Identitätskrisen und das vermeintlich Unsagbare doch Frischs Spezialgebiet (man denke nur an *Stiller*, *Sein Name sei Gantenbein* oder *Montauk*).[7] Eine Zusammenschau aller erhaltenen Erzählfassungen zeigt jedoch, dass es nicht so sehr der Inhalt gewesen ist, der Frisch änderungsbedürftig erschien.[8] Vielmehr lassen die verschiedenen Versionen von *Der Mensch erscheint im Holozän*, aber auch Tagebucheinträge und Notizen des Autors, erkennen, dass Frisch die Frage nach der passenden Erzählperspektive umtrieb. Im Gegensatz zu vorherigen Arbeiten steht im Zentrum dieses Texts

Das Verschwinden in Max Frischs Erzählung *Der Mensch erscheint im Holozän*." In: *Limbus* 8 (2015): 125–46. Voorgang, Juliane. "'Schlimm wäre der Verlust des Gedächtnisses'. Anthropologische und archäologische Archivierung in Max Frischs *Der Mensch erscheint im Holozän*." In: *Limbus* 8 (2015): 13–32.

6 Frisch, Max. *Der Mensch erscheint im Holozän*. In: Ders. *Gesammelte Werke in zeitlicher Folge. Sieben Bände: Vol. 7*. Ed. Hans Mayer. Frankfurt a.M.: Suhrkamp Verlag, 1986, 205–300. Im Folgenden wird der Titel mit *Holozän* sigliert und unter Angabe der jeweiligen Seitenzahl im laufenden Text zitiert. Zur Rekonstruktion der Textgenese vgl. De Vin, Daniel. "'Schlimm wäre der Verlust des Gedächtnisses': Zur Entstehung von Max Frischs Erzählung *Der Mensch erscheint im Holozän*." In: Eijiro Iwasaki (ed.). *Begegnungen mit dem ‚Fremden'. Grenzen – Traditionen – Vergleiche; Akten des VIII. internationalen Germanisten-Kongresses, Tokyo 1990: Vol. 9*. München: Iduicium Verlag, 1991, 494–98.

7 Zur Ähnlichkeitsbeziehung zwischen *Der Mensch erscheint im Holozän* und *Montauk* vgl. Hajduk. "Montauk erscheint im Holozän."

8 Alle erhaltenen Fassungen weisen große inhaltliche Überschneidungen auf. Selbst die ersten Vorarbeiten lassen die später ausgearbeitete Handlung erkennen und finden sich auch zu großen Teilen in der endgültigen Fassung wieder. Vgl. De Vin. "'Schlimm wäre der Verlust des Gedächtnisses'", 493.

nicht nur eine alternde, sondern eine demente Figur, deren Gedächtniseinbußen den Autor vor erzählerische Herausforderungen stellten. Darum bemüht, den Erinnerungsverlust adäquat darzustellen, änderte Frisch die Erzählperspektive immer wieder ab: So zeichnet sich das 1972 entstandene erste Textfragment *Regen* noch durch einen weitestgehend autodiegetischen Erzähler aus. In einer späteren Version wandelte Frisch diese Perspektivierung in eine ungewöhnlichere Erzählerposition um. Im *Fragment aus einer Erzählung* spricht eine namenlose Erzählerfigur den Protagonisten direkt an, indem sie dessen Tun und Denken kommentiert und den Protagonisten Geiser dabei stets siezt. Mal mahnend, mal aufmunternd sagt der Erzähler Sätze wie, „Sie erinnern sich oft an dasselbe, Herr Geiser."[9] Die ausgearbeitete Fassung mit dem Titel *Klima* wurde von Frisch 1974 kurz vor der Veröffentlichung zurückgezogen, heute liegt nur noch das zwölfseitige Fragment vor, das Eingang in die *Gesammelten Werke* gefunden hat.[10] Dass sich Frisch vor allem mit einer geeigneten Erzählperspektive auseinandersetze, lässt auch der 1975 erschienene autobiographische Text *Montauk* erkennen. Hierin fällt der vielzitierte Satz: „Eine literarische Erzählung, die im Tessin spielt, ist zum vierten Mal mißraten; die Erzähler-Position überzeugt nicht."[11] Im Jahr 1979 wird schließlich die heute vorliegende Fassung publiziert, die den Titel *Der Mensch erscheint im Holozän* trägt. Nach sieben Jahren ständiger Abänderungen befand der Autor die Erzählung für gelungen, ja hielt sie sogar für den eigentlichen Abschluss seines Gesamtwerks.[12]

---

9 Frisch, Max. "Fragment einer Erzählung." In: Ders. *Gesammelte Werke in zeitlicher Folge. Sechs Bände*: *Vol. 6.* Frankfurt a.M.: Suhrkamp Verlag, 1976, 529.

10 Max Frisch schreibt im März 1974 in seinem *Berliner Journal* über den Rückzug des Manuskripts aus dem Verlagsprogramm: „März: KLIMA (Erzählung) an den Verlag geschickt, dann in Frankfurt (6.3.) zum Geburtstag von Helene Ritzerfeld, Lektorat-Gespräche mit Unseld und Elisabeth Borchers freundlich. Es ist, glaube ich, schwierig für sie. Termine und alles vereinbart. Zwei Tage später, wieder in Berlin, ziehe ich das Manuskript zurück. Ich habe kein Urteil mehr." Frisch, Max. *Aus dem Berliner Journal.* Ed. Thomas Strässle, Margit Unser. Berlin: Suhrkamp Verlag, 2014, 165. Hervorhebungen im Original.

11 Frisch, Max. *Montauk*. In: Ders. *Gesammelte Werke in zeitlicher Folge. Sechs Bände*: *Vol. 6.* Frankfurt a.M.: Suhrkamp Verlag, 1976, 630.

12 Über seinen tatsächlich letzten Prosatext schreibt Frisch: „Das neue Buch ist gedruckt und käuflich, BLAUBART, der Umschlag ist blau und gefällig. Was habe ich geschrieben? Eine Fratze, eine gekonnte Grimasse – als letztes Buch? Das vorletzte [*Der Mensch erscheint im Holozän*] hätte verdient, das letzte zu sein." Frisch, Max. *Entwürfe zu einem dritten Tagebuch.* Ed. Peter von Matt. Berlin: Suhrkamp Verlag, 2010, 58. Hervorhebungen im Original.

In *Der Mensch erscheint im Holozän* werden die letzten Wochen im Leben des dreiundsiebzigjährigen, verwitweten Herrn Geiser erzählt, der in einer kleinen Ortschaft im Tessin vermutlich Ende der 1970er Jahre lebt. Anhaltende, ungewöhnlich heftige Sommergewitter haben hier Unheil angerichtet: Durch Erdrutsche sind Straßen verschüttet, sodass der Ort zeitweise von der Außenwelt abgeschnitten ist. Herr Geiser, der von zunehmendem Gedächtnisverlust beeinträchtigt ist, sieht in dieser vermeintlichen Naturkatastrophe seinen Gesundheitszustand gespiegelt. So setzt er die Erosionsprozesse, die sich in seiner Umgebung zutragen, mit seinem schwindenden Gedächtnis in Beziehung, indem er beispielsweise denkt:

> Offenbar fallen Hirnzellen aus.
> Bedenklicher als der Einsturz der Trockenmauer wäre ein Riß durchs Gelände, ein vorerst schmaler Riß, handbreit, aber ein Riß –
> (So fangen Erdrutsche an, wobei solche Risse lautlos entstehen und sich Wochen lang nicht erweitern oder kaum, bis plötzlich, wenn man nichts erwartet, der ganze Hang unterhalb des Risses rutscht und auch Wälder mit sich reißt und alles, was nicht Grundfels ist.
> Man muß auf alles gefaßt sein. (Frisch. *Holozän*, 232)

Um der verschiedenartigen ‚Erosionsprozesse' habhaft zu werden und ihnen entgegenwirken zu können, sammelt Geiser enzyklopädisches Wissen über erdgeschichtliche Phänomene, aber auch biblische Schilderungen der Sintflut. Er heftet zunächst handgeschriebene Zettel, später Ausschnitte aus Lexika und Sachbüchern an seine Wohnzimmerwände, denn „Wissen beruhigt" (Frisch. *Holozän*, 215).

Die Erzählung erstreckt sich über einen Zeitraum von ungefähr ein bis zwei Wochen, innerhalb derer Geisers Gedächtnisstörungen rapide zunehmen, er oftmals die zeitliche Orientierung verliert und irrational handelt.[13] Als der Dreiundsiebzigjährige schließlich von der Isolation und Hilflosigkeit seiner Situation übermannt wird, wagt er einen Ausbruch: Um in seine Stadtwohnung und zur Tochter nach Basel zu kommen, bricht er zu einer Wanderung über die Passhöhe in das benachbarte Maggiatal auf. Nach einem beschwerlichen Aufstieg kehrt er plötzlich wieder um. Unbemerkt in sein Haus zurückgekehrt, erleidet er anscheinend in Folge der Wanderung einen leichten Schlaganfall (hierauf weisen ein Zusammenbruch und das plötzlich herunterhängende Augenlid hin. Vgl. Frisch. *Holozän*, 283–84). Durch die daraufhin zunehmenden dementiellen Schübe

13 Die äußerst rapide Verschlechterung des Gesundheitszustands wird mit (vermutlich mehreren) Schlaganfällen in Zusammenhang gebracht, die Herr Geiser in dieser Zeit erleidet.

verliert der Protagonist zeitweise die Kontrolle über sein Handeln, findet sich kaum noch zurecht. Er vergisst die Namen seiner Enkel und hat kein Zeitgefühl mehr. Umso mehr bemüht er sich aber, alte Erinnerungen zu aktivieren (vgl. Frisch. *Holozän*, 289–94). Als die Straßen wieder befahrbar sind, kommt ihm die Tochter aus Basel zur Hilfe. Der letzte Lexikon-Ausschnitt thematisiert die Folgen eines Schlaganfalls, danach verstummen erlebte Rede und außenperspektivischer Gedankenbericht. Auf den folgenden zwei Seiten wird Herr Geiser nicht mehr erwähnt, wodurch dem Leser nahegelegt wird, dass der Protagonist verstorben ist. Bei den letzten Zeilen handelt es sich um eine Beschreibung des Tals, die sich aus bereits vorher verwendeten Sätzen speist. Der in diesem Zusammenhang erwähnte Käuzchenruf ist ein weiterer, wenn auch unterschwelliger Hinweis auf Geisers Tod (vgl. Frisch. *Holozän*, 299).[14]

Da die Hauptfigur keines ihrer Leiden klar benennt (auf den Schlaganfall wird nur durch einzelne Hinweise und den Lexikonausschnitt hingedeutet) und sich auch keiner ärztlichen Untersuchung unterzieht, bleibt offen, ob sie tatsächlich an Demenz leidet. Einige inhaltliche Aspekte weisen aber auf ein entsprechendes Krankheitsbild hin: So werden Geisers Gedächtniseinbußen mit mehreren Schlaganfällen in Verbindung gebracht, was einer vaskulären Demenz gleichkäme.[15] In jedem Fall ist der Protagonist der Erzählung durch eine Erkrankung derart beeinträchtigt, dass er sein zeitliches und räumliches Orientierungsvermögen verliert, sich Störungen des Kurz- und Langzeitgedächtnisses einstellen und er vordergründig irrationale Entscheidungen trifft (wenn er zum Beispiel grundlos ein Treppengeländer abmontiert oder seine Katze brät). Diese Symptome deuten darauf hin, dass Geiser an einem komplexen Störungsmuster leidet. Auf der Grundlage eines weiten, kultursemiotischen Verständnisses der Krankheit[16] kann in diesem Fall

---

14 Auf die Todesmetaphorik des Käuzchenrufs weist ebenfalls hin: Schneider, Sabine. "Stille Katastrophen. *Der Mensch erscheint im Holozän*." In: Daniel Nielaba, Yves Schumacher, Christoph Steier (eds.). *'Man will werden, nicht gewesen sein.' Zur Aktualität Max Frischs*. Zürich: Chronos Verlag, 2012, 229–46.

15 Vaskuläre Demenz-Formen sind gefäßbedingt und werden u.a. durch mehrere Mikroschlaganfälle ausgelöst. Vgl. Todica, Olga, Wiltfang, Jens, Hermann, Dirk. "Vaskuläre Demenz". In: Dirk Hermann, Thorsten Steiner, Hans-Christoph Diener (eds.). *Vaskuläre Neurologie*. Stuttgart/New York: Georg Thieme Verlag, 2010, 269–76. Dieses Krankheitsbild wurde in den 1970er Jahren mit dem Fachausdruck „Gehirnaterienverkalkung" bezeichnet. Vgl. Fn. 32.

16 Ein solch breites Krankheitsverständnis (ausgehend von den Symptomen) steht einer eng gefassten medizinischen Determination gegenüber, die im Fall einer literarischen Analyse nicht geleistet werden kann und auch nicht so sehr von Interesse ist. Statt einer

von einer Demenz-Darstellung gesprochen werden, ohne dass eine im engeren Sinne medizinische ‚Figurendiagnose' möglich (und auch nicht nötig) ist.

III. Die Semantik der Form: Das zersetzte Druckbild

Die typographische Gestaltung der Erzählung ist von der literaturwissenschaftlichen Forschung eingehend behandelt worden, wobei vor allem der Collagetechnik Aufmerksamkeit zuteil geworden ist.[17] Dieses narrative Verfahren setzt jedoch nicht gleich zu Beginn der Erzählung ein. Vielmehr wird der erste Leseeindruck durch das zergliederte Druckbild bestimmt: Absätze, die sich als weiße Lücken auf nahezu jeder Seite manifestieren, unterteilen die Textoberfläche in kurze, kohärente Passagen und freistehende, knappe Einzelsätze, was dem Satzspiegel eine zergliederte Struktur verleiht. Während die zusammenhängenden Textstellen meist Aufschluss über das Geschehen geben, bringen die isolierten Einzelsätze spontane Gedanken und Fragen des Protagonisten zum Ausdruck, die nicht notwendigerweise in erkennbarem Zusammenhang mit dem zuvor Gesagten stehen. Im Verlauf der Erzählung, insbesondere nach dem Schlaganfall des Protagonisten, mehren sich diese freistehenden Sätze. Allein eine längere Passage über den tödlichen Kletterunfall von Geisers Bruder fällt aus diesem Muster heraus (vgl. Frisch. *Holozän*, 289–94). Ansonsten vermengen sich in den kurzen, oft elliptischen Sätzen Assoziationen, Beobachtungen und Erinnerungen und zeugen von dem stetigen Zerfall des Gedächtnisses. Auf diese Weise wird dem Leser ein Einblick in unausgesprochene mentale Vorgänge gewährt: So lässt die zunehmende Auflösung des Druckbilds den stockenden Denkprozess und die voranschreitende Krankheit, die Geiser eigentlich zu verdrängen sucht, auf typographischer Ebene erkennen. Diese semantisch aufgeladene, formal komplexe Schreibweise erinnert an lyrische Gestaltungsformen, die sich in einem ähnlichen „Spannungsfeld zwischen dem Ausgesprochenen und dem Unausgesprochenen"[18] befinden und deshalb eines vergleichbar hohen Interpretationsaufwands (auch hinsichtlich des Druckbilds) bedürfen.

(nicht seriös durchführbaren) ‚Figurendiagnose' soll in diesem Aufsatz der Frage nach der literarischen Umsetzung von Sprachverlust und Vergessen nachgegangen werden.

17 Eine präzise Analyse der Textstruktur leistet Cohen, Robert. "Zumutungen der Spätmoderne. Max Frischs *Der Mensch erscheint im Holozän*." In: *Weimarer Beiträge. Zeitschrift für Literaturwissenschaft, Ästhetik und Kulturwissenschaften* 54,4 (2008): 541–56.

18 Crauwels, Geert. "Über die sprachlose Sprache. Modi memorandi und Collage als Kompositionstechnik in *Der Mensch erscheint im Holozän*." In: Daniel De Vin. *Max Frisch. Citoyen und Poet.* Göttingen: Wallstein Verlag, 2011, 114–15.

Diese Nähe zur Lyrik drückt sich auch in den zahlreichen Aufzählungen und durchnummerierten Listen aus, die an Günter Eichs reduktionistisches Gedicht "Inventur" erinnern.[19] Ähnlich dem lyrischen Ich dieses Gedichts subsummiert Geiser, was ihm noch geblieben ist. Darunter fallen Nahrungsvorräte (vgl. Frisch. *Holozän*, 211), Dokumente und persönliche Gegenstände (vgl. Frisch. *Holozän*, 253), ebenso mentale Fähigkeiten. Diese Bestandsaufnahmen werden meist in durchnummerierten Listen geleistet. Einzelne Sätze deuten aber auch darauf hin, dass Geiser fortwährend darüber Buch führt, was vorhanden ist und was eben nicht mehr funktioniert. Vordergründig wenig bedeutsame Feststellungen wie „Vergessen hat Herr Geiser die Thermos-Flasche. [...] Nicht vergessen hat Herr Geiser die Landkarte" (Frisch. *Holozän*, 268), lassen seine Angst vor dem gänzlichen Gedächtnis- und Kontrollverlust erahnen. Diese Furcht wird nicht offen ausgesprochen. Stattdessen weist, wie Karlheinz Rossbach bemerkt, die grammatische Struktur der Sätze darauf hin, dass Geiser die vergessene Thermoskanne nicht als Lappalie, sondern als Hinweis auf seinen fortschreitenden Gedächtnisverlust wertet.[20] Die häufigen Negationen und ungewöhnlichen Satzstellungen sind Ausdruck von Geisers Abwägungen darüber, wie prekär die Situation tatsächlich ist. Diese Zustandsdokumentation beginnt mit der Erfassung der vermeintlich alarmierenden Wetterlage und seiner Umgebung. Doch ebenso wie er diese äußeren Erosionsprozesse registriert, kommentiert er, wenn auch sehr spärlich, sein eigenes schwindendes Erinnerungsvermögen. So denkt er beispielsweise: „Schlimm wäre der Verlust des Gedächtnisses – [...]" (Frisch. *Holozän*, 210) und „Ohne Gedächtnis kein Wissen." (Ibid., 210) Schließlich stellt er verzweifelt fest: „Man verblödet – !" (Ibid., 224). Neben diesen wenigen, aber sehr konkreten Kommentaren zeugt der in die Erzählung montierte Lexikonausschnitt „Gedächtnisschwäche" von Geisers konkreter Auseinandersetzung mit seinem Leiden (ibid., 237–38).

IV. Die Semantik der Form: Die Collagetechnik

Während solche direkten Bemerkungen und Hinweise nur vereinzelt in den Text eingestreut sind, bringt die semantisch aufgeladene Form der Erzählung Geisers Sorgen zum Ausdruck. So weist unter anderem die komplex ausgearbeitete Collagetechnik auf seine Gefühlslage hin. Dieses narrative Verfahren ist

19 Vgl. Eich, Günter. "Inventur." In: Axel Vieregg (ed.). *Günter Eich. Gesammelte Werke in vier Bänden: Vol. 1. Die Gedichte. Die Maulwürfe*. Frankfurt a.M.: Suhrkamp Verlag, 1991, 35–36.

20 Vgl. Rossbach. "Lesevorgänge," 256.

zunächst inhaltlich motiviert: Um dem Schwinden seiner Erinnerung Einhalt zu gebieten, macht Geiser sich Notizen und schneidet Passagen, die ihm wichtig erscheinen, aus Sach- und Kinderbüchern, Lexika oder der Bibel aus. Bei diesen Ausschnitten handelt es sich um authentische Buchzitate, die am Ende der Erzählung durch ein Quellenverzeichnis belegt werden (vgl. Frisch. *Holozän*, 300). Die handschriftlichen Notizen sind fiktional und von Frisch verfasst worden, sie beziehen sich jedoch überwiegend auf die zitierten Sachbücher.[21] Eine Selektion dieser Textpassagen ist in Form von Collageelementen in die Erzählung eingepasst worden. Im Laufe des Texts finden sich über 70 Elemente, die teilweise thematisch aufeinander abgestimmt sind. Manche dieser zusammengestellten Informationen erwecken aber auch einen unsystematischen, zusammenhanglosen Eindruck (vgl. Frisch. *Holozän*, 225).

Das werkfremde Material zeichnet sich durch unterschiedliche Schriftarten – Fraktur, Antiqua und Handschrift – und verschiedene Schriftgrößen und Hervorhebungen aus, besticht aber auch durch Illustrationen. Diese Eigenschaften weisen die Collageelemente als unverändertes Fremdmaterial aus, das in seiner „typographischen Originalform"[22] belassen worden ist, was sich auch in der unterschiedlichen Hintergrundgestaltung ausdrückt: Wie Kopien oder Faksimiles authentischer Dokumente heben sich die Textausschnitte durch einen unterschiedlich getönten Hintergrund voneinander ab (beispielsweise sind die handschriftlichen Notizen auf kariertem Papier verfasst). Auf diese Weise integrieren sich die Collageelemente nicht in den Autortext, sondern sind deutlich als einmontierte Fremdtexte markiert worden. Diese Textgestaltung hat unter anderem dazu geführt, dass die Erzählung in der Forschung mit postmodernen Ästhetiken in Verbindung gebracht wird.[23] Frisch nimmt dabei die Rolle eines Arrangeurs ein, der neben eigenen Passagen textfremde Elemente auswählt und in einen

---

21 Indem Frisch die Notizen Geisers in seiner eigenen Handschrift verfasste und ebenso wie der Protagonist mit Fremdtexten arbeitete und diese aneinander montiert, begibt er sich in eine vergleichbare Position wie seine Figur. Vgl. Cohen. "Zumutungen der Spätmoderne," 545.

22 Cohen. "Zumutungen der Spätmoderne," 544.

23 Zur Postmodernität des Texts vgl. Evans, Tamara. "Lurch und Maßliebchen. Moderne und postmoderne Bestandsaufnahmen in Max Frischs *Der Mensch erscheint im Holozän* und Gerhart Meiers *Baur und Bindschädler*." In: *Amsterdamer Beiträge zur neueren Germanistik* 38/39 (1994): 353–68. Oder aber Bunge, Sophie. "'Der Mensch bleibt ein Laie'. (Post-)Kantische Auseinandersetzungen in Max Frischs *Der Mensch erscheint im Holozän*." In: *Text und Kritik* 47/48 (2013): 162–71. Oder: Cohen. "Zumutungen der Spätmoderne," 545.

größeren Zusammenhang neu einmontiert.[24] Dabei zersetzen die von ihm eingefügten Faksimiles den Text und führen dessen künstlerische Gestaltung vor Augen – eine Gestaltung, von der wiederum eine poetologische Aussage ausgeht. So stellt die stark durchkomponierte Textoberfläche einen Lösungsansatz dar, um das vermeintlich Unsagbare, die Sprachlosigkeit (hier in der konkreten Form der Demenz) erzählbar zu machen.[25] Schließlich wird in der für eine Collage typischen „Zerstückelung der Zusammenhänge" Geisers Hilflosigkeit gegenüber seiner Erkrankung erkennbar.[26] Auch der Protagonist setzt sich mit diesem Phänomen auseinander:

> Was Herr Geiser nicht bedacht hat: der Text auf der Rückseite, den Herr Geiser erst bemerkt, nachdem er die Illustration ausgeschnitten hat, wäre vielleicht nicht minder aufschlussreich gewesen; nun ist dieser Text zerstückelt, unbrauchbar für die Zettelwand. (Frisch. *Holozän*, 280)

Die Prozesse des Ausschneidens und Einklebens bringen es mit sich, dass eine Auswahl an Texten und Bildern getroffen werden muss, was einen zwangsläufigen Verzicht auf umfassende Information bedeutet. Die beschriebene Collagetechnik illustriert somit die Grenzen lexikalen Wissens, an die nicht nur die erkrankte Figur, sondern auch der Leser stößt. Statt einer Gedächtnisstütze oder Informationsquelle entsteht eine unüberschaubare Zettelwirtschaft, die von Fragmentierung und scheinbarer Zusammenhanglosigkeit gekennzeichnet ist. Vom Detailreichtum und offensichtlich veralteten Informationen der Collage überfrachtet, muss der Leser den Kontrollverlust und die Überforderung des Demenzkranken nachempfinden.[27] Die Collageelemente lassen jedoch nicht nur die krankheitsbedingten Verluste erkennen, sondern ermöglichen es andererseits auch, einen besseren Zugang zu den Gedankengängen des Protagonisten zu gewinnen. So zeugt die von Geiser getroffene Zettelauswahl von seiner allgemeinen Auseinandersetzung mit der Vergänglichkeit, die nicht nur das menschliche Schicksal berührt. Plötzliche Umbrüche, langsame Erosionsprozesse und unheilbare Krankheiten betreffen die Gesteins-, Tier- und Pflanzenwelten ebenso wie den Menschen. Im Kontext

---

24 Erstmals verweist Robert Cohen darauf, dass Frisch eine Doppelrolle – nämlich der des „Autor als Arrangeur" – zukomme. Vgl. Cohen. "Zumutungen der Spätmoderne," 548. Sabine Schneiders Erkenntnisse stimmen nicht nur in diesem Punkt mit Cohens Wortlaut überein. Vgl. Schneider. "Stille Katastrophen," 243.

25 Vgl. Schneider. "Stille Katastrophen," 237–38.

26 Kaiser, Gerhard. "Endspiel im Tessin. Max Frischs unentdeckte Erzählung *Der Mensch erscheint im Holozän*." In: *Schweizer Monatshefte für Politik, Wirtschaft, Kultur* 82/83 (2002/2003): 46–52, 48.

27 Vgl. Crauwels. "Über die sprachlose Sprache," 144.

dieser erdgeschichtlichen Fakten erkennt Herr Geiser, dass er sich diesen allumfassenden Prozessen nicht wird entziehen können (vgl. Frisch. *Holozän*, 295). Gleichzeitig führt ihm sein Wissen über Flora, Fauna und Gesteine vor Augen, welch untergeordnete – nämlich kurze – Rolle der Mensch auf der Erde spielt. Wie Georg Braungart in seinem Artikel treffend bemerkt, kommt diese Erkenntnis der vierten „Kränkung des Narzißmus neuzeitlicher Subjektivität" gleich.[28] So stößt sich Geiser vor allem an der im ausgehenden achtzehnten und neunzehnten Jahrhundert getätigten „Entdeckung der unermeßlichen Zeiträume durch die Geologen, Mineralogen und Paläontologen, in denen die Erde ohne den Menschen existiert haben musste."[29] Diese Erkenntnis empfindet der Protagonist (wie bereits viele Menschen vor ihm) als Relativierung der Relevanz der eigenen Spezies, was sich auch in einer von ihm ausgeschnittenen Abbildung ausdrückt: Die Illustration zeigt das Größenverhältnis eines menschlichen Skeletts gegenüber dem eines Dinosauriers, wobei der Knochenmann neben dem beleibten Spinosaurus erschreckend klein und unbedeutend wirkt (vgl. Frisch. *Holozän*, 282). Vor dem Hintergrund dieser Marginalisierung kommen Geiser seine Kategorisierungsversuche zwecklos vor. Resigniert gibt er seinen Kampf gegen das Vergessen und Vergessenwerden auf, indem er feststellt:

> Die Ameisen, die Herr Geiser neulich unter einer tropfenden Tanne beobachtet hat, legen keinen Wert darauf, daß man Bescheid weiß über sie, so wenig wie die Saurier, die ausgestorben sind, bevor der Mensch sie gesehen hat. Alle diese Zettel können verschwinden. Was heißt Holozän! Die Natur braucht keine Namen. Das weiß Herr Geiser. Die Gesteine brauchen sein Gedächtnis nicht. (Frisch. *Holozän*, 296)[30]

Mit dieser Aussage endet Geisers Gedankenbericht. Darauf folgen unkommentiert sieben Faksimiles, die die Themen Erosion, Kastanienbäume, Eschatologie, Kohärenz, Kastanienkrebs, die Bodenbeschaffenheit des Orts Locarno und den Schlaganfall behandeln (vgl. Frisch. *Holozän*, 296–98). Eine solche Zusammenstellung der Collageelemente zeugt einerseits von Geisers speziellen Interessen, die im konkreten Kontext seiner Erkrankung stehen. Andererseits lassen diese Faksimiles erneut seine Vorstellung erkennen, es bestünde ein Zusammenhang zwischen den Vorgängen in der Natur und seiner Krankheitsentwicklung (vor allem der

---

28 Braungart. "Katastrophen kennt allein der Mensch, sofern er sie überlebt," 33.

29 Braungart. "Katastrophen kennt allein der Mensch, sofern er sie überlebt," 33.

30 Dieses Zitat steht auch mit dem Titel der Erzählung im Zusammenhang. In der Forschung wurde bemerkt, dass es sich bei der Aussage, der Mensch erscheint im Holozän, um einen Irrtum Geisers handelt, schließlich leben die ersten Menschen bereits im Pleistozän. Zu dieser Verschiebung vgl. Kaiser. "Endspiel im Tessin," 47.

Ausschnitt über Kohärenz deutet auf eine von Geiser konstruierte Verbindung zwischen den unterschiedlichen Phänomenen hin). Dieser Zusammenhang wird nicht nur als fixe Idee Geisers dargestellt, vielmehr scheint die äußere Handlung diese Vorstellung zu bestätigen: Ebenso wie das Gedächtnis des Protagonisten ‚wegbricht' und von der Demenz-Erkrankung ‚unterspült' wird, lösen sich Erd- und Gesteinsschichten bei Unwettern und verschütten Straßen, ja manchmal ganze Täler. Wurde Geisers Geschichte häufig als Parabel auf menschheits- und erdgeschichtliche Entwicklungen gelesen,[31] lässt die Krankheitsdarstellung auch eine umgekehrte Lesart zu: Die Ereignisse in der Natur, also die starken Regenfälle, daraus resultierende Erdrutsche und Risse im Gelände, zeigen nach dem Prinzip des *totum pro parte* auf, was sich im Inneren Geisers abspielt. Genauso unvermeidlich wie sich Gesteinsablagerungen bilden, ‚verkalkt' Herr Geiser.[32] Genauso radikal wie die Gesteinsformationen durch die Witterung gespalten und abgetragen werden können, löschen Schlaganfälle ganze Hirnareale funktional aus. Herr Geisers Schicksal führt vor Augen, dass sich der Mensch als Teil der Natur nicht aus diesen Krankheitsprozessen und Umbrüchen herauszulösen vermag. Von der Hauptfigur wird dies gleichermaßen als Erlösung und als unerbittliches Schicksal empfunden.

V. Gesichts- und schonungslos: Die Erzählperspektive

Schon ein erster Blick ins Buchinnere lässt die geradezu ‚unebene' Textoberfläche erkennen. Die Listen und verschiedenen Schriftarten, die Collageelemente und die durch Majuskeln oder Kursierungen hervorgehobenen Sätze ähneln Frischs Tagebuch, das er von 1966 bis 1971 führte und ein Jahr nach Beendigung des Texts veröffentlichte. Neben den frappierenden gestalterischen Ähnlichkeiten weist dieses Selbstzeugnis auch inhaltliche Überschneidungen mit *Der Mensch erscheint im*

---

31 Vgl. Butler. "Die Dämonen an die Wand malen," 103.

32 Der Begriff ‚Verkalkung' fällt auch in *Der Mensch erscheint im Holozän*: Im einmontierten Lexikonartikel des *Großen Brockhaus* ist von „Gehirnarterienverkalkung" die Rede (Frisch. *Holozän*, 238). Während der Ausdruck ‚Verkalkung' heute als umgangssprachlich und diskreditierend empfunden wird, wurde er lange Zeit als medizinischer Fachausdruck verwendet und findet sich bis in die 1990 Jahre in einschlägigen medizinischen Lexika. Unter dem Krankheitsbild verstand man, dass vermeintlich kalkhaltige Ablagerungen die Gehirnarterien sukzessive verstopften, was zu Infarkten und infolgedessen zu vaskulärer Demenz führen könne. In der medizinischen Fachsprache wird dieses Krankheitsbild mittlerweile ‚Arteriosklerose' genannt. Vgl. Renz-Polster, Herbert, Krautzig, Steffen (eds.). *Basislehrbuch Innere Medizin*. München/Jena: Elsevier, Urban & Fischer, [4]2008, 218.

Holozän auf.[33] Nach dem Gestaltungsprinzip eines Mosaiks reiht Frisch in diesem Tagebuch unterschiedlich lange Passagen aneinander, die zwischen zeitgeschichtlicher Dokumentation, persönlichen Beobachtungen, fiktionalen Komponenten sowie poetologischen Aussagen changieren.[34] Statt einer linear-chronologischen Erzählabfolge wendet Frisch bei der Anordnung der verschiedenen Textpassagen das „Prinzip der assoziativen Verknüpfung" an, wobei es dem Leser obliegt, diese thematisch-motivischen Zusammenhänge zu rekonstruieren.[35] In der Forschung wurde bereits mehrfach auf diese Ähnlichkeitsbeziehung zwischen dem *Tagebuch 1966–1971* und der Erzählung *Der Mensch erscheint im Holozän* hingewiesen.[36] Dabei ist vor allem die inhaltliche Nähe zu den Textstellen der fiktiven „Vereinigung Freitod" herausgearbeitet worden.[37] Die Parallelen zwischen den beiden Texten sind nicht zu übersehen, darüber hinaus erinnern persönliche Notizen, zum Beispiel zu Frischs Skiausflug oder seine Schilderungen des Orts Brenzona, an Geisers Ausführungen.[38] Diese augenfälligen Überschneidungen könnten die Vermutung nahelegen, dass *Der Mensch erscheint im Holozän* als Tagebuchfiktion angelegt worden sei, was auch die Collageelemente plausibel erscheinen ließe. Frisch hat sich jedoch von einer Ich-Perspektive und infolgedessen auch von einer Tagebuchkonzeption distanziert. Auf Anregung von Uwe Johnson wandelte er die in seiner ersten Textfassung *Regen* verwendete autodiegetische Erzählhaltung ab, mit der Begründung: „Johnson hat recht, es liegt an der Optik; der Alte kann sich nicht selber darstellen."[39] Da ein Demenzkranker im vorgerückten Stadium seinen Gedanken nicht mehr vollumfänglich Ausdruck verleihen kann und manche seiner Befürchtungen auch möglicherweise verdrängen könnte, musste Frisch eine andere Perspektive entwickeln, die eine Innensicht ermöglicht. Er

33 Vgl. Frisch, Max. *Tagebuch 1966–1971*. Frankfurt a.M.: Suhrkamp Verlag, 1972.

34 Vgl. Heinrich-Korpys, Meike. *Tagebuch und Fiktionalität. Signalstruktur des literarischen Tagebuchs am Beispiel der Tagebücher von Max Frisch*. St. Ingbert: Röhrig Universitätsverlag, 2003, 117–18. Heinrich-Korpys verwendet im Zusammenhang mit Frischs literarischen Tagebüchern den Begriff des Mosaiks, um den fragmentarischen Charakter der Texte zu betonen. Dabei handelt es sich um einen abgeschwächten Montage-Begriff.

35 Heinrich-Korpys. *Tagebuch und Fiktionalität*, 180.

36 Vgl. Schneider. "Stille Katastrophen," 234. Cohen. "Zumutungen der Spätmoderne," 544–45.

37 Frisch entwickelt in seinem Tagebuch die fiktive „Vereinigung Freitod", deren Mitglieder für aktive Sterbehilfe und gegen eine überalterte Gesellschaft sind. Vgl. z.B. Frisch. *Tagebuch 1966–1971*, 90–95.

38 Vgl. Frisch. *Tagebuch 1966–1971*, 13 oder ibid., 75.

39 Frisch. *Aus dem Berliner Journal*, 105.

entschied sich für eine personale Erzählsituation – ein Verfahren, das der Autor für glaubwürdiger als die Autodiegese hielt, denn

> […] zu einer Figur gehört auch, was sie verhehlt, was sie selber im Augenblick nicht interessiert, was ihr nicht bewußt ist usw. … Im Sinne der Beicht-Literatur (maximale Aufrichtigkeit über sich selbst) vermag die ER-Form mehr.[40]

Aus diesem Grund werden dem Leser mittels erlebter Rede und einem außenperspektivischen Gedankenbericht Einblicke in Geisers Seelenleben gewährt, ohne dass diese kommentiert oder in einen größeren Rahmen eingeordnet würden. Die Erzählerfigur entwickelt keinerlei Persönlichkeitsprofil, sondern bleibt verborgen. Allein die Gestaltungsformen weisen auf eine arrangierende Instanz hin, die die Textoberfläche strukturiert und eine Auswahl der Collageelemente und Notizen getroffen haben muss. Aufgrund dieser Ausarbeitung hat die Forschungsliteratur den Erzähler als gesichts- und identitätslos, distanziert und merkwürdig beschrieben.[41] Tatsächlich handelt es sich um eine gewissermaßen ‚durchsichtige' Erzählposition, die den Leser durch die „Innenperspektive in Außenperspektive"[42] gerade soweit auf Distanz hält, dass eine unverstellte Betrachtung Geisers möglich wird. Gleichzeitig lässt diese Erzählhaltung eine Innensicht der Figur zu, die durch die Collageelemente und die typographische Gestaltung ergänzt wird, sodass ein plastisches Bild der Krankheit entsteht, das über die Figurensicht hinausgeht. Dabei erfährt man auch von Dingen, die der Demente lieber für sich behalten hätte: Während Geiser versucht, die Zettelwand oder seine abgebrochene Wanderung vor anderen zu verheimlichen, kann er sich den Blicken des Lesers nicht entziehen. Die Collageelemente und das Druckbild verweisen außerdem auf das Ausmaß des Gedächtnisverlusts. Auf diese Weise ermöglicht Frisch dem Leser einerseits, mehr über die Figur zu erfahren, als diese über sich selbst weiß, ohne dass eine kritisch deutende Erzählerfigur nötig wäre. Andererseits ist davon auszugehen, dass Geiser auch vieles denkt, was dem Leser verborgen bleibt. Der Text praktiziert somit eine Art Doppelstrategie zwischen Verstellung und Enthüllung, die die Qualität und Komplexität der Demenz-Darstellungen verdeutlicht. Schließlich bleibt bei der literarischen Verarbeitung der Krankheit immer ein konstitutiver Rest von narrativ Uneinholbarem, weil dieser sich dem durch die Lektüre bedingten Wissen entzieht.

---

40 Frisch. *Tagebuch 1966–1971*, 310.

41 Vgl. Schneider. "Stille Katastrophen," 240. Oder: Evans. "Lurch und Maßliebchen," 358.

42 Kaiser. "Endspiel im Tessin," 47.

VI. Zwischen Wissen und Nicht-Wissen-Können: Die Darstellung mentaler Zerrüttung

Diese zwischen Außen- und Innenperspektive changierende Erzählhaltung steht in der Traditionslinie eines zentralen Textes des neunzehnten Jahrhunderts, nämlich mit Georg Büchners *Lenz*.[43] Beide Texte beleuchten mental zerrüttete Figuren, wobei sich diese Zerrüttung auch auf die Textoberfläche überträgt. Um die Auswirkungen für den Betroffenen, aber auch für sein Umfeld sichtbar zu machen, haben sich sowohl Büchner als auch Frisch für eine Erzählhaltung entschieden, die eine „Parallelisierung von Außen- und Innenweltdarstellung" ermöglicht.[44] So gibt eine heterodiegetische Erzählinstanz Lenz' Geschichte wieder, die mittels interner Fokalisierung Einblicke in die inneren Vorgänge und das subjektive Erleben der Figur gewährt. Dabei lässt sich die Stimme des Erzählers oft nicht von Lenz' eigener Stimme unterscheiden; die Vermittlungsinstanz ist – vergleichbar mit der von Frisch gestalteten Erzählerfigur – neutral, ja geradezu abwesend. Dieses Verfahren ermöglichte Büchner eine unvermittelt wirkende Darstellung der Krankheit, die sich überwiegend aus sich selbst heraus zu erzählen scheint. Frisch lehnte sich mit der Gestaltung seiner Erzählung erkennbar daran an. So deuten neben der Erzählerfigur zahlreiche weitere Aspekte darauf hin, dass Büchners *Lenz* als intertextuelle Folie für *Der Mensch erscheint im Holozän* zu betrachten ist. Gleich dem Prätext wird in Frischs Erzählung immer wieder davon berichtet, was sich tagein, tagaus ereignet: Wieder und wieder schneidet Geiser Zettel aus, studiert das Wetter, vervollständigt Listen. Eine solche iterative Zustandsbeschreibung verdeutlicht das Ausmaß der Krankheiten, die weder Lenz noch Geiser ruhen lassen und beide dazu treiben, in Ritualen Halt zu suchen. Die wohl auffälligste Parallele zwischen den Texten besteht jedoch darin, dass ebenso wie Lenz auch Geiser seinen Gemütszustand in der Natur spiegelt, wobei der Raum psychisch aufgeladen wird. So lässt sich aus der Schilderung der Umgebung und der Wetterlage die Stimmung der Figur ablesen, wobei sich die Beschreibungen der schroffen Bergwelt in beiden Erzählungen auffallend ähneln.[45] Speziell in seinen Naturdarstellungen entspricht

---

43 Auf diese Parallelen hat bereits Michael Butler im Jahr 1987 hingewiesen. Eine nähere Analyse dieser intertextuellen Referenzen ist jedoch ausgeblieben. Vgl. Butler. "Die Dämonen an die Wand malen," 98.

44 Neuhuber, Christian. "'Siehe die Briefe'. Büchners *Lenz* und der Verzicht auf die Brieffiktion." In: Gideon Stiening, Robert Vellusig (eds.). *Poetik des Briefromans. Wissens- und mediengeschichtliche Studien*. Berlin/Boston: De Gruyter, 2012, 319–37, 319.

45 Für einen Vergleich der Naturschilderungen bieten sich die Wanderung Geisers und der Beginn von Büchners Novelle an.

Der Mensch erscheint in Holozän auch Goethes *Die Leiden des jungen Werther*, an den sich Büchner seinerseits angelehnt hatte. Die Nähe zu Büchners *Lenz*, aber auch intertextuelle Verweise auf Shakespeares *Hamlet*[46] und Goethes *Werther* weisen darauf hin, dass die Erzählung *Der Mensch erscheint im Holozän* in der Tradition literarischer Wahnsinns- und Innerlichkeitsdarstellungen steht. Dieser Traditionsbezug leuchtet auch insofern ein, als Frischs Erzählung Elemente, die an Tagebuchfiktionen erinnern, aufgreift, was gleichzeitig auf das mit dem Tagebuch eng verwandte Genre des Briefromans hindeutet.[47] Dennoch unterscheidet sich Geiser deutlich sowohl von Werther als auch von Lenz. Anders als der zwischen Pathos, Angst und Liebe schwankende Werther oder der ruhelose, mal tiefreligiöse, mal gotteslästernde Schriftsteller Lenz wirkt Geiser trotz seiner Krankheit überaus rational. Um seiner Beunruhigung entgegenzuwirken, betätigt er sich als eine Art Archivar des Wissens und weist eine eher skeptische Haltung gegenüber Kunst und Glauben auf. In dieser Haltung ähnelt die Figur dem Protagonisten aus Frischs Roman *Homo Faber*.[48] Während sich Lenz und Geiser durch ihre Figurenzeichnung unterscheiden, kann jedoch die narrative Gestaltung der Erzählung *Der Mensch erscheint im Holozän* als Umsetzung des von Lenz (und auch Büchner) geforderten Fundamentalrealismus gedeutet werden.[49] Dieser Zusammenhang mag auf den ersten Blick widersprüchlich scheinen, handelt es sich doch bei Frischs Erzählung um einen hochartifiziellen Text, der seine künstlerische Überformung offen kommuniziert und dabei das Entgleiten des dementiellen Bewusstseins in die Erzählstruktur überträgt. Diese Umsetzung steht einer umfassenden „Schaffung von Ordnung in Literatur“[50] gegenüber und scheint deshalb auch

---

46 Der von Geiser mehrfach getätigte Ausspruch, „Bereitsein ist alles“, stellt eine Referenz auf Shakespeares Hamlet dar, der den berühmten Satz in der zweiten Szene des fünften Akts spricht. Vgl. Shakespeare, William. *Hamlet*. In: Apel, Friedmar (ed.). *27 Stücke von William Shakespeare in der Übersetzung von Erich Fried*. Berlin: Verlag Klaus Wagenbach, 1989, 457.

47 Vgl. Keller, Renate. *Der Tagebuchroman als literarische Gattung*. Berlin/Boston: De Gruyter, 2015, 18.

48 Vgl. Probst, Hans Ulrich. “Zwischen Resignation und republikanischer Alters-Radikalität. Spuren des Citoyen Max Frisch im Spätwerk.” In: Daniel de Vin (ed.). *Leben gefällt mir – Begegnung mit Max Frisch*. Brüssel: Literarischer Treffpunkt, 1992, 27–57, 45.

49 Zum Begriff des Fundamentalrealismus vgl. Schmidt, Jochen. *Die Geschichte des Genie-Gedankens in der deutschen Literatur, Philosophie und Politik 1750–1945. Vol. 2: Von der Romantik bis zum Ende des Dritten Reichs*. Heidelberg: Winter, ³2004, 49.

50 Koopmann, Helmut, Perraudin, Michael (eds.): *Formen der Wirklichkeitserfassung nach 1848. Deutsche Literatur und Kultur vom Nachmärz bis zur Gründerzeit in europäischer Perspektive*: *Vol. 1*. Bielefeld: Aisthesis Verlag, 2003, 8.

realistischen bzw. naturalistischen Gestaltungsformen zuwiderlaufen. Und doch lässt sich Frischs Schreibweise als Ausdruck eines gesteigerten Mimesis-Verständnisses deuten: Schließlich gehen Erzählverfahren, die auf Kohärenz und Ordnung abzielen, an der Realität vorbei, wenn sie zur Darstellung eines disparaten und zersetzenden Phänomens wie Demenz genutzt werden. Indem Frisch die Grenzen diegetisch-narrativer Ordnungen aufbricht, kommt er Büchners Forderung nach, selbst den Wirklichkeitszerfall erzählbar zu machen. Dabei gelingt es ihm, anhand der formalen wie inhaltlichen Fragmentierung der Erzählung die vermeintliche Innensicht eines Demenz-Kranken zu entwerfen und dem Leser gleichzeitig vor Augen zu führen, dass es sich hierbei um ein Kunstprodukt handelt, das notwendigerweise unvollständig bleiben muss. Auf diese Weise verleihen die Lücken, Listen und Lexikonausschnitte in der Erzählung dem Nicht-Wissen über die Selbstwahrnehmung eines Demenz-Kranken Ausdruck.

Bibliographie

Bauer Pickar, Gertrude. "'Es wird nie eine Pagode': Frisch's *Der Mensch erscheint im Holozän.*" In: *Seminar. A Journal of Germanic Studies* 19,1 (1983): 33–56.

Bergengruen, Maximilian, Müller-Wille, Klaus, Pross, Caroline (eds.). *Neurasthenie. Die Krankheit der Moderne und die moderne Literatur.* Freiburg i.Br./Berlin/Wien: Rombach Verlag, 2010.

Braungart, Georg. "'Katastrophen kennt allein der Mensch, sofern er sie überlebt'. Max Frisch, Peter Handke und die Geologie." In: Carsten Dutt, Roman Luckscheiter (eds.). *Figurationen der literarischen Moderne.* Heidelberg: Universitätsverlag Winter, 2007, 23–41.

Büchner, Georg. *Lenz.* In: Henri Poschmann, Rosemarie Poschmann (eds.). *Georg Büchners sämtliche Werke, Briefe und Dokumente in zwei Bänden: Vol. 1.* Frankfurt a.M.: Deutscher Klassiker Verlag, 1992, 225–50.

Butler, Michael. "Die Dämonen an die Wand malen. Zu Max Frischs Spätwerk: *Triptychon* und *Der Mensch erscheint im Holozän.*" In: *Text und Kritik* 47/48 (1983): 88–107.

Charbon, Rémy. "Zeit und Raum, Zeit-Raum in Max Frischs Erzählung *Der Mensch erscheint im Holozän.*" In: Dariusz Komorowski (ed.). *Jenseits von Frisch und Dürrenmatt. Raumgestaltung in der gegenwärtigen Deutschschweizer Literatur.* Würzburg: Königshausen & Neumann, 2009, 15–24.

Cohen, Robert. "Zumutungen der Spätmoderne. Max Frischs *Der Mensch erscheint im Holozän.*" In: *Weimarer Beiträge. Zeitschrift für Literaturwissenschaft, Ästhetik und Kulturwissenschaften* 54,4 (2008): 541–56.

Crauwels, Geert. "Über die sprachlose Sprache. Modi memorandi und Collage als Kompositionstechnik in *Der Mensch erscheint im Holozän*." In: Daniel De Vin (ed.). *Max Frisch. Citoyen und Poet*. Göttingen: Wallstein Verlag, 2011, 114–15.

De Vin, Daniel. "'Schlimm wäre der Verlust des Gedächtnisses': Zur Entstehung von Max Frischs Erzählung *Der Mensch erscheint im Holozän*." In: Eijiro Iwasaki (ed.). *Begegnungen mit dem ‚Fremden'. Grenzen – Traditionen – Vergleiche; Akten des VIII. internationalen Germanisten-Kongresses, Tokyo 1990: Vol. 9*. München: Iduicium Verlag, 1991, 494–98.

Eich, Günter. "Inventur." In: Axel Vieregg (ed.). *Günter Eich. Gesammelte Werke in vier Bänden: Vol. 1. Die Gedichte. Die Maulwürfe*. Frankfurt a.M.: Suhrkamp Verlag, 1991, 35–36.

Evans, Tamara. "Lurch und Maßliebchen. Moderne und postmoderne Bestandsaufnahmen in Max Frischs *Der Mensch erscheint im Holozän* und Gerhart Meiers *Baur und Bindschädler*." In: *Amsterdamer Beiträge zur neueren Germanistik* 38/39 (1994): 353–68.

Frisch, Max. *Tagebuch 1966–1971*. Frankfurt a.M.: Suhrkamp Verlag, 1972.

Frisch, Max. "Fragment einer Erzählung." In: Ders. *Gesammelte Werke in zeitlicher Folge. Sechs Bände*: *Vol. 6*. Ed. Hans Mayer. Frankfurt a.M.: Suhrkamp Verlag, 1976, 522–34.

Frisch, Max. *Montauk*. In: Ders. *Gesammelte Werke in zeitlicher Folge. Sechs Bände*: *Vol. 6*. Ed. Hans Mayer. Frankfurt a.M.: Suhrkamp Verlag, 1976, 617–754.

Frisch, Max. *Der Mensch erscheint im Holozän*. In: Ders. *Gesammelte Werke in zeitlicher Folge. Sieben Bände*: *Vol. 7*. Ed. Hans Mayer. Frankfurt a.M.: Suhrkamp Verlag, 1986, 205–300.

Frisch, Max. *Entwürfe zu einem dritten Tagebuch*. Ed. Peter von Matt. Berlin: Suhrkamp Verlag, 2010.

Frisch, Max. *Aus dem Berliner Journal*. Ed. Thomas Strässle, Margit Unser. Berlin: Suhrkamp Verlag, 2014.

Hajduk, Stefan. "Montauk erscheint im Holozän. Literarisches Schreiben und Altern bei Max Frisch." In: *Limbus. Australisches Jahrbuch für germanistische Literatur- und Kulturwissenschaft* 8 (2015): 67–84.

Heinrich-Korpys, Meike. *Tagebuch und Fiktionalität. Signalstruktur des literarischen Tagebuchs am Beispiel der Tagebücher von Max Frisch*. St. Ingbert: Röhrig Universitätsverlag, 2003.

Helbig, Holger. s.v. "Alzheimer-Krankheit." In: Bettina v. Jagow, Florian Steger (eds.). *Literatur und Medizin: Ein Lexikon*. Göttingen: Vandenhoeck & Ruprecht, 2005, 46–50.

Kaiser, Gerhard. "Endspiel im Tessin. Max Frischs unentdeckte Erzählung 'Der Mensch erscheint im Holozän'." In: *Schweizer Monatshefte für Politik, Wirtschaft, Kultur* 82/83 (2002/2003): 46–52.

Keller, Renate. *Der Tagebuchroman als literarische Gattung. Thematologische, poetologische und narratologische Aspekte.* Berlin/Boston: De Gruyter, 2015.

Neuhuber, Christian. "'Siehe die Briefe.' Büchners *Lenz* und der Verzicht auf die Brieffiktion." In: Gideon Stiening, Robert Vellusig (eds.). *Poetik des Briefromans. Wissens- und mediengeschichtliche Studien.* Berlin/Boston: De Gruyter, 2012, 319–37.

Probst, Hans Ulrich. "Zwischen Resignation und republikanischer Alters-Radikalität. Spuren des Citoyen Max Frisch im Spätwerk." In: Daniel de Vin (ed.). *Leben gefällt mir – Begegnung mit Max Frisch.* Brüssel: Literarischer Treffpunkt, 1992, 27–57.

Renz-Polster, Herbert/Krautzig, Steffen (eds.). *Basislehrbuch Innere Medizin.* München/Jena: Elsevier, Urban & Fischer, ^{4}2008.

Röthinger, Julia. "'Erosion ist ein langsamer Vorgang.' Das Verschwinden in Max Frischs Erzählung 'Der Mensch erscheint im Holozän'." In: *Limbus* 8 (2015): 125–46.

Rossbach, Karlheinz. "Lesevorgänge. Zu Max Frischs Erzählung 'Der Mensch erscheint im Holozän'." In: Paul Lützeler (ed.). *Zeitgenossenschaft. Zur deutschsprachigen Literatur im 20. Jahrhundert.* Frankfurt a.M.: Athenäum Verlag, 1987, 252–65.

Seling-Dietz, Carolin. "Büchners *Lenz* als Rekonstruktion eines Falls ‚religiöser Melancholie'." In: *Georg Büchner Jahrbuch 9* (1995–1999): 188–236.

Schmidt, Jochen. *Die Geschichte des Genie-Gedankens in der deutschen Literatur, Philosophie und Politik 1750–1945: Vol. 2: Von der Romantik bis zum Ende des Dritten Reichs.* Heidelberg: Winter, ^{3}2004.

Schneider, Sabine. "Stille Katastrophen. 'Der Mensch erscheint im Holozän'." In: Daniel Nielaba, Yves Schumacher, Christoph Steier (eds.). *'Man will werden, nicht gewesen sein'. Zur Aktualität Max Frischs.* Zürich: Chronos Verlag, 2012, 229–46.

Shakespeare, William. *Hamlet.* In: Apel, Friedmar (ed.). *27 Stücke von William Shakespeare in der Übersetzung von Erich Fried.* Berlin: Verlag Klaus Wagenbach, 1989, 377–461.

Sontag, Susan. *Krankheit als Metapher.* Frankfurt a.M.: Fischer Taschenbuchverlag, 1981.

Todica, Olga, Wiltfang, Jens, Hermann, Dirk. "Vaskuläre Demenz." In: Dirk Hermann, Thorsten Steiner, Hans-Christoph Diener (eds.). *Vaskuläre Neurologie.* Stuttgart/New York: Georg Thieme Verlag, 2010, 269–76.

Vedder, Ulrike. "Erzählen vom Verfall. Demenz und Alzheimer in der Gegenwartsliteratur." In: *Zeitschrift für Germanistik* 22,2 (2012): 274–89.

Voorgang, Juliane. "'Schlimm wäre der Verlust des Gedächtnisses.' Anthropologische und archäologische Archivierung in Max Frischs 'Der Mensch erscheint im Holozän.'" In: *Limbus* 8 (2015): 13–32.

Dementia in the Media/ Mediale Repräsentationen

Jarmila Mildorf (Paderborn)

Negotiating Vulnerable Subjects: Margaret Thatcher's Dementia in Film and Media

Abstract: This article examines in how far the representation of Margaret Thatcher's dementia in the media raises philosophical and ethical questions concerning illness, identity and self-determination. By analysing newspaper reports and the movie *The Iron Lady*, the article identifies to what extent these representations are socially shaped but perhaps also shape social perceptions and thus potentially perpetuate stereotypes and the stigma attached to dementia.

1a) "Thatcher's battle with dementia" (*The Sydney Morning Herald*)
b) "Dementia: Margaret Thatcher's Death 'Merciful,' says Norman Tebbitt" (*International Business Times*)
c) "Lady Thatcher's final days cheered by puppy antics and tales of former PMs" (*The Guardian*)
d) "Thatcher dementia fight revealed" (*BBC*)
e) "Margaret Thatcher too frail for Queen's visit" (*Express*)
f) "Old Iron Lady: Thatcher cuts a frail figure on park bench" (*Mirror*)
g) "'She didn't get who David Cameron was': Former Tory minister Jonathan Aitken on Margaret Thatcher's dementia" (*Mail Online*)
h) "The one agonising battle even she could not win: How the cruel dimming of her awesome mental powers tested the great love between her and Denis to the limit" (*Mail Online*)

These headlines provide only a few examples of how newspaper articles dealing with the former British Prime Minister Margaret Thatcher's dementia sought to catch readers' attention. They are typical in that they use common strategies to make the presented news item both interesting and trustworthy. Examples (1b) and (1g), for instance, create credibility through eyewitness reports by quoting Conservative politicians who commented on Thatcher's illness and who – the implication is – must have had authoritative knowledge concerning the issue. The headline in (1h), which introduces an excerpt from Robin Harris' biography as published in the *Daily Mail*, even promises a glimpse into more intimate or private details surrounding Thatcher's illness and family life. Harris in this article (and in his biography) seemingly speaks as an authority on this matter because he was Thatcher's confidant for thirty years. These headlines also present Thatcher's dementia in ways that are reminiscent of the war metaphor frequently used by people when talking about illness more generally[1]: Thatcher's illness is seen as a "fight" (1d) or a "battle" (1a) which was "agonising" and "cruel" (1h) and which even Thatcher "could not win" (1h). This latter comment implicitly refers to the clichéd image of Thatcher as the "Iron Lady" (see also 1f), a metaphor which the media have employed as a shortcut to summarize what they perceived as Thatcher's typical epithets: she was seen as a powerful, strict and rigorous politician, perhaps even ruthless, tough and unfeminine. Against this background, her illness became even more note- and newsworthy, and the contrast is often already highlighted in the headlines. Examples (1e) and (1f) present Thatcher as "old" and "frail" and as no longer able to attend public functions. There may even be a pun in (1f) hinging on the fact that this politician, who for the largest part of her life was quite at home on the political benches of Parliament, had been diminished to cutting "a frail figure" on a park bench in the end. Thatcher's life in its final stage had been reduced to trivialities, as the headline in (1c) suggests. The fact that Thatcher was "cheered by puppy antics and tales of former PMs" presupposes that her life with dementia was no longer cheerful – an assumption that made her former colleague Tebbitt call her death "merciful", as we learn in example (1b).

These examples tell us not only something about the presentation of Margaret Thatcher's dementia but also about the way this problem, which increasingly affects families and societies worldwide due to growing life expectancy, is perceived and discursively constructed by the news media more generally: patients are presented as people to be pitied; dementia is seen as a loss and a state that is largely undesirable. This has ramifications for people's perceptions of dementia – if one assumes that the media not only reflect and give voice to but also shape public opinion. "The world is as we imagine it", says Maximilian Gottschlich in the title of his book on our media society[2] and uses this expression as a starting point for mounting an argument about why we ought to approach the media from a cultural-critical perspective. If we think of dementia the way it is presented to us through the media – and for most laypersons newspapers and magazines will be resources alongside internet fora and TV reportage – then we need to pay closer attention to what exactly these sources present and how they do it. Scholars of Critical Discourse Analysis maintain that

---

1 See Sontag, Susan. "Illness as Metaphor." In: David Rieff (ed.). *Essays of the 1960s & 70s*. New York: Library of America, 2013 [1978], 675-729.

2 Gottschlich, Maximilian. *Die Welt ist, wie wir sie denken: Zur Kulturkritik der Mediengesellschaft*. Wien: Springer, 1999.

> discourse is socially *constitutive* as well as socially shaped: it constitutes situations, objects of knowledge, and the social identities of and relationships between people and groups of people. It is constitutive both in the sense that it helps to sustain and reproduce the social status quo, and in the sense that it contributes to transforming it.[3]

In this chapter I look at the stories surrounding Margaret Thatcher's illness with a view to identifying to what extent they are socially shaped but perhaps also shape social perceptions and thus potentially perpetuate stereotypes and the stigma attached to dementia. As we shall see, the newspaper reports also raise philosophical and ethical questions concerning illness, identity and self-determination.

In a second step I will discuss the prize-winning 2011 film *The Iron Lady* by Abi Morgan (dir. Phyllida Lloyd) starring Meryl Streep as Margaret Thatcher.[4] The film, which narrates Thatcher's life story from the vantage point of her state of dementia, received controversial reviews and discussions, not least because it was shot and shown while Thatcher was still alive. One question that arises is whether the fact that the film is an aesthetic artefact, which conveys Thatcher's illness in an artistically mediated way, changes the ethical implications for this particular illness narrative. To answer this question I will draw on G. Thomas Couser's concept of "vulnerable subjects".[5] Couser defines "vulnerable subjects" as "persons who are liable to exposure by someone with whom they are involved in an intimate or trust-based relationship but are unable to represent themselves in writing or to offer meaningful consent to their representation by someone else".[6] What happens if the person whose illness narrative is told has been a public figure and is thus inevitably also appropriated by the media and, as in my example, by the film industry?

I. Thatcher's Illness in the News Media

In order to discuss the presentation of Thatcher's case in the news media it is important to briefly reflect on the role of the press in Britain first. British newspapers have for a long time now enjoyed the worst reputation among European

3 Fairclough, Norman, Jane Mulderrig, Ruth Wodak. "Critical Discourse Analysis." In: Teun A. van Dijk (ed.). *Discourse Studies: A Multidisciplinary Introduction*. Los Angeles: Sage, 2011, 357–78, 358.

4 *Die eiserne Lady*. Screenplay: Abi Morgan, dir. Phyllida Lloyd, perf. Meryl Streep, Jim Broadbent, Richard E. Grant. DVD. Concorde, 2012.

5 Couser, G. Thomas. *Vulnerable Subjects: Ethics and Life Writing*. Ithaca: Cornell University Press, 2004.

6 Couser. *Vulnerable Subjects*, xii.

newspapers. Professional transgressions by British journalists have repeatedly resulted in a call for more control. Attempts at providing institutional control from within the profession, e.g., through a code of honour issued by the National Union of Journalists or through more independent ethics commissions such as the Press Complaints Commission (PCC) or the Broadcasting Standards Council (BSC) did not have the wished-for results.[7] The debate on ethics and journalism in Britain has primarily hinged on the question of legal control since – unlike in other European countries – there has been no legislation specifically geared towards the press and broadcasting. More recently, the debate was fanned again by the so-called Leveson Inquiry, which led its key investigator, Lord Justice Brian Leveson, to recommend the implementation of an independent regulator, whose power of control should be established in law.[8] This point was disputed by David Cameron, among others, who emphasized the importance of free speech and a free press. Against this background, it is interesting to see how a topic like dementia, and in this example a very specific illness narrative, is treated in the news media and what ramifications this might have for the ethical debate concerning both the media and medicine.

II. Comparisons and Contrasts: Dementia and the Self

As I already mentioned, one striking feature in most of the newspaper articles is that they present Thatcher's illness in terms of a dichotomy between her former self and what she was like as a result of her illness. A good example is an article published in *The Star*, which draws its information from British newspapers such as the *Daily Mail* and *The Guardian*. The article repeatedly juxtaposes Thatcher's 'old' and 'new' selves by starting sentences with the complex noun phrase "the woman who..." and ending them with epithets describing her condition towards the end of her life:

2a) In her final days, **the woman who once took Britain to war** and was known everywhere as the Iron Lady was reduced to many levels of loneliness – intellectual, physical and also in terms of her severely curtailed independence. Her condition brought not just mental deprivation but conversational ineptitude as well.

---

7 See Thomaß, Barbara. *Journalistische Ethik: Ein Vergleich der Diskurse in Frankreich, Großbritannien und Deutschland*. Opladen: Westdeutscher Verlag, 1998, 188–89.

8 For more information on the investigation, see the official website: <http://www.levesoninquiry.org.uk/>

b) So **the woman who spent her political life surrounded by people** in various positions of power spent her last months in the constant care of those who were employed to look after her.
c) **The woman who never flinched from a challenge** could not go anywhere without a walking stick to keep herself steady and the arm of at least one person to keep her stable.[9]

Similarly, an article in the *Mirror* uses contrasts to depict Thatcher as an "Old Iron Lady":

3a) Only the famous hooded eyes and steely gaze betray the fact that this frail, white-haired lady **was once one of the most powerful – and hated – politicians in the world**.
b) **The killer-heels that once click-clacked menacingly through the corridors of power** have been replaced by comfy, brown slip-on shoes.
c) And at her side, where **terrified grey-suited men once hung on her every word**, female carers are ready to catch her if she stumbles.[10]

The opposition created in these two articles is between being powerful, fearless, independent, and at the centre of everyone's attention on the one hand and being intellectually deprived, dependent, frail and lonely on the other. These dichotomies are based on stereotypes and clichés, both as far as the image of the Iron Lady and the presentation of dementia are concerned.[11] The *Mirror* article in particular linguistically creates a very vivid picture of a threateningly powerful, almost *femme fatale*-like politician who instilled fear in everyone. The result is a simplified account of who Thatcher was before ("once") and after the onset of her illness rather than a characterization that acknowledges the emotional, psychological and behavioural complexity of human beings. The juxtaposition of two types also raises fundamental, philosophical questions concerning what the 'self' is and

9 McMahon, David. "The Final Days of Margaret Thatcher." *The Star Online*, 17 April 2013. <http://www.thestar.com.my/lifestyle/features/2013/04/17/the-final-days-of-margaret-thatcher/> (last access: 02.03.2017). My emphasis.

10 Bletchly, Rachael. "Old Iron Lady: Thatcher Cuts a Frail Figure on Park Bench." *Mirror*, 20 March 2012. <http://www.mirror.co.uk/news/uk-news/margaret-thatcher-cuts-a-frail-figure-766463> (last access: 30.08.2016). My emphasis.

11 With regard to the perception of people as types, Theo van Leeuwen writes: "What makes people into types in this world? Essentially four things: professional and leisure activities, gender, race and age" (Van Leeuwen, Theo. *Discourse and Practice: New Tools for Critical Discourse Analysis*. Oxford: Oxford University Press, 2008, 156). In the newspaper accounts on Margaret Thatcher, three of these facets are drawn upon and contrasted: her professional activity, i.e., her role as former Prime Minister, her gender, and her age, more specifically, her role as an elderly woman suffering from dementia.

how we want to define the notion of 'person'.[12] The newspaper articles with their typified presentations and clear-cut oppositions suggest a break in personality: Thatcher's ill self is radically different from her former self. Moreover, Thatcher's dementia is described with negative words which connote an undesirable form of living. References to physical "frailty" and to the "loss" of Thatcher's faculties as well as the frequently recurring theme of loneliness abound in the news reports.

Interestingly, the articles also often try to mitigate this purely negative assessment by mentioning incidents where residues of Thatcher's former self resurfaced in conversations. In this context, the articles typically draw on eyewitness narratives. John Hooper, Nicholas Watt and Robert Booth, for example, drew on personal anecdotes by people who had met Thatcher in various contexts and wrote in their article in *The Guardian*: "Although illness had already largely swamped Lady Thatcher's famously sharp mental faculties, such flashes of her old drive were common in the final stretch of her life, friends said on Wednesday".[13] The authors also quote Lord Forsyth, the former Scottish secretary as saying, "Even when she appeared to be having a difficult day she was absolutely capable of coming back with a very incisive and clever response".[14] Lady Jenkin, wife of Bernard Jenkin MP, who made a similar comment, is also quoted directly: "Her very strong beliefs were still there; they were still bubbling down underneath".[15] The metaphors used in these quotes – "flashes of her old self", Thatcher "coming back" and her beliefs "bubbling down underneath" – suggest a conception of dementia as merely covering up or hiding the real self, which, however, is still present somewhere 'inside' or 'underneath' the surface of the ill persona.

---

12 The question of personhood has gained new momentum in debates surrounding bioethics and biolaw, which ultimately also have practical implications for medicine and the life sciences. One can distinguish between two main positions: the "separationist" position distinguishes between 'human beings' and 'persons' and consequently values life not in itself but only if certain qualitative criteria are met; the "personalist" position argues that personhood and being human cannot be separated and that human life therefore has to be preserved and protected at all costs. (Carpi, Daniela. "Introduction." In: Daniela Carpi (ed.). *Bioethics and Biolaw through Literature*. Berlin: de Gruyter, 2011, 1–19, 4).

13 Hooper, John, Watt, Nicholas, Booth, Robert. "Lady Thatcher's Final Days Cheered by Puppy Antics and Tales of Former PMs." *The Guardian*, 10 April 2013. <http://www.theguardian.com/politics/2013/apr/10/margaret-thatcher-final-days> (last access: 30.08.2016).

14 Hooper et al. "Lady Thatcher's Final Days Cheered by Puppy Antics and Tales of Former PMs."

15 Hooper et al. "Lady Thatcher's Final Days Cheered by Puppy Antics and Tales of Former PMs."

What these comments show is not so much that there seems to be a tacit belief in a core self that continues over a lifespan no matter what happens to a person but, more importantly, that people seem to *wish* to believe in such a core self. For people observing a demented person from the outside it can be difficult to accept the fact that the illness gradually changes that person's familiar pattern of behaviour and ways of interacting with others. It is probably also hard to imagine how this person might feel, what she thinks, how she relates or does not relate to her illness. As Daniel L. Schacter contends, it "is excruciating for family members to witness a patient's painful awareness of his own vanishing memory".[16] However, research has also shown that patients who suffer from Alzheimer's or other forms of dementia "become progressively less aware of the extent, or even the existence, of their deficits".[17] The fact that friends, colleagues and family members continued to seek, and took pleasure in 'catching a glimpse of', the 'real' Margaret Thatcher in the ill persona suggests that we have to take this human factor into account when thinking more generally about the question of personhood, for example.

Philosopher Robert Spaemann argues that debilitated and disabled people create a test case for humanity because they require help from others.[18] Starting from the assumption that human beings are special creatures since they must be 'had' or 'owned' by other human beings and cannot simply 'be',[19] Spaemann maintains that healthy people's willingness to help disabled people indicates their tacit assumption that even disabled people are and remain persons, regardless of their apparent or visible characteristics. We are never only the sum of our characteristic features, Spaemann writes, and every human being creates an enigma. The recognition of this enigma even in people with whom we can never hope to approximate, let alone resolve, the enigma – because they cannot communicate their inner lives or because we have no clues as to whether there is still an intentional inner life – constitutes the most significant proof that humanity is a community of persons. This community is based on respect for others and thus in turn forms the basis of self-respect.

---

16 Schacter, Daniel. *Searching for Memory: The Brain, the Mind, and the Past*. New York: Basic Books, 1996, 160.

17 Schacter. *Searching for Memory, 160.*

18 See Spaemann, Robert. *Personen: Versuch über den Unterschied zwischen ‚etwas' und ‚jemand'*. Stuttgart: Klett-Cotta, 1996, 259–61.

19 Spaemann writes: "Menschen sind Wesen einer Art, deren Natur es erfordert, ‚gehabt' zu werden, nicht einfach zu sein"; see Spaemann, *Personen*, 260. He probably refers to the fact that humans are social beings who have an awareness of their sociality and the moral responsibilities implied by this.

III. 'Eye Witness' Reports and Personal Anecdotes: Dementia and Gossip

One may ask whether respect for others is perhaps missing precisely in those newspaper accounts that trade on stereotypes. As I mentioned, most of the articles I surveyed portray Thatcher's dementia in a simplified, if not clichéd way. In some articles those clichés are even used for ridicule, whether explicitly or implicitly, or they expose Thatcher's seemingly diminished life. Tabloid newspapers in particular made every effort to foreground the specifically negative aspects of Thatcher's illness. Since her case did not involve sex or violence – the stuff of which tabloid journalism is made as it focuses on sensationalism and the spectacular – the only newsworthy point was to stress her mental and physical decline. One article published in the *Daily Mail*, for example, already mentions in its headline what a former cabinet member, Jonathan Aitken, revealed in an interview with the *Sunday Telegraph* about Thatcher's attendance of a formal dinner at his house: "She didn't get who David Cameron was".[20] The colloquial phrase "she didn't get [it]" is repeated verbatim twice in the actual article, and its proposition is repeated another three times in the phrases "Iron Lady was confused when cabinet member mentioned Prime Minister's name", "Mrs Thatcher seemed to be unaware of who the current Prime Minister was", and "her confused state-of-mind was peppered with moments of clarity". In this latter phrase, one can see again the strategy of pinpointing what is still 'left' of the former Margaret Thatcher, but overall the article foregrounds Thatcher's inability to remember something as important and universally known as who the current Prime Minister is. Aitken's colloquial phrase puts this news item on a discursive level that is reminiscent of the everyday language used among people sharing a certain familiarity. The news item thus becomes a piece of gossip, just as if neighbours, for example, shared the news of a common acquaintance's failing mental capacities.

Typically, this gossipy style also involves providing direct quotations from people who are either specified in the article or remain generalized, e.g., "a friend". An article in the *Express*, for example, quotes Lord Bell as saying "I'm afraid she is not very lucid now" and a "former Cabinet colleague" is reported to have said: "Often things don't make sense to her". What is revealed about Thatcher's condition thus assumes the quality of hearsay. This discursive strategy of hearsay is

---

20 Mcqueeney, Kerry. "'She Didn't Get Who David Cameron Was': Former Tory Minister Jonathan Aitken on Margaret Thatcher's Dementia." *Mail Online*, 15 January 2012. <http://www.dailymail.co.uk/news/article-2086941/Margaret-Thatcher-dementia-The-Iron-Lady-didnt-know-David-Cameron-was.html> (last access: 30.08.2016).

sometimes employed to further undermine whatever positive image persisted through Thatcher's illness. Thus, the *Star* article I mentioned above – which presents what one could call a 'parade of witnesses' to buttress the image it creates of Thatcher – also draws on one such allegedly authoritative voice to introduce another piece of gossip:

> Conservative lawmaker Conor Burns revealed that Mrs Thatcher did have one particular preference when he visited her on as many Sunday evenings as possible. 'We would have a couple of what she called 'proper ones' – stiff gins,' he said. But along with that lighter revelation came the corollary that he was often her only visitor on an entire weekend.[21]

Again, Burns' authority as a witness of Thatcher's illness is stressed by the fact that he was a regular visitor. It does not matter that the sentence "he visited her on as many Sunday evenings as possible" is in fact ambiguous since the visits could still have been rare. The word "many" in itself is likely to create an impression of frequency in the reader's mind. What is most interesting here, however, is the particular anecdote Burns relates. Presenting Thatcher as someone who enjoyed the occasional drink is somewhat extraneous to a report on her "final days". Furthermore, the way that Burns talks about Thatcher's attitude towards alcohol suggests that it may have been a bit more of an issue. For example, "a couple of" drinks could refer to two or more drinks, at any rate more than one. The fact that Thatcher herself allegedly called her occasional "stiff gins" "proper ones" suggests that she must have been quite used to consuming strong alcohol.

This image of a drinking Margaret Thatcher is also reinforced in an excerpt from Robin Harris' biography, which was published in *Mail Online* and thus already received wide circulation.[22] Harris relates how Thatcher still tried to keep up a regular life as long as it was possible, and as part of that she "also entertained, and was the model of a charming hostess. Indeed, she was somewhat better company than in the past because she did not dominate every conversation, and nowadays never drank excessively".[23] The wording of the second sentence is very interesting because it juxtaposes the past with the present and subtly points to Thatcher's tendency to "dominate" conversations and to her "excessive" drinking. The fronted

---

21 McMahon. "The Final Days of Margaret Thatcher."

22 See Harris, Robin. "The One Agonising Battle Even She Could Not Win: How the Cruel Dimming of Her Awesome Mental Powers Tested the Great Love between Her and Denis to the Limit." *Mail Online*, 13 April 2013.<http://www.dailymail.co.uk/news/article-2306583/Margaret-Thatcher-The-cruel-dimming-mental-powers-tested-limit.html> (last access: 30.08.2016).

23 Harris. "The One Agonising Battle Even She Could Not Win."

temporal adverbial "nowadays" is marked and thus presupposes a contrast to the past, in which – the implication is – Thatcher drank a lot. Harris' article divulges similarly intimate details of Thatcher's family life, e.g., the marital problems she had or the financial pressure that her illness had incurred for her children. His comments are highly but subtly judgmental. For example, he gives away his dislike for Thatcher's daughter, Carol, when he explains why Thatcher approved of Carol's participation in the TV reality show *I'm a Celebrity ... Get Me out of Here!*: "Despite Lady Thatcher's image, she was not averse to vulgarity if it went with success and rewards – as in this case it did".[24] Carol Thatcher is indirectly presented as a vulgar person, and even Thatcher's own image is refashioned here and brought into association with vulgarity.

Articles like this one and Carol Thatcher's own memoir *A Swim-on Part in the Goldfish Bowl* are problematic to the extent that they undermine more positive or respectful presentations of Thatcher's illness. More importantly, they were published at a time when Thatcher herself was no longer able to react to these presentations. The question of autonomy and illness is central here, and it creates a paradox, as Couser argues:

> Vulnerable subjects are more likely to have their autonomy violated in practice precisely because what makes them vulnerable—whether their extreme youth or age or their physical or mental impairment—may be thought inconsistent with their autonomy; those perceived to have diminished autonomy are often, for that reason, treated in a way that may reduce whatever autonomy they do have. There is a further danger. In some cases, such as those of limited mental capacity or cognition, the very cause of subjects' vulnerability to exploitation may seem to make them invulnerable to certain kinds of harm—such as psychic pain or harm to reputation. [...] Ironically, then, the assumption of their invulnerability to harm may make them all the more prone to abuse.[25]

The thought that one can write about a person whatever one likes simply because one assumes this person will not be hurt by it anymore suggests a loss of the notion of personhood in Spaemann's sense. Thatcher's illness narrative can thus be used to illustrate an additional facet to Couser's concept: In the case of more prominent public personae, media talk about them renders the subjects not only doubly, but even multiply vulnerable. Not only did gossipy reports by friends, colleagues and family members make Thatcher vulnerable both on account of her illness and because she could no longer control their representation of her. Thatcher's story also assumed a life of its own when turned public, providing its recipients

24 Harris. "The One Agonising Battle Even She Could Not Win."
25 Couser. *Vulnerable Subjects*, 23.

with a precarious sense of ownership and seemingly intimate knowledge. Just as information becomes magnified and twisted when disseminated through gossip, the same mechanism might be in place when people read about someone like Thatcher as if she was their next-door neighbour. Such effects are of course difficult to verify, let alone quantify. And yet, the fact that the press especially in Britain caters towards people's voyeuristic inclinations and uses a 'gossipy' style even across the boundaries of tabloid and broadsheet papers suggests that such a mechanism must be in place.

IV. Further Facets: Voyeurism, Education and Politics

Voyeurism is also invited in the articles through the use of photographic material. Frequently, the articles featured photographs of Thatcher both when she was still politically active and as a retiree, thus underlining the dichotomies exploited in the text. Tabloid press articles such as those in the *Mirror* or the *Daily Mail* typically chose less flattering photos of Thatcher – for example, as she is being propped up by helpers. The images reinforce the stereotype of an elderly woman in need of support and also reduce Thatcher to a figure that comes closer to what people perceive in their own life-world surroundings. As the *Mirror* article has it, Thatcher "is one of many well-heeled pensioners taken around the park by their carers".[26] The distance between an unreachable public persona and the very public within which she played a prominent role is thus seemingly reduced.

Some articles also used Thatcher's specific case to then reflect more generally on the problem of dementia or even to give further information on this illness. For example, an article published in the *Los Angeles Times* on 08 April, 2013 – the day Thatcher died – discusses the question whether her death might have been related to the physical effects of dementia and then goes on to explore this nexus by citing specialists working on this problem.[27] An article in the *Sydney Morning Herald* provides an informative paragraph on the four basic types of dementia and a reference to the association Alzheimer's Research UK, whose patron Margaret Thatcher had been for many years.[28] In this regard, the news media can even be

---

26 Bletchly. "Old Iron Lady: Thatcher Cuts a Frail Figure on Park Bench."

27 See Healy, Melissa. "Margaret Thatcher's Dementia: Cause of Death or Unrelated Factor?" *Los Angeles Times*, 08 April 2013. <http://articles.latimes.com/2013/apr/08/news/la-heb-thatcher-dementia-cause-death-20130408> (last access: 30.08.2016).

28 See Anonymous. "Thatcher's Battle with Dementia." *The Sydney Morning Herald*, 09 April 2013. <http://www.smh.com.au/world/thatchers-battle-with-dementia-20130408-2hhsg> (last access: 30.08.2016).

said to assume an educational function, providing useful information to people who are interested in or affected by this problem. Whether it is acceptable to use a prominent person's specific case as an eye-catcher to then pursue other ulterior motives is of course another question.

An article posted by Jane Gross on the *New York Times* blog "The New Old Age" in reaction to Carol Thatcher's publication of her memoir discusses precisely such ethical questions surrounding the debate of dementia in the public domain.[29] Gross argues that, although one could evaluate public discussions about Thatcher's illness as a violation of her privacy, this illness also renders Thatcher's image more human and links her case to similar cases affecting many other families. In this sense, Thatcher's case may help break "one of the great taboos of our time", as Gross says, and work towards preventing the "conspiracy of silence", in which sufferers, their friends and families commonly engage.[30] I agree with Gross, but I would caution against a position which focuses on making things public at all costs and without due attention paid to *how* things are made public. If an article on Thatcher quite openly criticizes her on the grounds of her policies, for example, this at least gives readers a chance to recognize that viewpoint and to then either agree or disagree. However, many of the newspapers I surveyed have a slant that is not so easily recognizable at first. Moreover, by verbally insinuating or suggesting things rather than spelling them out and by reinforcing stereotypical images of dementia, they may contribute to the perpetuation of misconceptions rather than educate their readers.

The discourse I have hitherto looked at is largely based on, or at least purports to be based on factual information. The question of ethics and of patients' vulnerability shifts to another level, I would argue, once it involves an aesthetic remediation of these patients' life stories.

V. *The Iron Lady*: Margaret Thatcher's Illness on Film

From a point of view of artistic presentation, Morgan's film is quite remarkable. It presents Thatcher's life with dementia not from the outside perspective of close observers but from Thatcher's very own vantage point. The story is focalized through Thatcher, and so we are allowed an insight into this 'other' world she inhabits as an ill persona – a world that no-one can usually enter. The film shows

---

29 See Gross, Jane. "Margaret Thatcher's Open Secret." *The New York Times*, 02 September 2008. <http://newoldage.blogs.nytimes.com/2008/09/02/margaret-thatchers-open-secret/?_php=true&_type=blogs&_r=2> (last access: 30.08.2016).

30 Gross. "Margaret Thatcher's Open Secret."

how Thatcher slides in and out of her memories, how different memories fade into one another and, more importantly, how Thatcher's thoughts and memories motivate her actions, which to her daughter and carer, for example, remain incomprehensible and are merely a sign of Thatcher's dwindling faculties. Then we also see Thatcher interact with her husband, Denis, even though he has been dead for many years. These scenes are probably the most interesting ones because they are presented in a realistic mode, as if Denis was really there with his wife. There is no change in lighting or background colouring or a shift from high to low resolution or similar camera techniques to indicate a contrast between reality and fantasy life. The implication is that for Thatcher both the world around her and her inner world have the same status; they naturally blend into one another and do not cause any ruptures, except when other people react with incredulity or lack of comprehension. Because Thatcher's interactions are presented from her perspective, we are invited to share her special world with her and not to dismiss her fantasies as nonsense. This creates an interesting tension as it is frequently the characters surrounding Thatcher who appear not to be able to see or understand, and not Thatcher herself. To use a phrase from one of the newspaper articles, Thatcher's family, doctors, friends and carers are shown to be the ones who "do not get it".

More importantly, the scenes between husband and wife present a largely romanticized picture of their marriage. The two interact in a way that demonstrates their mutual trust, caring love and shared laughter. In fact, a lot of those intimate scenes are funny because Denis Thatcher is portrayed as a good-humoured, natural comedian, who manages to make his wife laugh and thus to defuse tense situations. His impersonation of Charlie Chaplin when going out, which Thatcher observes lovingly from her window, or the scene where he presents himself with some kind of self-fashioned turban and is then admonished by his wife for lying on her bed make Thatcher's fantasy life rich and hilarious – quite in contrast to the common discourse of dementia that often presents patients' lives as being marked by loss, deprivation and emptiness. Only occasionally are problems alluded to, for example, when Denis Thatcher is upset about his wife's decision to pursue her career further and to compromise her family life for this, or when he urges his wife to go to bed because it is "ten to three" in the morning. Often, as in the latter example, such moments of marital tension mesh with critical historical and political moments, thus signalling how much of Thatcher's life was taken up by her political role. Denis Thatcher's request that his wife eventually come to bed is juxtaposed with Thatcher watching news reports on terrorist bombings in Madrid, which are in turn interlaced with her memories of how she experienced a series of IRA bombings during her premiership. When Thatcher finally rises from her comfy chair to announce that "one must not give in to terrorism", we cannot help but admire her for her courage and principles – instead of seeing her as a deranged old lady who is merely confused about the events taking place around her.

This and similar moments create an image of Thatcher that suggests continuity rather than a break in personality. In fact, the way her memories of the past are inserted into Thatcher's current trains of thought – all of them visualized – is not in any way different from the way one might portray any other person's memories. One important function of these memories in the film is to show Thatcher's development and how these memories themselves also contribute to Thatcher's sense of who she is – a sense of self that is presented as very strong and vibrant despite Thatcher's illness. The visual semiotics in this film contributes to this impression of continuity – often in very subtle ways. Thus, we at one point see Thatcher talk to her secretary, for example, and Thatcher is captured by the camera from the vantage point of the other woman. Interestingly, she is shown standing near the window, and when looking at her we see a portrait of her in her garter gown on the wall behind her as well as a photo on a little cupboard showing her and Denis Thatcher. The visual presentation of three different instantiations of Thatcher in one camera shot suggests the continuity and contemporaneity of different facets of her and her life, symbolizing that, despite her illness, these facets are still present. Thatcher's tone of voice accomplishes something similar on the aural semiotic level. Thus, when Thatcher criticizes her daughter for fussing too much about her after Thatcher had gone out on her own to buy some milk, the irritation expressed in Thatcher's sentence "I'm not for the knacker's yet" reminds one of the famous line "This lady is not for turning" because a similar intonation contour and vocal intensity are used. Here, again, it is Thatcher who appears as the strong character, and her defiance of how the others treat her seems almost entirely justified and sensible.

The film *The Iron Lady* raises a number of ethical questions surrounding the presentation of a vulnerable subject. On the one hand, one has to acknowledge a certain degree of artistic license. Abi Morgan's film is a biopic and thus aims at showing a person's life. At the same time, this presentation is not simply meant to be realistic; instead, it creates meaning by drawing on conventions and forms of presentation typical for the specific medium, in this case film. As a piece of art, the film also allows for elements that would be impossible in real life. Thus, we are given an insight[31] into Thatcher's mind and how she perceives the world. The

31 We are quite literally allowed to *see* what Thatcher thinks and imagines because the film medium provides us with concrete pictures.

film also visualizes her frailty by having her walk about with sloping shoulders or holding a glass with trembling hands and the like. Overall, however, the film seems to diminish some of the problems involved in dementia, e.g., as regards the often difficult dynamics between the patient and her family. This has mainly to do with the chosen perspective, namely Thatcher's own. In contrast to much of the press coverage, which was largely negative, the film seems to carry Thatcher's portrayal to the other extreme by being overly positive. It is debatable how much of this poetic license will be reflected on by average viewers when watching the film. In other words, one may suspect that at least some people may have actually seen the film as more or less accurately reflecting Thatcher's life with dementia. In this case, the film could be criticized for romanticizing the problem. Another point of criticism could be that the film's focus on Thatcher's private life depoliticizes her and draws attention away from the role Thatcher played in British politics. One can of course argue that, from the perspective of an artist, it is legitimate to ignore the question of possible reception. What one cannot ignore, however, is the fact that the object of one's artistic presentation is a real-life person who is no longer able to react to and control her presentation. As one reviewer put it angrily, the film to a certain degree makes us voyeurs of Thatcher's life.[32]

VI. Conclusion

The values and concepts that are at the heart of much philosophical debate – respect, dignity, privacy, autonomy – are key to what has been discussed in this paper. I explored the representation of Margaret Thatcher's dementia across a range of newspaper articles and online news channels as well as in the film *The Iron Lady*. Using the analytical framework of Critical Discourse Analysis, I discussed to what extent a medium's general agenda and internal conditions and conventions influenced the depiction of Thatcher's illness. The newspapers can be said to offer a biased picture and thus to either support or refute a certain public image of Thatcher by drawing on existing stereotypes and by creating an atmosphere of gossip and hearsay. The ethical implications are further complicated, I argued, if that representation is based not only on an allegedly truthful exposure through persons intimately related to Thatcher but also on a fictive and fictionalized

32 See Pemberton, Max. "The Iron Lady and Margaret Thatcher's Dementia: Why this Despicable Film Makes Voyeurs of us All." *The Telegraph*, 14 January 2012. <http://www.telegraph.co.uk/news/politics/margaret-thatcher/9013910/The-Iron-Lady-and-Margaret-Thatchers-dementia-Why-this-despicable-film-makes-voyeurs-of-us-all.html> (last access: 30.08.2016).

account of her life. The film *The Iron Lady*, as interesting as it may be from a film critical perspective, becomes problematic in its almost euphemistic portrayal of dementia and in the fact that it chose as an object of presentation someone who was a "vulnerable subject".

References

Carpi, Daniela. "Introduction." In: Daniela Carpi (ed.). *Bioethics and Biolaw through Literature*. Berlin: de Gruyter, 2011, 1–19.

Couser, G. Thomas. *Vulnerable Subjects: Ethics and Life Writing*. Ithaca: Cornell University Press, 2004.

Die eiserne Lady. Screenplay: Abi Morgan, dir. Phyllida Lloyd, perf. Meryl Streep, Jim Broadbent, Richard E. Grant. DVD. Concorde, 2012.

Fairclough, Norman, Jane Mulderrig, and Ruth Wodak. "Critical Discourse Analysis." In: Teun A. van Dijk (ed.). *Discourse Studies: A Multidisciplinary Introduction*. Los Angeles: Sage, 2011, 357–78.

Gottschlich, Maximilian. *Die Welt ist, wie wir sie denken: Zur Kulturkritik der Mediengesellschaft*. Wien: Springer, 1999.

Schacter, Daniel. *Searching for Memory: The Brain, the Mind, and the Past*. New York: Basic Books, 1996.

Sontag, Susan. "Illness as Metaphor." In: David Rieff (ed.). *Essays of the 1960s & 70s*. New York: Library of America, 2013 [1978], 675–729.

Spaemann, Robert. *Personen: Versuch über den Unterschied zwischen ‚etwas' und ‚jemand'*. Stuttgart: Klett-Cotta, 1996.

Thomaß, Barbara. *Journalistische Ethik: Ein Vergleich der Diskurse in Frankreich, Großbritannien und Deutschland*. Opladen: Westdeutscher Verlag, 1998.

Van Leeuwen, Theo. *Discourse and Practice: New Tools for Critical Discourse Analysis*. Oxford: Oxford University Press, 2008.

Newspaper articles surveyed:

Anonymous. "Margaret Thatcher 'Suffering from Dementia." *Independent*, 24 August 2008. <http://www.independent.co.uk/news/uk/home-news/margaret-thatcher-suffering-from-dementia-907478.html> (last access: 30.08.2016).

Anonymous. "Thatcher Dementia Fight Revealed." *BBC News*, 24 August 2008. <http://news.bbc.co.uk/2/hi/uk_news/politics/7579352.stm> (last access: 30.08.2016).

Anonymous. "Thatcher's Battle with Dementia." *The Sydney Morning Herald*, 09 April 2013. <http://www.smh.com.au/world/thatchers-battle-with-dementia-20130408-2hhsg> (last access: 30.08.2016).

Bletchly, Rachael. "Old Iron Lady: Thatcher Cuts a Frail Figure on Park Bench." *Mirror*, 20 March 2012. <http://www.mirror.co.uk/news/uk-news/margaret-thatcher-cuts-a-frail-figure-766463> (last access: 30.08.2016).

Gross, Jane. "Margaret Thatcher's Open Secret." *The New York Times*, 02 September 2008. <http://newoldage.blogs.nytimes.com/2008/09/02/margaret-thatchers-open-secret/?_php=true&_type=blogs&_r=2> (last access: 30.08.2016).

Harris, Robin. "The One Agonising Battle Even She Could Not Win: How the Cruel Dimming of Her Awesome Mental Powers Tested the Great Love between Her and Denis to the Limit." *Mail Online*, 13 April 2013. <http://www.dailymail.co.uk/news/article-2306583/Margaret-Thatcher-The-cruel-dimming-mental-powers-tested-limit.html> (last access: 30.08.2016).

Healy, Melissa. "Margaret Thatcher's Dementia: Cause of Death or Unrelated Factor?" *Los Angeles Times*, 08 April 2013. <http://articles.latimes.com/2013/apr/08/news/la-heb-thatcher-dementia-cause-death-20130408> (last access: 30.08.2016).

Helliker, Adam. "Margaret Thatcher Too Frail for Queen's Visit." *Express*, 20 May 2012. <http://www.express.co.uk/comment/columnists/adam-helliker/321356/Margaret-Thatcher-too-frail-for-Queen-s-visit> (last access: 30.08.2016).

Hinsliff, Gaby. "Thatcher's Dementia Battle Revealed in Book." *The Guardian*, 24 August 2008. <http://www.theguardian.com/politics/2008/aug/24/margaret thatcher.conservatives> (last access: 30.08.2016).

Hooper, John, Watt, Nicholas, Booth, Robert. "Lady Thatcher's Final Days Cheered by Puppy Antics and Tales of Former PMs." *The Guardian*, 10 April 2013. <http://www.theguardian.com/politics/2013/apr/10/margaret-thatcher-final-days> (last access: 30.08.2016).

McMahon, David. "The Final Days of Margaret Thatcher." *The Star Online*, 17 April 2013. <http://www.thestar.com.my/lifestyle/features/2013/04/17/the-final-days-of-margaret-thatcher/> (last access: 30.08.2016).

Mcqueeney, Kerry. "'She Didn't Get Who David Cameron Was': Former Tory Minister Jonathan Aitken on Margaret Thatcher's Dementia." *Mail Online*, 15 January 2012. <http://www.dailymail.co.uk/news/article-2086941/Margaret-Thatcher-dementia-The-Iron-Lady-didnt-know-David-Cameron-was.html> (last access: 30.08.2016).

Osborne, Hannah. "Dementia: Margaret Thatcher's Death 'Merciful', says Norman Tebbitt." *International Business Times*, 08 April 2013. <http://www.ibtimes.co.uk/baroness-margaret-thatcher-death-highlights-stigma-surrounding-454782> (last access: 30.08.2016).

Owen, David. "Thatcher's Disciples Do Her No Favours by Covering up Her Illness." *Independent*, 07 January 2012. <http://www.independent.co.uk/voices/

commentators/david-owen-thatchers-disciples-do-her-no-favours-by-covering-up-her-illness-6286244.html> (last access: 30.08.2016).

Pemberton, Max. "The Iron Lady and Margaret Thatcher's Dementia: Why This Despicable Film Makes Voyeurs of Us All." *The Telegraph*, 14 January 2012. <http://www.telegraph.co.uk/news/politics/margaret-thatcher/9013910/The-Iron-Lady-and-Margaret-Thatchers-dementia-Why-this-despicable-film-makes-voyeurs-of-us-all.html> (last access: 30.08.2016).

Swinford, Steven. "Margaret Thatcher: Final Moments in Hotel without Her Family by Her Bedside." *The Telegraph*, 08 April 2013. <http://www.telegraph.co.uk/news/politics/margaret-thatcher/9980269/Margaret-Thatcher-final-moments-in-hotel-without-her-family-by-her-bedside.html> (last access: 30.08.2016).

Wessely, Simon. "Dementia and Mrs Thatcher." *The Lancet* 379.9812 (2012): 210. <http://www.thelancet.com/journals/lancet/article/PIIS0140-6736(12)60089-0/fulltext> (last access: 30.08.2016).

Wolff, Michael. "Iron Can't Shield Us from Everything." *USA Today*, 14 April 2013. <http://www.usatoday.com/story/money/columnist/wolff/2013/04/14/dementia-robbed-thatcher-of-voice/2082517/> (last access: 30.08.2016).

Philosophical Issues/ Philosophische Fragen

Katharina Bauer (Bochum/Groningen)

Selbst-Vergessen. Über den Umgang mit demenzbedingten Erfahrungen des Selbstverlusts

Abstract: One of the most threatening effects of dementia is the experience of forgetting or losing one's self. How can patients and their caregivers cope with this experience? Based on the example of Arno Geiger's narrative about his father this paper suggests aiming at a joint re-interpretation of the patient's personality. For this purpose it is essential to respect the patient as a person with practical significance.

I. Erfahrungen des Selbstverlusts

Demenzerkrankungen erscheinen unter anderem deshalb als Bedrohung, weil sie mit einer Erfahrung des Selbstverlusts verbunden sind. Es geht in letzter Instanz nicht nur darum, *etwas* (wenn auch beispielsweise etwas für die Bewältigung des Alltags Essentielles) zu vergessen, sondern es droht die Aussicht darauf, *sich selbst* zu vergessen. Es findet eine grundlegende Entfremdung von der eigenen Identität statt. Was genau ist ein ‚Selbstverlust'? Liegt er vor, wenn die eigene Selbstkontrolle bzw. Selbstbestimmtheit bis zu einem gewissen Grad oder vollständig verloren geht? Geht es eher um einen Verlust des eigenen Selbstbildes, um eine Verschiebung in der Selbstwahrnehmung? Oder ist das, was als Selbstverlust wahrgenommen wird, letztlich ein Verlust der eigenen Selbstzufriedenheit? Da ich erfassen möchte, wie sich das ‚Selbst-Vergessen' in der Demenzerkrankung als Erfahrung des Selbstverlusts aus der Perspektive der Betroffenen darstellt, bezieht sich mein Gedankengang im Folgenden primär auf frühe und mittlere Stadien einer Demenzerkrankung, in denen die damit verbundenen Verlusterfahrungen noch bewusst zum Ausdruck gebracht werden können. Ich werde auf eine literarische Quelle zurückgreifen, in der Äußerungen eines Demenzkranken dokumentiert werden. Es handelt sich dabei um Arno Geigers Auseinandersetzung mit der Demenzerkrankung seines Vaters in *Der alte König in seinem Exil.* In Geigers Darstellung werden die Dimensionen der mit der Krankheit verbundenen Verlusterfahrung besonders greifbar. Das Vergessen wird dabei zwar sehr deutlich, aber nicht ausschließlich als Bedrohung empfunden. Insofern über den Identitätsverlust *erzählt* wird, drängt es sich auf, die Identität, die auf dem Spiel steht, als narrative Identität zu erfassen. Das Konzept der narrativen Identität wird aber letztlich, sowohl in der literarischen Quelle als auch in meiner Interpretation, auf eine dialogisch-poetische Ebene sowie auf eine Ebene der praktischen Interaktion erweitert.

Cheshire Calhoun bietet eine Definition dafür an, was es heißen könnte, sich selbst zu verlieren:

> One may lose one's self [*a*] by being disabled from enacting one's core identity, [*b*] by becoming disconnected from one's normative outlook as a whole, [*c*] or by being disabled from planning.[1]

Calhouns Ausgangspunkt für diese Definition ist nicht die Auseinandersetzung mit Demenz, sondern mit anderen Arten der Entfremdung vom eigenen Leben, insbesondere durch Depressionen, die allerdings wiederum häufig eine Begleiterscheinung von Demenzerkrankungen bilden. Die drei verschiedenen Aspekte des Selbstverlusts, die sie anspricht, lassen sich aber durchaus auch mehr oder weniger treffend mit Demenzerkrankungen in Verbindung setzen:

a) *being disabled from enacting one's core identity:* Man ist nicht mehr in der Lage, den Kern der eigenen Identität bzw. des eigenen Selbstverständnisses in seinem Handeln aktiv und kontrolliert zu realisieren.

Vorausgesetzt ist mit dieser Idee der *core identity* eine Orientierung an Harry G. Frankfurt. Er geht davon aus, dass die individuelle Identität einer Person im Kern dadurch konstituiert und geformt wird, dass man sich mit bestimmten Wünschen identifiziert und Wünsche zweiter Ordnung entwickelt. Man legt also fest, was man tatsächlich selbst ‚wollen will'. Ein mit Demenzerkrankungen einhergehender Verlust von Selbstkontrolle scheint Personen eher in die Position eines *wantons* zurückzuversetzen – das ist bei Frankfurt derjenige, der seinen Impulsen unkontrolliert folgt und von einem Wunsch zum anderen wechselt, ohne eine klare Hierarchie der eigenen Wünsche und damit eine strukturierte Identität und ein eindeutig geformtes Selbstverständnis herstellen zu können.[2]

b) *becoming disconnected from one's normative outlook as a whole*: Man wird von seiner eigenen normativen Weltsicht abgetrennt oder kann sich nicht mehr damit identifizieren.

---

1 Calhoun, Cheshire. "Losing One's Self." In: Kim Atkins, Catriona Mackenzie (eds.). *Practical Identity and Narrative Agency*. New York, London: Routledge, 2008, 193–211, 198.

2 Vgl. Frankfurt, Harry. "Autonomie, Nötigung und Liebe." In: Monika Betzler, Barbara Guckes (eds.). *Harry G. Frankfurt. Freiheit und Selbstbestimmung*. Berlin: Akademie Verlag, 2001, 166–83.

Hier ist weniger eindeutig, ob dieser Aspekt des Selbstverlusts auf an Demenz erkrankte Personen zutrifft. Es geht um die Erfahrung, nicht mehr zu schätzen, was man in seinem Leben eigentlich wertgeschätzt oder als Ideale oder Ziele verfolgt hat. Z.T. sind auch bei Demenzpatienten starke Persönlichkeitsveränderungen im Hinblick auf den Umgang mit eigenen Überzeugungen zu beobachten oder eine Veränderung dessen, was man wertschätzt.[3] Dies gilt zunächst unabhängig vom Verlust der Fähigkeit, abstrakte Normen und Werte zu formulieren. Zu beobachten sind auch Abweichungen von alltäglichen Normen und Regeln der Kommunikation und des Umgangs miteinander.

c) *being disabled from planning*: Dieser Verlust der Selbstkontrolle im Sinne von kontrollierten und zielführenden Planungen des eigenen Handelns scheint eindeutig mit der Symptomatik von Demenzerkrankungen verbunden – und zwar ganz konkret im Bezug auf Planungen alltäglicher Handlungen und Verrichtungen – was mache ich als nächstes, wo gehe ich hin, wie soll mein Tag ablaufen… Es wird einem nicht durch äußere Bedingungen ‚unmöglich gemacht' zu planen und seine Pläne zu realisieren, sondern man verliert die *Fähigkeit* dazu.

Es ist mit Calhouns Definition des Selbstverlusts vereinbar, festzuhalten, dass an Demenz erkrankte Personen sich früher oder später im Verlaufe ihrer Erkrankung selbst verlieren. Das würde bedeuten, dass sie dann quasi ‚ohne sich selbst' weiterleben, also ‚sich selbst überleben'. Das wirft zahlreiche Fragen auf: Wie radikal ist ein solcher Selbstverlust? Gilt der Selbstverlust nur aus der eigenen Sicht der Betroffenen, insofern sie nicht mehr in der Lage sind, sich selbst zu identifizieren, sich an sich selbst zu erinnern oder insofern sie unter der Erfahrung leiden, sich selbst zu entgleiten – oder erfolgt ein Selbst- bzw. Identitätsverlust auch nach externen Kriterien und aus der Sicht anderer Personen (*das ist nicht mehr mein Vater/meine Mutter*)? Sind Personen, die sich selbst verlieren (bzw. ihr ‚Selbst' verlieren), dann auch nicht mehr ‚als sie selbst' zu behandeln?

Ich möchte mich hier vor allem auf die Frage konzentrieren, ob und inwieweit sich der Selbstverlust oder das Selbst-Vergessen, das mit Demenzerkrankungen einhergeht, eventuell bis zu einer gewissen Grenze in eine Veränderung umdeuten lässt. Das Selbst geht dann nicht ‚verloren', es verändert sich lediglich – wenn auch möglicherweise radikal. Eine Verlusterfahrung der bisherigen Identität lässt sich zwar im Rahmen von Demenzerkrankungen nicht vollständig vermeiden. Das muss aber nicht eine vollständige ‚Selbstaufgabe', einen vollständigen Identitätsverlust oder gar einen Verlust des Status der Personalität bedeuten.

---

3 Vgl. Jaworska, Agnieszka. "Respecting the Margins of Agency: Alzheimer's Patients and the Capacity to Value." In: *Philosophy and Public Affairs*. 28,2 (1999): 105–38.

II. Selbstverlust, Persönlichkeits*wechsel* oder Persönlichkeits*entwicklung*?

Greift man auf die Terminologie Michael Quantes zurück, so erfolgt in Fällen von Demenzerkrankungen nicht ein Selbstverlust, sondern ein Persönlichkeits*wechsel*, der jedoch auch wesentlich radikaler und weniger autonom vollzogen wird als eine Persönlichkeits*entwicklung*.

Quantes Auseinandersetzung mit dem Phänomen des Persönlichkeitswechsels steht im Zusammenhang seiner Untersuchungen zum Begriff der Person. In der philosophischen Debatte über diesen Begriff geht es zumeist um die Bestimmung von Kriterien der Zugehörigkeit zur Klasse der Personen und um Fragen nach der Identität einer Person – im Sinne einer synchronen und diachronen (Re-) Identifizierbarkeit und Einheit. Ausgangspunkt hierfür ist John Lockes klassische Definition der Person als ein „denkendes, verständiges Wesen, das Vernunft und Überlegung besitzt und sich selbst als sich selbst betrachten kann. Das heißt, es erfaßt sich als dasselbe Ding, das zu verschiedenen Zeiten und an verschiedenen Orten denkt."[4] Das Kriterium der Einheit der Person ist damit also im Selbstbewusstsein anzusiedeln. Eine wesentliche Rolle spielt dabei für Locke die Fähigkeit, sich zu erinnern.[5]

Während sich nun für Quante die *Persönlichkeit* im Verlauf von Demenzerkrankungen verwandelt, oder sie eben ‚gewechselt wird', geht der Status als *Person* dabei gerade nicht verloren oder wird verändert. Denn Quante bindet die Persistenz der Person, anders als die Kontinuität der Persönlichkeit, an die biologischen Gegebenheiten des menschlichen Organismus, zu denen sich aber wiederum die einzelne Persönlichkeit jeweils individuell verhalten kann. Den Begriff der *Persönlichkeit* bezieht Quante auf ein Selbstverständnis in einem biographischen Zusammenhang, und zwar „im Sinne eines evaluativ-normativen Selbstverhältnisses" (Quante. *Person*, 8). Es geht nicht um die Klassifizierung von Persönlichkeitstypen, sondern um die individuelle Ausprägung einer *Lebensführung* als Person.

Während Personalität in der Regel ein Schwellenwertkonzept impliziert, also zumindest das Bestreben besteht, eine möglichst klare Grenze der Zugehörigkeit

---

4 Locke, John. *Versuch über den menschlichen Verstand*. Buch II. Hamburg: Meiner, [5]2000, 419.

5 Quante hebt hervor, dass es Locke um eine nicht-metaphysische und von theologischen Voraussetzungen unabhängige Theorie der Person geht, die nicht unmittelbar normativ ist, aber dennoch ganz wesentlich darauf ausgerichtet, die Frage zu beantworten, wer in der ethischen Praxis als Adressat von Lohn und Strafe zu betrachten ist.

zur Klasse der Personen festzulegen, ist das Konzept der Persönlichkeit graduell zu verstehen. So unterscheiden wir auch in unserem Alltagsverständnis zwischen schwachen und starken Persönlichkeiten. Und wir gehen vermutlich auch ganz intuitiv davon aus, dass sich die Identität einer Persönlichkeit im Laufe der Zeit stark verändern kann, ohne dass dadurch die Kontinuität des Selbstseins immer schon in Frage gestellt würde.

Die Strukturen einer Persönlichkeit werden laut Quante weder aus der Perspektive der ersten Person noch aus einer neutralen Beobachterperspektive adäquat erfasst. Entscheidend ist dafür die *Teilnehmerperspektive*. Das heißt, eine Persönlichkeit kann nur in einem „hermeneutische[n] Zusammenspiel von Ich und Wir" adäquat beschrieben werden (Quante. *Person*, 189).

Quante setzt voraus, dass sich Personalität prinzipiell in sozialen Beziehungen wechselseitiger Interpretation und Anerkennung konstituiert (vgl. Quante. *Person*, 31),[6] und zwar darin,

> sich selbst und anderen Personen gegenüber die teilnehmende Perspektive einzunehmen, Rationalität zu unterstellen sowie nach evaluativen und anderen Sinnzusammenhängen Ausschau zu halten (Quante. *Person*, 138).

Zudem hebt Quante die diachrone Persistenz hervor, die sich in der Ausrichtung auf Lebenspläne und in der rückblickenden Einordnung von Erlebnissen in eine biographische Erzählung der eigenen Geschichte manifestiert. Wesentlich sind die Aspekte einer aktiven Lebensführung und Gestaltung der eigenen Persönlichkeit und das „Bestreben nach Kohärenz in Sinne einer sinnhaften Einheit" (Quante. *Person*, 147). Ebenso geht er von einer grundlegenden *Expressivität* aus: „Eine menschliche Person drückt in ihrer Persönlichkeit aus, wer sie ist und wer sie sein will" (Quante. *Person*, 170). Quante versucht also einen Vorschlag dafür zu entwickeln, wie sich zwischen einem vollständigen und radikalen Persönlichkeits*wechsel* und einer kontinuierlicheren Persönlichkeits*entwicklung* unterscheiden lässt. Ihm gelingt es dabei nicht, harte und eindeutig nachprüfbare Kriterien zu entwickeln. Ein solcher Eindeutigkeitsanspruch wäre aber, wie er selbst betont,

---

6 Auch Robert Spaemann weist dem Anerkennungsverhältnis eine wesentliche Funktion zu, kritisiert allerdings die Vorstellung, dass der Status des Personseins erst durch den Vollzug realer Anerkennungsbeziehungen etabliert würde. Für Spaemann ist „die Anerkennung von Personen […] die Anerkennung eines unbedingten Anspruchs" und es „kann und darf nur ein einziges Kriterium für Personalität geben: Die biologische Zugehörigkeit zum Menschengeschlecht". Spaemann, Robert. *Personen. Versuche über den Unterschied zwischen ‚etwas' und ‚jemand'*. Stuttgart: Klett-Cotta, 1996, 262, 264.

dem komplexen und interpretationsbedürftigen Phänomen der Persönlichkeit auch nicht angemessen (vgl. Quante. *Person*, 175).

Es gibt nun für Quante trotz einer solchen Komplexität ‚persönlicher Kontinuität' dennoch eindeutig bestimmbare Veränderungen, die sich aus der Perspektive eines aktiv-gestaltenden, normativ-evaluativen und biographisch-interpretierenden Selbstverhältnisses „nicht verständlich machen lassen" (Quante. *Person*, 155). Sie lassen sich nicht „als Dynamik dieser bestimmten Persönlichkeit", sondern nur „als Verlust einer Persönlichkeit und gegebenenfalls als Entstehung einer neuen Persönlichkeit" deuten (ibid.), also als Persönlichkeits*wechsel*.

Für die Bestimmung einer Persönlichkeits*entwicklung* hält er hingegen letztlich folgende Formel fest:

> Entscheidend ist, dass sich die Veränderung der Persönlichkeit für die jeweilige Person selbst und für die interpretierenden Subjekte als aktives Erzeugen einer biografischen Kohärenz durch Identifikation mit gegenwärtigen, vergangenen (beim Erinnern) und zukünftigen (beim Antizipieren) Eigenschaften und Wünschen verständlich machen lässt. (Quante. *Person*, 174)

Eine Persönlichkeitsentwicklung, die kein Persönlichkeitswechsel ist, setzt also, noch einmal zusammengefasst, diachrone Kohärenz voraus und eine aktive Gestaltung, die – auch hier ausgehend von Harry Frankfurt – wesentlich eine aktive Identifikation mit Wünschen, Entscheidungen und Handlungen der Persönlichkeit oder aber auch mit Interpretationsvorschlägen anderer verlangt. Es handelt sich also um eine selbstbestimmte und in die eigene biographische Identität integrierte Veränderung. Der Persönlichkeitswechsel wiederum unterscheidet sich von der Persönlichkeitsentwicklung dadurch, dass die Person sich nicht mehr als sie selbst verstehen kann und von anderen nicht mehr als sie selbst verstanden wird (nach dem Muster ‚*das bist doch nicht du*').

Fälle von Persönlichkeitsstörungen bilden für Quante den „*lebensweltliche[n] Testfall*" und die „negative Ersatzprobe" für das Kriterium einer Persistenz der Persönlichkeit (Quante. *Person*, 173). In diesem Zusammenhang verweist er explizit darauf, dass wir im Falle einer Demenzerkrankung die Krankheitssymptome als Persönlichkeits*verlust* betrachten. Es erfolgt zugleich ein Persönlichkeits*wechsel*, weil die aktive Herstellung der eigenen biographischen Kohärenz nicht mehr funktioniert, also keine Identifikation mit der bisherigen Persönlichkeit mehr gelingt. Die gegen die Erkrankung gerichteten Bemühungen des Patienten, ‚er selbst zu bleiben', würde man wiederum eher als Aspekt einer Persönlichkeits*entwicklung* deuten. Interessant ist hier, dass es in diesem Kampf zumeist nicht nur darum geht, gegen den Verlauf der Krankheit anzugehen, sondern auch darum, die alte, intakte Identität vor anderen zu verteidigen, indem die Patienten – oft mit großem Geschick – versuchen, die Symptome zu verbergen oder zu überspielen.

Ich möchte jedoch zeigen, dass nicht nur das Ankämpfen *gegen* die Krankheit, sondern auch Versuche des Patienten, aktiv *mit* den Krankheitssymptomen und Persönlichkeitsveränderungen umzugehen, sie zu akzeptieren und in sein Selbstverständnis zu integrieren, als Teil einer Persönlichkeits*entwicklung* deutbar sind. Man muss dann allerdings den Punkt der Herstellung einer ‚biographischen Kohärenz', etwas zurücknehmen – also die Fähigkeit, die eigene Geschichte in einer sinnvollen chronologischen Ordnung zu erzählen und sich damit zu identifizieren. Damit stellt sich die Frage, wie eine andere Form der Herstellung einer dennoch in sich bedeutungsvollen und sinnvollen Einheit als Persönlichkeit aussehen könnte.

Um eine sinnvolle Neudeutung der Persönlichkeit zu ermöglichen, ist in jedem Fall die Unterstützung durch andere Personen entscheidend, die die Herstellung der biographischen Kohärenz zum Teil übernehmen und zu einem Prozess interpersonaler Verständigung über das durch den Krankheitsverlauf veränderte Selbst beitragen. Das interpretierende Zusammenspiel zwischen Ich und Wir verlagert sich also vom Ich zum Wir.

III. Interpersonale Verständigungen über ein ‚anderes Selbst'

Im Falle eines pathologischen Persönlichkeitsverlusts wird im interpretierenden Zusammenspiel von Ich und Wir, in dem die Identität der Persönlichkeit gedeutet wird, die Position des Ichs geschwächt. Daher sind die Bezugspersonen des Erkrankten – also ‚andere interpretierende Subjekte' – aufgefordert, den Selbstverlust zumindest teilweise durch einen intersubjektiven Prozess der Verständigung über die Identität einer ‚neuen Persönlichkeit' aufzufangen. Es ist ein erstrebenswertes Ideal, einen Selbstverlust in der interpersonalen Kommunikation mit dem Betroffenen zumindest *so weit wie möglich* zu einer Persönlichkeits*entwicklung* umzudeuten. Dies stellt keinen paternalistischen Übergriff dar, solange es sich um einen gemeinsamen Interpretationsprozess handelt. Die Grenzen zwischen Selbstdeutung und Fremdbestimmung sind hier allerdings sicherlich fließend. Bei der Umdeutung von Erfahrungen des Selbstverlusts in integrierbare Erfahrungen der Veränderung und der Re-Interpretation der Persönlichkeit des Erkrankten ist daher in jedem Fall besondere Sensibilität geboten.

Ein gelungenes Beispiel für dieses schwierige Unterfangen findet sich in Arno Geigers Buch *Der alte König in seinem Exil*. Geiger setzt sich darin literarisch mit der Alzheimererkrankung seines Vaters auseinander und dokumentiert Gespräche, die er mit diesem führt. Er beschreibt die letzten Lebensjahre und

Veränderungen seines Vaters, der nach und nach die wichtigsten Kenntnisse für alltägliche Verrichtungen, die Menschen und Erfahrungen seines Lebens und am Ende wohl auch sich selbst vergisst. Der Erzähler setzt seinem Vater ein literarisches Denkmal, das aber gerade nicht darauf abzielt, ihn gesund und als intakte Persönlichkeit in Erinnerung zu behalten.

Der Weg ins Vergessen und die damit verbundene Verletzlichkeit werden schonungslos aufgezeigt als eine spürbare Bedrohung, die sich auf den Leser überträgt. Es drohen ein Kontrollverlust, Orientierungslosigkeit, Verzweiflung, tiefe Trauer darüber, nirgendwo mehr zuhause zu sein, weil es keinen Ort gibt, an den man sich erinnert. Beschrieben wird das, was Paul Ricœur als einen „Marsch in Richtung auf den Verlust alles Errungenen, alles Erworbenen" bezeichnet.[7] Als ein existenzielles Unglück wird dieses Vergessen, sofern man es nicht unmittelbar selbst erfährt, in der künstlerischen bzw. literarischen Darstellung besonders deutlich fassbar. Ricœur unterscheidet verschiedene Formen des Vergessens, die teilweise eher auf historische Ereignisse als auf individuelle Selbsterfahrungen bezogen sind. Sehr treffend erscheint aber als Darstellung der Bedrohung durch Demenzerkrankungen seine Definition des unerbittlichen Vergessens:

> Es beschränkt sich nicht darauf, das Abrufen von Erinnerungen (›Wie war doch gleich ihr Name?‹) zu verhindern (oder zu beeinträchtigen); es zielt darauf ab, die Spur dessen, was man gelernt oder gelebt hat, *auszulöschen*.[8]

Die Unerbittlichkeit liegt also darin, dass nicht nur einzelne Erinnerungen verloren gehen oder einzelne Aspekte der eigenen Identität, sondern alles, was von dem, „was man gelernt oder gelebt hat" (s.o.), übrigbleibt. Eine solche Verlusterfahrung wird in Geigers Darstellung sehr greifbar. In seinem literarisch-dokumentarischen Text manifestieren sich zwei verschiedene Aspekte einer Bedrohung durch das Vergessen, die sich jeweils als *Selbstverlust* bezeichnen lassen: Beschrieben wird ein *pathologisches Vergessen* als Verlust des Erinnerungsvermögens und aller damit verbundenen kognitiven Kompetenzen. Dieses Vergessen untergräbt das Selbstverständnis der Person und ihre Fähigkeiten als aktives, bewusstes Handlungssubjekt. Das Subjekt ist einem Selbstverlust als Verlust seiner Selbstkontrolle oder Selbstbeherrschung ausgeliefert. Performativ vollzogen (und auch explizit reflektiert) wird durch die Erzählung zugleich ein Kampf gegen die Bedrohung des *Vergessenwerdens*. Unterschieden werden kann hier also zwischen einem

7 Ricœur, Paul. *Das Rätsel der Vergangenheit. Erinnern, Vergessen, Verzeihen*. Übers. v. Andris Breitling u. Henrik R. Lesaar. Göttingen: Wallstein, 2004, 132.

8 Ricœur. *Das Rätsel der Vergangenheit*, 131–32; Hervorhebung im Original.

Selbstverlust, der vom Subjekt selbst ausgeht, und einem Verlust, der darin besteht, dass ein individuelles, personales Selbst von anderen vergessen wird.

Eingewoben in das Erzählen *über* seinen Vater und dessen Erkrankung dokumentiert Geiger, wie bereits erwähnt, auch Dialoge *mit* ihm. Geiger gibt an, diese nicht literarisch bearbeitet zu haben. Die dokumentierten Gespräche entsprechen nicht den Regeln einer vernünftigen Kommunikation, sie gelingen aber, wenn Geiger auf die z.T. sehr poetische, fragmentierte Redeweise des Vaters eingeht. Dabei wird der Selbstverlust durchaus explizit thematisiert, aber nicht (nur) als eine tragische Ausweglosigkeit, sondern eher als eine Veränderung, die trotz ihrer Bedrohlichkeit und dem damit verbundenen Leid auch Möglichkeiten zu einer neuen Art des Umgangs miteinander und zu einer neuen Wahrnehmung der Umwelt und des eigenen Selbst ermöglicht. Der Selbstverlust wird hier also nicht nur im ‚Erzählen gegen das Vergessen' aufgehoben, sondern auch dialogisch in Prozessen interpersonaler Verständigung aufgefangen.

Zwar verliert die eigene Persönlichkeit für den Betroffenen ihre biographische Kohärenz. Es fällt ihm schwer, sich mit „vergangenen (beim Erinnern) und zukünftigen (beim Antizipieren) Eigenschaften und Wünschen" zu identifizieren (Quante. *Person*, 174). Es bleiben aber doch Momente – quasi poetische Augenblicke jenseits der narrativen, diachronen Ordnung – in denen er ganz bei sich zu sein scheint, in denen er sich ganz intensiv mit Wünschen und Eigenschaften identifiziert und seine individuelle Persönlichkeit ganz deutlich zum Ausdruck bringt. Er scheint darin dann nicht *weniger* er selbst zu sein, als vorher – als gesunde Person –, sondern eben anders. Diese Momente in Bezug zur Kohärenz seiner gesamten Biographie zu setzen obliegt dann wiederum anderen, in diesem Fall seinem Sohn.

Wenn, wie für Paul Ricœur, die Identität von Personen als eine narrative Identität in der Erzählung zu erfassen ist, dann ist von vornherein klar, dass unsere Lebensgeschichte allein aus der Ich-Perspektive niemals vollständig erzählt werden kann, weil niemand den Anfang und das Ende seiner eigenen Lebensgeschichte – seine Geburt, ebenso wie seine frühe Kindheit, und seinen Tod, ebenso wie möglicherweise Phasen der Krankheit davor, – selbst aktiv erinnern und erzählen kann. Zugleich gilt mit Marya Schechtman: „infancy and dementia are part of the structure of a standard life story" (Schechtman. *Staying Alive*, 107).

Persönlichkeiten sind also in ihrem Selbstverständnis vom Vergessenwerden bedroht, und sie sind dabei immer darauf angewiesen, von anderen weitererzählt ebenso wie auch ‚mitinterpretiert' zu werden. Über die bis hierher entwickelte Idee einer interpersonalen Dimension der narrativen Identität soll jedoch noch ein Schritt hinausgegangen werden – ebenso wie über Quantes Ansatz des Verstehens von Persönlichkeiten im hermeneutischen Zusammenspiel von ‚Ich und Wir'. So wichtig diese Verständigungsprozesse sind, lässt sich auch stark machen, dass die Identität einer Person als eine praktische Identität nicht nur in gemeinsamen Denk-, Interpretations- oder Kommunikationsprozessen determiniert wird. Sie wird auch ganz konkret in der gemeinsamen Interaktion geformt und bestimmt.

Diese Vorstellung prägt Schechtmans Konzeption des ‚Überlebens' als Interaktionspartner auch angesichts von Bedrohungen des Selbstverlusts. Unter dem Titel *Staying Alive* erörtert Schechtman, was es heißt, *als Person* zu überleben – und zwar u.a. auch angesichts der Bedrohung durch Demenzerkrankungen. Schechtman will den Begriff der Person bewusst weiter fassen als in klassischen, an Locke orientierten Positionen. Sie hält fest:

> [T]he continuity of a human person consists in the interactions among the different biological, psychological, and social attributes and functions, which support and mutually reinforce one another in everday life (Schechtman. *Staying Alive*, 201–2).

Da nun das Zusammenspiel dieser verschiedenen Faktoren die Kontinuität einer menschlichen Person ausmacht, können Verluste einzelner sowie auch mehrerer Faktoren durchaus überlebt werden, ohne dass durch diese Verluste die Person selbst verloren ginge:

> [A] person can in principle survive the loss of almost any of the standard functions and relations that make up a paradigmatic life if enough remain [...] to maintain an integrated unit of action. (Schechtman. *Staying Alive*, 202)

Schechtman betont, dass Personen nicht aufhören und letztlich sogar gar nicht aufhören können, andere Personen als Interaktionspartner zu betrachten, auch dann nicht, wenn ihr aktiver, selbstbestimmter Part sowohl im Hinblick auf ihre Selbstkonstituierung als auch im Hinblick auf die Interaktion stark eingeschränkt ist: „we do see (and cannot help seeing) one another as unified targets of interpersonal interaction" (Schechtman. *Staying Alive*, 202).

Wenn Angehörige oder Freunde einen Demenzpatienten weiter besuchen und sich um ihn kümmern, obwohl sie gar nicht mehr erkannt werden, dann deshalb, weil sie seine Geschichte kennen und selbst Teil dieser Geschichte sind (vgl. Schechtman. *Staying Alive*, 106). Die Identität als Person (und das Überleben als Person) ist an deren praktische Bedeutung für andere Personen gebunden: „a person's identity is bound up with her practical significance" (Schechtman. *Staying Alive*, 204).

Ich möchte ergänzen, dass sich die genaue Ausdeutung der praktischen Bedeutung in den Veränderungen einer Persönlichkeit stark verändern kann, ohne dass dies einen kompletten ‚Bedeutungsverlust' darstellen muss. Auch wenn jemand über die erkrankte Person sagt ‚*sie ist nicht mehr sie selbst, das ist nicht mehr meine Mutter/meine Partnerin/Schwester etc.*' wird man damit ganz und gar nicht automatisch meinen: ‚*sie bedeutet mir nichts mehr*' und auch nicht ‚*sie kann für mich überhaupt keine Interaktionspartnerin mehr sein*' – auch hier wird eben eine *Umdeutung* der Bedeutung und des Platzes in der Interaktion notwendig.

Es lassen sich letztlich drei Möglichkeiten einer interpersonalen Zusammenarbeit aufzeigen, das ‚Selbst-Vergessen' von an Demenz erkrankten Personen nicht in einen radikalen Selbstverlust münden zu lassen bzw. in die Situation, sich quasi selbst zu überleben, ohne weiterhin man selbst zu sein:

1) ein interpersonales Weitererzählen der biographischen Kohärenz
2) eine interpersonale Vergegenwärtigung und Neuinterpretation der Persönlichkeit
3) eine Behandlung des Erkrankten als Interaktionspartner mit einer ‚praktischen Bedeutung' (wenn auch vielleicht mit einer anderen als vor der Erkrankung).

Im Hinblick auf die anfänglich ausgehend von Calhoun dargestellten Aspekte des Selbstverlusts wäre, um den Selbstverlust aufzufangen, folgendes anzustreben:

a) eine gemeinsame Neu-Deutung der (noch) realisierbaren, in Handlungen und Verhaltensweisen ausdrückbaren Identität
b) eventuell auch eine gemeinsame Neubestimmung der normativen Weltsicht bzw. eine schlichte Akzeptanz veränderter Normen oder des veränderten Umgangs mit Normen und Konventionen
c) der Patient sollte so weit wie möglich in seinen eigenen Planungen und deren Umsetzung unterstützt werden, auch wenn diese sich nur auf kleine, überschaubare Schritte beziehen.

Zu beachten ist allerdings, dass all diese Momente einer interpersonalen Verständigung über ein ‚anderes Selbst' der Verlusterfahrung und Bedrohung der Demenzerkrankung sicherlich abhängig vom Krankheitsverlauf (angesichts von keineswegs zu verharmlosenden Symptomen wie Unruhe, Rastlosigkeit, Depressionen, Aggression) nur begrenzt entgegentreten können.

IV. Selbst-Vergessenheit ... Ein Ausblick

Wie bedrohlich ist letztlich das *Vergessen*, das an Demenzerkrankungen so gefürchtet wird? Ricœur betont, dass dem Vergessen als Fehlfunktion des rationalen Subjekts ein *selektives Vergessen* gegenübersteht, das sogar als Bedingung des funktionierenden Gedächtnisses vorauszusetzen ist.[9] Würden wir permanent alles

9 Ricœur. *Gedächtnis, Geschichte, Vergessen*. Übers. v. Hans-Dieter Gondek, Heinz Jatho u. Markus Sedlaczek. München: Wilhelm Fink, 2004, 652.

Erlebte unwiderruflich in unserem Gehirn abspeichern, wären wir überfordert damit, dieses Erlebte später wieder als Erinnerung zu reaktivieren und uns im Archiv unseres Gedächtnisses zu orientieren. Zudem würden irgendwann die natürlichen Grenzen der Speicherkapazität erreicht.

Die Fähigkeit zu einem selektiven Vergessen ist in diesem Sinne ein großes Glück. Für Ricœur müssen daher *ars oblivionis* und *ars memoriae*, die Kunst des Vergessens und die Kunst des Erinnerns, Hand in Hand gehen. Im Regelfall ist aber die Auswahl dessen, was man vergisst und woran man sich erinnert, nicht vollständig bewusst zu steuern. Deshalb bleibt das Vergessen, so Ricœur, immer eine Bedrohung für die Selbstkontrolle des Subjekts und für „*die* hybris *der totalen Reflexion*".[10] Die Anerkennung der Tatsache, dass wir notwendig vergessen müssen, um überhaupt sinnvoll erinnern zu können,[11] ist eine Bedrohung für den Anspruch, alles reflexiv und rational beherrschen zu können. Die Anerkennung der Tatsache, dass das Vergessen nicht immer schon per se negativ sein muss, kann aber auch deutlich machen, dass das Vergessen, selbst wenn es nicht steuerbar ist, man also nicht vergessen will, nicht *nur* eine Bedrohung darstellen muss.

Arno Geiger gelingt es – bei aller Bedrohlichkeit des Vergessens –, zu zeigen, wie der nach und nach verschwindende Mann, den er portraitiert, zugleich in manchen Momenten auf eine verwirrende Art und Weise viel präsenter und viel mehr bei sich selbst, aber auch bei den ihm nahestehenden anderen zu sein scheint, als vor seiner Erkrankung. Seine Äußerungen sind durch ein Zerbrechen narrativer und logischer Strukturen gekennzeichnet, sie generieren aber dennoch Sinn und zeugen von einem tiefer liegenden, anderen Verständnis der Welt und der eigenen Identität. Vielleicht lässt sich hier eine ‚poetische', expressive, eher augenblickliche als kontinuierliche Sinneinheit der Person bzw. der Persönlichkeit als Alternative zur verlorenen diachronen Kohärenz des Selbstseins denken.

Vermittelt wird in Geigers Darstellung eine durchaus bewusste Wahrnehmung des eigenen Vergessens, das eben *auch*, aber nicht *nur* als Bedrohung empfunden wird. Da heißt es dann etwa:

> Nee – –nee. – – Es geht alles daneben. Wobei ich aber durchaus nicht unglücklich bin, dass ich manches nicht mehr beherrsche. Es ist einfach vorbei. Ich kann noch Freude haben, wenn anderen etwas gelingt. Aber meine Federn, die sind fort. (Geiger. *Der alte König in seinem Exil*, 158)

---

10 Ricœur. *Gedächtnis, Geschichte, Vergessen*, 634.

11 Anknüpfungspunkt ist hier noch tiefergehend auch Heideggers Voraussetzung, dass erst „auf dem Grund des Vergessens" überhaupt Erinnerung möglich wird. Vgl. Ricœur. *Gedächtnis, Geschichte, Vergessen*, 674.

Es ist ganz sicher kein Glück des Vergessens, das Geiger beschreibt, aber trotz des Vergessens, trotz des existenziellen Unglücks, das es mit sich bringt, bleiben Augenblicke des Glücks möglich: Es muss eben nicht mehr alles beherrscht und geplant werden, weder in der Reflexion noch im Handeln. Der Anspruch des Gelingens und der Kontrolle wird ebenso wie der Anspruch der Kohärenz anderen überlassen. Es bleiben Augenblicke einer *Selbstvergessenheit* als *Sorglosigkeit*, die kein Selbst*verlust* ist.[12] Und die Person, die sich selbst vergisst und alles vertauscht und verwechselt, bleibt dennoch eine eigenständige und unverwechselbare Persönlichkeit und sollte von anderen Personen zweifellos auch als eine solche behandelt werden.

Bibliographie

Calhoun, Cheshire. "Losing One's Self." In: Kim Atkins, Catriona Mackenzie (eds.). *Practical Identity and Narrative Agency*. New York/London: Routledge, 2008, 193–211.

Frankfurt, Harry. "Autonomie, Nötigung und Liebe." In: Monika Betzler, Barbara Guckes (eds.). *Harry G. Frankfurt. Freiheit und Selbstbestimmung*. Berlin: Akademie Verlag, 2001, 166–83.

Geiger, Arno. *Der alte König in seinem Exil*. München: Hanser, 2011.

Jaworska, Agnieszka. "Respecting the Margins of Agency: Alzheimer's Patients and the Capacity to Value." In: *Philosophy and Public Affairs* 28, 2 (1999): 105–38.

Locke, John: *Versuch über den menschlichen Verstand*. Buch II. Hamburg: Meiner, [5]2000, 419.

Quante, Michael. *Person*. Berlin/New York: de Gruyter, 2007.

Ricœur, Paul. *Das Rätsel der Vergangenheit. Erinnern, Vergessen, Verzeihen*. Übers. v. Andris Breitling u. Henrik R. Lesaar. Göttingen: Wallstein, 2004.

Ricœur, Paul. *Gedächtnis, Geschichte, Vergessen*. Übers. v. Hans-Dieter Gondek, Heinz Jatho u. Markus Sedlaczek. München: Wilhelm Fink, 2004.

Schechtman, Marya. *Staying Alive. Personal Identity, Practical Concerns, and the Unity of Life*. Oxford: Oxford University Press, 2014.

Spaemann, Robert. *Personen. Versuche über den Unterschied zwischen ‚etwas' und ‚jemand'*. Stuttgart: Klett-Cotta, 1996.

12 Zur These vom Glück des Vergessens als Glück der Selbstvergessenheit und Sorglosigkeit vgl. Ricœur. *Gedächtnis, Geschichte, Vergessen*, 775.

Daniela Ringkamp (Magdeburg)

Dementia, Autonomy and Practical Selfhood

Abstract: This paper argues for a weak understanding of diachronic unity as a basic element of personal identity. With reference to Jeff McMahan's notion of time-relative interests, it shows that dementia patients up to the second stage of the disease are able to perform the requirements that constitute this concept and that the discussions about prolonged and current autonomy in dementia can be enriched by it.

In addition to physical and psychological symptoms and in contrast to other mental diseases as for example schizophrenia, a permanent coma or a temporary disturbance of cognitive abilities, dementia is characterized by a gradual, but irreversible loss of mental capacities. These characteristics constitute major challenges concerning nursing issues and everyday care of dementia sufferers: Especially in the second and third stages of the disease a patient's interests and requirements may hardly be identified, and this problem can only partly be resolved if the patient has passed an Advance Directive before showing serious symptoms. Due to these difficulties, it is not surprising at all that much effort has been made to analyze the decision-making abilities of dementia sufferers. There is a series of studies which discusses the possibilities and limits of self-determination performed by dementia patients from an empirical viewpoint.[1] These investigations are correlated with examinations concerning the moral status of the patients, the justification of patient autonomy in dementia and possible interventions into the decision-making of the patients concerned.[2]

1 See for example Hughes, Julian C. "Assessment of Competency and Advanced Directives." In: Gabriela Stoppe (ed). *Competence Assessment in Dementia*. Wien: Springer, 2008, 77–84, van der Vorm, Anco, Olde Rikkert, Marcel GM. "Informed Consent in Dementia Research." In: Gabriela Stoppe (ed). *Competence Assessment in Dementia*. Wien: Springer, 2008, 85–91, Schütz, Holger, Heinrichs, Bert, Fuchs, Michael, Bauer, Andreas. "Informierte Einwilligung in der Demenzforschung. Eine qualitative Studie zum Informationsverständnis von Probanden." In: *Ethik in der Medizin* 28,2 (2016): 91–106.

2 The literature on this subject is indeed very extensive. See i.a. Jongsma, Karen. *Advanced Directives in Dementia Research. A Medical Ethical Inquiry*. Rotterdam: Erasmus University, 2016. De Grazia, David. *Human Identity and Bioethics*. New York: Cambridge University Press, 2005, 159–202, Birnbacher, Dieter. "Patientenverfügungen und Advance Care Planning bei Demenz und anderen kognitiven Beeinträchtigungen." In:

Comparatively few emphasis, however, has been placed on underlying assumptions about the personhood of dementia sufferers.[3] At first glance, this may not be surprising. In applied ethics, the ascription of personhood is – among other factors – used to address properties and abilities which explain a particular moral status of an entity, and the abilities which are mentioned in this respect are those which disappear in dementia: The capacity for self-consciousness, rational decision-making, a sense of one's biographical past and future, and others. From this perspective, a discussion of the personhood of dementia sufferers may be a futile endeavor at all. There are, however, two starting points for a meaningful examination of the personhood of dementia patients. First of all, the loss of mental capacities decreases gradually, in a process which is interrupted by stages of nearly full accountability, and there may be moments within the disease which provide a solid basis for ascribing the status of personhood to an individual patient. Secondly, a patient's previous interests, especially if they are articulated in an Advance Directive, cannot only be used to identify a patient's wishes, but also define person-making characteristics of the individual who has become ill, and which may even be valid during the disease. So an investigation of the personhood of dementia sufferers concerns – at least in part – central ethical problems and should be at issue in a philosophical engagement with the disease.

Ethik in der Medizin, First Online 01 April 2016, DOI: 10.1007/s00481-016-0388-6, Holm, Søren. "Autonomy, Authenticity, or Best Interest: Everyday Decision-making and Persons with Dementia." In: *Medicine, Health Care and Philosophy* 4,2 (2001): 153–59.

3 Some investigations in this regard are undertaken by Engelhardt and McMahan. For Engelhardt, dementia patients should be regarded as persons in a social sense. In contrast to persons in a strict sense, who qualify as full moral agents, persons in a social sense should be treated "as if they were persons." (Engelhardt, H. Tristram Jr. *The Foundation of Bioethics*. New York: Oxford University Press, ^{2}1996, 147). As social persons, dementia patients "do not have intrinsic moral standing", but are embedded in social practices which may also include utilitarian or consequentialist considerations (ibid.). McMahan holds that dementia sufferers could be seen as post-persons, "that begin to exist immediately upon the ceasing to exist of the person and continue [ ] to exist in association with the organism until the organism ceases to be capable of supporting consciousness and mental activity." (McMahan, Jeff. *The Ethics of Killing. Problems at the Margins of Life*. New York: Oxford University Press, 2002, 47) McMahan's position is indeed more complex than outlined here and will be analyzed in the second part of this paper. In addition, a connection between personhood and patient autonomy of dementia sufferers is drawn by Julian Hughes. See for this Hughes, Julian C. *Thinking Through Dementia*. Oxford: Oxford University Press, 2011.

The aim of this paper is to fill this gap between ethical investigations and the status of personhood to a minimal degree. In connection with approaches concerning their status of personhood, it seeks to analyze the decreasing potential for self-determination and decision-making of dementia sufferers. In doing so, it is motivated by the idea that at least in the first and second stages of the disease, the patients can still execute *some* of those capabilities which allow for ascribing the status of personhood to a human being. A central starting point in this context is the idea of diachronic identity as a basic ontological element of being a person in the course of time. By considering the special circumstances dementia patients are in, I will refer to abilities which enable a patient to perform a *weaker* sense of diachronic identity as it is demanded in more advanced accounts, and which is sufficient for performing self-determination within the disease. Due to the illness, however, a point will be reached at which even these person-making characteristics will have disappeared. The ascription of personhood to a dementia patient can therefore only be maintained for a specific period of the disease: Personhood is a phase-sortal which can be attributed to a human being for a certain period of time and maybe nearly for a lifetime, but no human being is a person throughout his or her whole life, and some human beings will never be a person at all.[4]

In the first part of the paper, I will show in how far questions concerning the personhood of dementia sufferers arise in practical situations. In this context, I will briefly point to the debate between Ronald Dworkin and Rebecca Dresser about the tension between prolonged and actual autonomy performed by dementia patients. As I would like to demonstrate, Dresser's account leads to a specific problem, which cannot be solved by those approaches favoured by Dworkin or other proponents of prolonged autonomy, and it is precisely at this point, in which an investigation about a patient's status of personhood is of importance. This is why a special concept of personal identity will be outlined in the second part – namely the position of Jeff McMahan: His account provides fundamental elements for elaborating a weaker concept of diachronic identity as a basic feature of personhood. In the third and last part of the paper, the impact of McMahan's position will be traced back to the notion of patient autonomy: It will be outlined

4 This does not mean that those human beings (and other animals), who cannot be regarded as persons, do not award any moral or legal protection at all. Ascribing the status of personhood to an entity is only one option for justifying moral protection. Further possibilities can be illustrated by referring to basic needs or a right to adequate care, which aims at securing the moral demands of these persons. To be discussed adequately, however, these issues require a separate discussion, which cannot be achieved in this paper.

how to conceive best the autonomy of dementia patients and in how far it can be extended to a concept of practical selfhood.

I. Prolonged and Actual Autonomy and the Examination of Personhood

Ronald Dworkin: Critical and Experiential Interests

Dworkin's analysis about autonomy and personhood of dementia patients is characterized by the distinction between critical and experiential interests, which can be applied to the former and actual situation of dementia sufferers.[5] A patient in later stages of the illness has so-called experiential interests, for example an interest in being nourished, an interest in experiencing pleasant emotions and closeness to others. Experiential interests presuppose emotional abilities, for instance the ability to perceive pleasant experiences, and can be faced by caring issues. Dworkin illustrates experiential interests by referring to Margo, a dementia patient in the later stages of the disease, who is visited by Andrew Firlik, a medical student. Dworkin holds that

> [t]he apartment had many locks to keep Margo from slipping out at night [...]. Margo said she knew who Firlik was each time he arrived, but she never used his name and he suspected that this was just politeness. She said that she was reading mysteries, but Firlik noticed 'that her place in the book jumps randomly from day to day.' [...] Margo attended an art class for Alzheimer's victims – they all, including her, painted pretty much the same picture every time, except near the end, just before death, when the pictures became more primitive. Firlik was confused, he said, by the fact that 'despite her illness, or somehow because of it, Margo is undeniable one of the happiest people I have ever known.' He reports, particularly, her pleasure at eating peanut-butter-and-jelly sandwiches [...]. (Dworkin. *Life's Dominion*, 221–22)

Margo still has got experiential interests – she feels pleasure at eating peanut butter sandwiches and is satisfied with painting pictures. This illustrates that experiential interests are given in the current stage of the disease and do not require enhanced mental capabilities. They correspond to a right of adequate care, by which they can be met, but do not respond to questions of autonomy and self-determination.

In contrast to experiential interests, critical interests require advanced rational abilities, for example the ability of situating the self in past, present and future, of self-determination and of realizing why certain values and options are preferred,

5 Dworkin, Ronald. *Life's Dominion. An Argument About Abortion, Euthanasia, and Individual Freedom*. New York: Random House, 1994, 201–08.

whereas others are rejected.[6] Critical interests express a person's concept of life, they enable us to place ourselves in our social environment and to perform our life according to the values we approve of. As they no longer possess the relevant abilities, critical interests cannot actively be maintained by dementia patients.[7] Nevertheless, critical interests *outlast* a patient's mental state. This is why – even though they are not actively perceived – former critical interests are still present in the later stages of dementia. They govern and control a patient's status with regard to his or her former opinions. According to this concept, self-determination of patients suffering from dementia is only possible with regard to their *former* decisions, as a particular type of *prolonged* autonomy, but not in their current situation, which misses the conditions for advanced autonomy and for articulating sustainable preferences.[8]

The distinction between critical and experiential interests leads to remarkable consequences if applied to specific situations. For Dworkin, only critical interests can be used in questions of patient autonomy, because only preferences which have been articulated in a state of advanced mental capabilities allow for self-determination. If Margo had established an advance directive before turning ill, and if this directive entailed that she does not want to receive medical treatment if she gets another, life-threatening disease, because life in a state of dementia is not compatible with her understanding of dignity and self-worth, then a medical treatment of a further disease has to be omitted, even if Margo shows signs of enjoying life. Nevertheless, Margo may receive pain relieving medications, for this is consistent with her positive experiential interests. Experiential interests, however, cannot override critical interests and cannot be used to answer questions which require a higher standard of rational abilities. This does not necessarily mean that relatives and medical professionals are obliged to act according to the directive. There may be other reasons for overriding it, but in doing so, Margo's autonomy would be disrespected:

> Should we really deny a person like that the routine medical care needed to keep her alive? Could we ever conceivably *kill* her? We might consider it morally unforgivable not to try to save the life of someone who plainly enjoys her life, no matter how demented she is, and we might think it beyond imagining that we should actually kill her. We might hate living in a community whose officials might make or license either of such a decision. We might have other good reasons for treating her as she now wishes, rather than, as, in my

6 Dworkin. *Life's Dominion*, 202–08, 215.
7 Dworkin. *Life's Dominion*, 232.
8 Dworkin. *Life's Dominion*, 226.

> imaginary case, she once asked. But still, that violates, rather than respects her autonomy. (Dworkin. *Life's Dominion*, 228–29)[9]

Rebecca Dresser: Emphasizing the Current Situation

Dworkin's position has frequently been criticized for its failure to observe the current state of dementia patients. One of the first and clearest criticism is from Rebecca Dresser. Dresser points out that critical and experiential interests cannot easily be distinguished from one another. Most of all, she criticizes that Dworkin devaluates experiential interests and does not consider changes between former and current preferences.[10] For her, the quality of life of the affected patients "is substantially dependent on their social and physical environments, as opposed to the neurological condition itself."[11] As a result, Dresser emphasizes the value of emotional engagement and argues for a right of self-determination, which is based on the current experiential preferences a dementia patient recognizes, even though the disease is already in an advanced state. Concerning Margo's case, Dresser comes to a different conclusion:

> Although substantially impaired, Margo retains capacities for pleasure, enjoyment, interaction, relationships and so forth. I believe her continued ability to participate in the life she is living furnishes a defensible basis for state limitations on the scope of her precedent autonomy, as well as on the choices her intimates make on her behalf. Contrary to Dworkin, I believe that such moral paternalism is justified when dementia patients have a quality of life comparable to Margo's. (Dresser. "Dworkin on Dementia," 36)

This argument in favour of Margo's current state is linked with a criticism on Dworkin's understanding of personal identity.[12] According to Dresser, Dworkin does not consider Margo as a person whose preferences may change within the course of life. For her, Dworkin adheres to a concept of personal identity which overestimates rational abilities. His view of identity is merely static and does not respect the special conditions of dementia. Preferences which are articulated

9 The first two questions in this quotation seem to combine the different aspects of actively killing a person and of letting a person die. This equation raises several conceptual and ethical problems and is frequently discussed in Medical Ethics. As I am primarily concerned with the conditions of autonomy performed by dementia patients and not with the distinction between active and passive euthanasia, I would only like to draw attention to this question without going into detail.

10 Dresser, Rebecca. "Dworkin on Dementia. Elegant Theory, Questionable Policy." In: *The Hastings Center Report* 25,6 (1995): 32–38, 34.

11 Dresser. "Dworkin on Dementia," 34.

12 Dresser. "Dworkin on Dementia," 35.

against the background of full mental capacities are still obligatory in a state in which they cannot be perceived at all: It is not possible to waive an adopted position and to withdraw from personal aims and wishes previously expressed.[13]

In contrast, Dresser argues that performing an identity must not necessarily be based on rational abilities. Rather, experiential interests of patients suffering from dementia have to be considered, even though they disagree with previous critical interests and are articulated in a state of decreasing mental acquirements. In this case, the loss of a person's intellectual faculties has to be managed by a concept of relational, extended autonomy, which demands other persons' activities.[14]

Regarding this, it becomes apparent that Dresser's understanding of personhood entails essentialist assumptions, according to which every human being has to be regarded as a person during his or her whole life.[15] Due to his anthropological constitution as a person situated in social contexts, passing the status of personhood is impossible. A central feature of being a person is to be integrated into a social environment, which is encouraged to uphold and to secure the basic interests of the impaired person. Waiving this social embeddedness is impossible both for the members of a social community as well as for the affected dementia

---

13 In doing so, Dresser argues for a response shift performed by dementia patients. A response shift is defined "as the change in self-evaluation of QoL [Quality of Life, D.R.] as a result of a change in 1) the respondent's internal standards of measurement [...], 2) the respondent's values [...] or 3) the meaning of QoL [...] by the respondent" (Jongsma. *Advance Directives in Dementia Research*, 67). The changes within preferences and wishes in the state of dementia, as they are observed by Dresser, could be regarded as a form of response shift. Jongsma, however, denies the possibility of articulating response shifts by dementia sufferers. Next to questions concerning validity and reliability she holds that especially in advanced stages dementia patients "are cognitively unable to provide self-reports of their QoL." (Ibid., 70)

14 Dresser. "Dworkin on Dementia," 37.

15 A main characterization of person essentialism is that if "we are essentially persons, then we cannot exist as nonpersons" (De Grazia, *Human Identity and Bioethics*, 12). Concerning this approach, personhood has to be understood as a necessary property of a being insofar as this thing or being cannot exist without having the property of personhood at all (ibid. 25). Dresser seems to support this account, because for her being a person does not depend on mental capabilities, but belongs to every member of the human species as such. It should be conceded that even Dworkin classifies his approach in the terms of person essentialism. As critical interests still hold for those cases in which they are not yet understood by a patient, they are still present even in the later stages of the disease and cannot be rejected. This is why "personal identity does survive even the most serious dementia." (Dworkin, Ronald. "Autonomy and the Demented Self." In: *The Milbank Quarterly* 64,2 (1986): 4–16, 5.

sufferer.[16] It therefore depends on the relatives, carers and medical professionals to make decisions which meet the best interests of a person. What may be in the best interest of a patient has to be determined from case to case by taking into consideration a person's former wishes, but also by valuing the current situation. In the case of Margo, Dresser points out that Margo's best interest would be met by a medical treatment of the further, life-threatening disease, even if this contradicts with her former wishes.

Even though some of the objections to Dworkin's distinction between critical and experiential interests may be justified, Dresser's position also causes problems. Whereas Dworkin does not consider the actual state of dementia patients, Dresser ignores their former state and those interests and values which have been important for a person before he or she suffered from the disease. But what is more important is that Dresser makes the mistake to conclude from the bare existence of positive experiential interests to a general interest in living on. However, an interest to live on presupposes an understanding of one's future existence, a minimal sense of time and how one would like to live with the disease in a couple of months, a year, or two.[17] It is this understanding of one's future existence and one's own relation to dementia disorders which cannot necessarily be ascribed to every dementia patient with positive experiential interests. In this case, Dworkin's account is more convincing.

To face the self-determination of dementia patients in an adequate way, it is necessary to balance the moral requirements of previous and actual autonomy. Unlike Dworkin, it must be considered that the mental abilities of patients suffering from dementia do not decrease suddenly, but are still partly given in the later stages of the disease. Contrary to Dresser, however, actual autonomy is limited by these decreasing cognitive capacities, which make a complex decision-making

16 Some proponents of this position also emphasize the embeddedness of embryos and fetuses as beings with a status of personhood, because they descend from human parents: From the moment of procreation on, every biological member of the human species has to be regarded as a person with an advanced moral status. See e.g. Spaemann, Robert. "Gezeugt, nicht gemacht." *Die Zeit* 18.1.2001. <http://www.zeit.de/2001/04/200104_klon.xml> (last access 07.09.2016).

17 This is also pointed out by Ralf Jox, who objects that the existence of positive experiential interests should not be confounded with an interest to live on: For him, there is a couple of very elderly people who state that they are feeling well but nonetheless refuse life-extending medical treatment. Concerning this see Jox, Ralf J. "Der 'natürliche Wille' bei Kindern und Demenzkranken. Kritik an einer Aufdehnung des Autonomiebegriffs." In: Claudia Wiesemann, Alfred Simon (eds.). *Patientenautonomie. Theoretische Grundlagen, Praktische Anwendungen.* Mentis, 2013, 329–39, 335.

more difficult than it is anticipated by her. An adequate approach has to consider both aspects: It should be sensitive if there is a sound basis for rejecting a person's former wishes, but it should also respect those preferences, which have been established in a process of prolonged decision-making. The abilities which are necessary within these deliberations transcend experiential interests and should at least imply a relation to oneself and an understanding of the future. When it comes to answering questions that concern a person's survival in a couple of years, this person should be able to grasp what it means to live on with the impairments of the illness and to react to it.

II. Personhood and Evaluative Self-Relations

It has been shown that the ability to understand and to evaluate one's future constitute an essential condition to confirm or to withdraw those views previously expressed in a state of full mental capacities. In the following part of the paper, two positions will be discussed which regard the relation to one's future as a fundamental element of ascribing the status of personhood to an entity. At first glance, it seems as if both approaches require advanced rational abilities to perform this relation. On closer examination, however, it becomes clear that the positions can be maintained even if they only presume a weaker sense of diachronic identity instead of a strong one.

Person-making Characteristics: Prudential Unity Relation and Concern for the Future

Numerical identity – understood as the synchrone and diachrone unity of an entity at one resp. two different instants of time – is a central element of ontological investigations concerning the status of personhood. Within this discourse, it was Derek Parfit's provocative[18] proposal to separate the idea of identity from issues which "matter"[19] – for Parfit the survival of an entity, which could be demonstrated

18 This is the terminology of Michael Quante, who describes Parfit's position as provocative in comparison to former accounts concerning identity understood as diachronic unity in the course of time. See Quante, Michael. *Person*. Berlin: De Gruyter, [2]2012, 116.

19 Parfit concedes that the diachronic identity of a person in the course of time does not contribute to the question about what matters – about what is important in life. For Parfit, what matters is a person's survival. Survival is bound to psychological connectedness and psychological continuity as strong chains of psychological connections. Parfit develops his approach by introducing several thought experiments which aim at showing that hypothetical cases like brain splitting and implementing someone's brain

without referring to the concept of identity at all. Jeff McMahan adopts central elements of this approach: Like Parfit, he distinguishes between the idea of identity and those issues which are, beyond a mere ontological framework, of fundamental importance for every person. But whereas Parfit regards psychological continuity (and not the numeric identity of an organism) as the essential factor for living on, McMahan points to the "egoistic concern about the future"[20] resp. the so-called "prudential unity relations"[21] as central factors for continuing in life. These factors also constitute person-making characteristics: Being a person is bound to the existence of prudential unity relations as a central element of an individual's concern for his or her future.

Following McMahan, the relation which is constitutive for identity is "sufficient physical and functional continuity of the areas of the brain in which consciousness is realized in order for those areas to retain the capacity to support consciousness".[22] Identity is a relation of all or nothing, which does not occur in degrees: There are either sufficient functioning parts of the brain which constitute consciousness, or the cerebrum is so severely damaged that consciousness cannot be sustained. Prudential unity relations, in contrast, occur in degrees: Their strength and weakness can be determined in a process of consideration, but particularly they constitute egoistic concern for one's future, which is an essential characterization for persons.[23] As for Parfit, this "separation of the theory of identity and the theory of egoistic concern"[24] is of special importance even for McMahan. It illustrates the different scope between substantial and psychological elements. What matters for us is established by a psychological framework, by our concern for our future existence, which is a matter of degree.

Starting point for identifying the strength of a psychological unity relation are so-called time-relative interests. Time-relative interests are understood as those interests of a person which are given at a particular time in past or present, but which are related to a person's future.[25] They balance the anticipated value of future

into another body should be regarded as a form of survival and not as death. In this line of argument, a person's survival does not depend on numerical identity understood as continuity of the body, but only on psychological continuity. See Parfit, Derek. *Reasons and Persons*. New York: Oxford University Press, 1984, 255, 262, 289.

20 McMahan. *The Ethics of Killing*, 83.
21 McMahan. *The Ethics of Killing*, 74.
22 McMahan. *The Ethics of Killing*, 79.
23 McMahan. *The Ethics of Killing*, 42.
24 McMahan. *The Ethics of Killing*, 43.
25 McMahan. *The Ethics of Killing*, 80.

situations and the consequences of current actions and decisions for prospecting living-conditions. The strength of prudential unity relations depends on the strength of time-relative interests – the stronger the latter, the stronger are the prudential unity relations, which connect a person with his or her future existence. Transferred to the notion of egoistic concern for the future, this framework implies a proportional correlation between the strength of prudential unity relations and future concern.

Prudential unity relations can be given to a greater or lesser extend and can refer to one's future in different degrees. In addition, they do not require an advanced concept of psychological continuity but are also observable in at most loose connections between successive mental sequences. Prudential unity relations illustrate an evaluative attitude to oneself and one's individual future. With regard to dementia it should be considered that even dementia patients are able to obtain prudential unity relations:

> But cases involving deprogramming or progressive dementia suggest that neither [...] psychological connectedness nor [...] psychological continuity is *necessary* for egoistic concern. A person in the early stages of Alzheimer's disease has reason to be egoistically concerned about what may happen to his body even in the final phases in which the mental life associated with his body will no longer be even weakly psychologically connected from day to day. (McMahan. *The Ethics of Killing*, 66–67)

The expression of an egoistic concern for one's future, however, is not only possible for patients at the onset but also for dementia sufferers in the later stages of the disease:

> There seems to be a minimal basis for egoistic concern for the future even when the structural organization of the brain that underlies psychological connectedness and continuity will be destroyed – as often happens over the course of progressive dementia. If this is right, organizational continuity is not a necessary condition of rational egoistic concern. (McMahan. *The Ethics of Killing*, 74)

Even in the later stages of Alzheimer's, when essential rational capacities can no longer be performed and the continuity between mental episodes decreases, a patient suffering from dementia is able to carry out prudential unity relations and – to a certain extend – to face his or her future from an evaluative position.

It is important to note that, in contrast to Dworkin, McMahan's approach does not necessarily presuppose a diachronic unity of a person's mental life as a continuum between past and future psychological connections. Egoistic concern for one's future can be realized without a deeper connection to a person's biographical past: Its main characterization is an evaluative attitude to current or future states. Besides this, an evaluation of one's future is also possible on the basis of only little or decreased rational skills. In how far a person is able to understand former wishes and if he or she is motivated by rational considerations is unimportant, as long as decisions are guided by an evaluative assessment of future situations or even of one's future existence at all. As the persons involved are discharged from advanced rational skills, a weaker concept of a person's diachronic unity, which relates current experiences to one's future existing without referring to the biographical past, is sufficient for performing an egoistic concern for the future.

Nevertheless – and this is important – developing an egoistic concern for one's future requires the presence of consistent volitions to a minimal degree. A permanent change of preferences does not only complicate the identification of stable expressions, it also shows that the person involved does not seem to have a clear understanding of his or her biographic future. This, however, is true, but it should be considered that at least up to a certain point in the disease the performance of almost consistent prudential unity relations is possible. To show this, the following section aims at illustrating in how far egoistic concern for the future as a central attitude of persons can be maintained in dementia. It will be illustrated that a central element of patient autonomy performed by dementia sufferers does not depend on advanced rational skills, but on evaluative judgements about the future.

Autonomy and the Capacity to Value

Considering the importance of egoistic concern for the future as a central element of an individual's status of personhood, it should be noted that the patient autonomy of dementia sufferers is not best expressed by cognitive skills, but by evaluative assessments. An example in how far evaluative elements can be integrated into a concept of patient autonomy is given by reference to the so-called capacity to value, as it is outlined by Agnieszka Jaworska. Core principle of this account is the distinction between critical interests and the capacity to value. This capacity is given if a dementia patient has lost most of his or her rational abilities, but is still able to perform normative judgements on a smaller scale. Exercising a capacity to value does not require to consider one's own life as a whole, as a continuity between past, present and future, as it is claimed by Dworkin.[26] Rather, it fills the gap between previous critical interests and experiential interests by addressing current preferences, which may be tied back or distinct from previous critical interests, but which allow for modelling *less* complex interests. These less complex interests cannot be equated with experiential or with former

26 Jaworska, Agnieszka. "Respecting the Margins of Agency. Alzheimer's Patients and the Capacity to Value." In: *Philosophy and Public Affairs* 28,2 (1999): 105–138, 113.

critical interests. They constitute an own category of interests, which illustrate the declining rational capacities of dementia sufferers, but are, nonetheless, linked to a certain degree of rationality, especially to evaluative attitudes. This is outlined by several examples. Dr. B., for instance, a dementia patient who could not recall the day of the week, the month or year, decided to participate in a study about Alzheimer's disease because his self-esteem was greater than it would be if he participated in regular group activities for dementia sufferers.[27] Another patient who had great difficulties in answering questions about what he did that day described and evaluated the decline of his mental abilities with the comment "Here you can see Alzheimer's at work."[28] In both cases, the patients situate themselves in their social environment and value their current situation. They show an engagement which goes far beyond the scope of experiential interests and which – at least in the case of Dr. B. – extends into their future.

In spite of this all, performing a capacity to value does not require developing a concept of one's life as a whole, about the similarities and differences to one's previous life. It allows, unlike Dworkin's position, changes between former critical interests and those current interests which are articulated on the basis of valuing. As such, it constitutes a minimal condition for performing autonomy:

> [P]ossessing the capacity to value does not guarantee that the person can exercise autonomy to a full degree. Full-blown autonomy involves not only acting on one's own principles and convictions, but also the ability to scrutinize these principles and convictions and to revise them in light of critical evaluation, so that they are well-articulated and robust. The capacity to value merely makes possible the most minimal and basic level of autonomy; other capacities are necessary to further develop and perfect autonomy. (Jaworska. "Respecting the Margins of Agency," 130)

As it exemplifies a basic level of autonomy, the capacity to value implies more than desiring, for example craving for food items. Values are distinct from mere wishes, habits and positive or negative sentiments, which are the core issue in experiential interests. According to Jaworska, there is a central difference between values and wishes: Values are situated "in a larger normative framework"[29] and "express the person's concern with something fully independent of himself".[30] Although even values are articulated in current situations, they are more abstract than wishes or desires, because they presuppose an identification with norms or conditions

27 Jaworska. "Respecting the Margins of Agency," 118.
28 Jaworska. "Respecting the Margins of Agency," 114.
29 Jaworska. "Respecting the Margins of Agency," 115.
30 Jaworska. "Respecting the Margins of Agency," 116.

which are supported or disliked. Losing the ability to perform values would be regretted differently than the nonfulfillment of desires. Values are linked with a sense of self-worth and practical identity:

> Another mark of valuing as opposed to mere desiring is that a person's values are usually entangled with her sense of self-worth: A person values *herself* in terms of how well she lives up to her values. [...]. Anyone who has a conception of herself, a set of ideals that she wants to live up and in virtue of which she assesses her own value, is no doubt a valuer. (Jaworska. "Respecting the Margins of Agency," 115–16)

It is this practical identity which marks the difference between valuing and desiring as the core principle in experiential interests. Valuing enables a patient to situate him- or herself in a normative position to the disease: Most of the examples Jaworska introduces to outline the capacity to value discuss a patient's attitude to dementia as such. It is important to note that this self-reference of a patient concerning his or her illness allows, at least indirectly, for indicating an interest in living on: If the current stage of illness is evaluated positively, there are good reasons to assume that a dementia sufferer shows an interest in a further existence, even though he or she has rejected medical treatment in an advanced directive before turning ill. An example for this distance from previous interests can be seen in the case of Walter Jens, who, before turning ill, stated that he does not want to receive medical treatment with life-extending effects if he should ever suffer from dementia. As his wife and his son report, Walter Jens, who died at the age of 90 in an advanced state of dementia, expressed his withdrawal from former decisions: "Nicht töten"[31] – don't kill – he claimed in a condition in which he was already severely influenced by his Alzheimer's disease.

A situation like this would allow for exercising medical treatment, even though a dementia sufferer has rejected it before in an advance directive: It is the positive evaluation of one's future existence, which indicates an interest to live on. In this regard, the positive assessment of one's future is one form of perceiving prudential unity relations, which tie a patient to his or her prospective existence and which express egoistic concern for their future. Prudential unity relations as a core element of performing selfhood and the capacity to value constitute a relation between personhood and autonomy, between a patient's sense of self and self-governing expressions, which go beyond experiential interests.

---

31 Koelbl, Herlinde. "Er versank vor meinen Augen buchstäblich im Nichts." Interview with Inge Jens. *Die Zeit* 6.2.2014 <http://www.zeit.de/2014/07/rettung-inge-jens/komplettansicht> (last access 07.09.2016).

III. Prospective Considerations: Dementia and Practical Selfhood

The capacity to value and the ability to perform prudential unity relations can be extended to a concept of practical selfhood as an indication for the existence of personhood at all. In his book *Sources of the Self* from 1989 Charles Taylor outlines an understanding of human selfhood which grounds on concerns about the meaningfulness of one's life. Taylor holds that "living with [...] qualified horizons is constitutive of human agency, [...] stepping outside these limits would be tantamount to stepping outside what we would recognize as integral, that is, undamaged human personhood."[32] A qualified horizon is maintained by a person if he or she articulates moral judgements, intuitions or reactions and performs a moral response[33] to situations in the social environment or other challenges he or she has to cope with. The main feature for maintaining a relation to oneself is a sense of self-worth and of situating oneself in a moral space of qualitative decision-making. This concept of selfhood corresponds both to prudential unity relations as well as to the capacity to value. Being a person who performs prudential unity relations and exercises the capacity to value presupposes a relation to oneself, and, in some cases, even a relation to one's disease.

In contrast to Dworkin, self-referential attitudes can also be established on the basis of a weak concept of diachronic unity. The main element of exercising self-reflective judgements, as they are outlined by Taylor, is the ability to evaluate situations and living conditions and to relate oneself to them. These achievements do not need to be embedded in a person's biographic past; they only require an understanding about the scope of one's actions and decisions for the immediate future. The ability to express self-referential actions ends with the incapability of representing at least temporarily consistent opinions and may therefore only be performed by dementia sufferers in the first and second but not in the third stage of their illness. Nevertheless, Taylor's understanding of selfhood is *not only* applicable for describing the self-relation of persons *without* mental diseases. Providing "the horizon within which we know where we stand",[34] these relations can be maintained *without* referring to more advanced rational capacities. Keeping a relation to oneself as a valuer and valuing one's living conditions in and with dementia already fulfils the conditions for developing a sense of selfhood

32 Taylor, Charles. *Sources of the Self: The Making of Modern Identity*. Cambridge: Cambridge University Press, 1989, 27.

33 Taylor. *Sources of the Self*, 26.

34 Taylor. *Sources of the Self*, 29.

and self-worth. As far as these notions are given, we have good reasons to regard patients suffering from dementia as persons.

References

Birnbacher, Dieter. "Patientenverfügungen und Advance Care Planning bei Demenz und anderen kognitiven Beeinträchtigungen." In: *Ethik in der Medizin*, First Online 01 April 2016, DOI: 10.1007/s00481-016-0388-6.

De Grazia, David. *Human Identity and Bioethics*. New York: Cambridge University Press, 2005.

Dresser, Rebecca. "Dworkin on Dementia. Elegant Theory, Questionable Policy." In: *The Hastings Center Report* 25,6 (1995): 32–38.

Dworkin, Ronald. *Life's Dominion. An Argument About Abortion, Euthanasia, and Individual Freedom*. New York: Random House, 1994.

Dworkin, Ronald. "Autonomy and the Demented Self". In: *The Milbank Quarterly* 64,2 (1986): 4–15.

Engelhardt, H. Tristram, Jr. *The Foundation of Bioethics*. New York: Oxford University Press, ^{2}1996.

Holm, Søren. "Autonomy, Authenticity, or Best Interest: Everyday Decision-making and Persons with Dementia." In: *Medicine, Health Care and Philosophy* 4,2 (2001): 153–59.

Hughes, Julian C. "Assessment of Competency and Advanced Directives." In: Gabriela Stoppe (ed). *Competence Assessment in Dementia*. Wien: Springer, 2008, 77–84.

Hughes, Julian C. *Thinking Through Dementia*. Oxford: Oxford University Press, 2011.

Jaworska, Agnieszka. "Respecting the Margins of Agency. Alzheimer's Patients and the Capacity to Value." In: *Philosophy and Public Affairs* 28,2 (1999): 105–38.

Jongsma, Karen. *Advanced Directives in Dementia Research. A Medical Ethical Inquiry*. Rotterdam: Erasmus University, 2016.

Jox, Ralf J. "Der ‚natürliche Wille' bei Kindern und Demenzkranken. Kritik an einer Aufdehnung des Autonomiebegriffs." In: Claudia Wiesemann, Alfred Simon (eds.). *Patientenautonomie. Theoretische Grundlagen, Praktische Anwendungen*. Münster: Mentis, 2013, 329–39.

Koelbl, Herlinde. "Er versank vor meinen Augen buchstäblich im Nichts." Interview with Inge Jens. *Die Zeit* 6.2.2014 <http://www.zeit.de/2014/07/rettung-inge-jens/komplettansicht> (last access 07.09.2016).

McMahan, Jeff. *The Ethics of Killing. Problems at the Margins of Life*. New York: Oxford University Press, 2002.

Parfit, Derek. *Reasons and Persons*. New York: Oxford University Press, 1984.

Quante, Michael. *Person*. Berlin: De Gruyter, [2]2012.

Schütz, Holger, Heinrichs, Bert, Fuchs, Michael, Bauer, Andreas. "Informierte Einwilligung in der Demenzforschung. Eine qualitative Studie zum Informationsverständnis von Probanden." In: *Ethik in der Medizin* 28,2 (2016): 91–106.

Spaemann, Robert. "Gezeugt, nicht gemacht." *Die Zeit* 18.1.2001 <http://www.zeit.de/2001/04/200104_klon.xml> (last access 07.09.2016).

Taylor, Charles. *Sources of the Self: The Making of Modern Identity*. Cambridge: Cambridge University Press, 1989.

van der Vorm, Anco, Olde Rikkert, Marcel GM. "Informed Consent in Dementia Research." In: Gabriela Stoppe (ed). *Competence Assessment in Dementia*. Wien: Springer, 2008, 85–91.

Oliver Hallich (Duisburg-Essen)

Dementia and the Principle of Precedent Autonomy

Abstract: Defenders of the view that advance directives are morally binding for dementia patients often invoke the principle of precedent autonomy to support their view. In this article, I contend that this principle provides no justificatory basis for overriding the current interests of the demented patient. This is why my answer to the question if advance directives in dementia are morally binding is a qualified "No".

Dementia has become a central problem for health care in modern societies. Currently, 47.5 million people worldwide have the disease, and it is projected that 75.6 million people will have it in 2030. The number of cases of dementia is estimated to more than triple by 2050.[1] Against this background, the question of the binding force of advance directives in dementia will be of growing importance in future years. Defenders of the view that dementia advance directives are morally binding often invoke the *principle of precedent autonomy* to support their view. According to this principle, it is the right of a competent individual to make decisions for a later time when competence has been lost. It is a specification of the more general principle of autonomy. Broadly speaking, the principle of autonomy claims that it is the right of the individual to make choices and take actions that reflect her own values and beliefs and that are free from controlling influences that determine her actions.[2] Extended over time and applied to cases of end-of-life decision-making,

1 These figures draw on estimations of the World Health Organisation, "10 Facts on Dementia," http://www.who.int/features/factfiles/dementia/en/ (last access 11.10.2015). The Alzheimer's Association, "Alzheimer's Disease Facts and Figures," *Alzheimer's & Dementia* 2015, <http://www.alzheimers.org.uk/site/scripts/documents_info.php?documentID=412.> (last access 11.10.2015) provides detailed U.S.-related data on the prevalence of dementia. For its prevalence in the U.K., see the annual report of the Alzheimer's Society, "Dementia 2014 Report. Statistics," http://www.alz.co.uk/research/statistics (last access 11.10.2015). For a general overview on the prevalence of dementia, see Jennings, Bruce. "Alzheimer's Disease: Quality of Life and the Goals of Care." In: John Arras, Elizabeth Fenton, Rebecca Kukla (eds.). *The Routledge Companion to Bioethics*. New York/London: Routledge, 2015, 437–48, 437.

2 For a classical exposition of the principle of autonomy, see, e.g., Feinberg, Joel. *Harm to Self. The Moral Limits of the Criminal Law 3*. Oxford: Oxford University Press, 1986, 27–97 (chap. 18, 19); Faden, Ruth, Beauchamp, Tom. *A History and Theory of Informed*

it requires respecting every individual's right to determine treatment in later stages of her life, including stages in which she has lost competence.[3]

In this article, I will cast a critical light on the principle of precedent autonomy. Though I will not dismiss it as wrong *sans phrase*, I contend that it does not have the justificatory role for medical decisions that many philosophers ascribe to it. In particular, I argue that it provides no justificatory basis for overriding the current interests of the demented patient if these run counter to the interests the

---

Consent. Oxford: Oxford University Press, 1986, 235–73 (chap. 7); Beauchamp, Tom, Childress, James. *Principles of Biomedical Ethics.* Oxford: Oxford University Press, [7]2013, 101–49 (chap. 4).

3 The most prominent defenders of the principle of precedent autonomy are Rhoden, Nancy. "The Limits of Legal Objectivity." In: *North Carolina Law Review* 68 (1990): 845–65; Dworkin, Ronald. *Life's Dominion. An Argument about Abortion, Euthanasia, and Individual Freedom.* New York: Vintage, 1994, 218–41 (chap. 8); Cantor, Norman. "Prospective Autonomy: On the Limits of Shaping One's Postcompetent Medical Fate." In: *Journal of Contemporary Health Law & Policy* 8 (1992): 13–48; Cantor, Norman. *Making Medical Decisions for the Profoundly Disabled.* Boston, MA: MIT Press, 2005, 27–8; Quante, Michael. *Personales Leben und menschlicher Tod. Personale Identität als Prinzip der biomedizinischen Ethik.* Frankfurt: Suhrkamp, 2002, 268–95 (chap. 7); Davis, John. "The Concept of Precedent Autonomy." In: *Bioethics* 16 (2002): 114–33; Davis, John. "Precedent Autonomy and Subsequent Consent." In: *Ethical Theory and Moral Practice* 7 (2004): 267–91; Davis, John. "Precedent Autonomy, Advance Directives, and End-of-Life Care." In: Bonnie Steinbock (ed.). *Oxford Handbook of Bioethics.* Oxford: Oxford University Press, 2009, 349–74; King, Nancy. *Making Sense of Advance Directives.* Washington: Georgetown University Press, 2007, 76–107 (chap. 3). The most persistent critics of the principle of precedent autonomy are Rebecca Dresser and John Robertson; see Dresser, Rebecca. "Bound to Treatment: The Ulysses Contract." In: *The Hastings Center Report* 14 (1984): 13–16; Dresser, Rebecca. "Life, Death, and Incompetent Patients: Conceptual Infirmities and Hidden Values in the Law." In: *Arizona Law Review* 28 (1986): 373–405; Dresser, Rebecca. "Missing Persons: Legal Perceptions of Incompetent Patients." In: *Rutgers Law Review* 46 (1994): 609–719; Dresser, Rebecca. "Dworkin on Dementia: Elegant Theory, Questionable Policy." In: *The Hastings Center Report* 25 (1995): 32–8; Dresser, Rebecca, Robertson, John. "Quality of Life and Non-Treatment Decisions for Incompetent Patients: A Critique of the Orthodox Approach." In: *Law, Medicine & Health Care* 17 (1989): 234–44; Robertson, John. "Second Thoughts on Living Wills." In: *The Hastings Center Report* 21 (1991): 6–9; see also Buchanan, Allen, Brock, Dan. *Deciding for Others. The Ethics of Surrogate Decision Making.* Cambridge: Cambridge University Press, 1990, 101–12. Instead of "precedent autonomy", some authors use terms like "prospective autonomy", "future-oriented autonomy" (Cantor, "Prospective Autonomy") or "prolonged autonomy" (Quante, *Personales Leben und menschlicher Tod*, 268–95).

patient formerly expressed in her advance directive. In part (1), I pave the way for a criticism of the principle of precedent autonomy by laying bare its fundamental premiss, which I shall call the "dominance thesis", according to which in cases of a conflict between critical and experiential interests, the former override the latter. In part (2), I distinguish between various ways in which critical and experiential interests may relate to each other, and I argue that the dominance thesis holds true only with regard to some, not all of these constellations. In part (3), I focus on a specific scenario in which the dominance thesis turns out to be false: in some cases of a conflict between critical and experiential interests, the latter ones negate the normative authority of the former ones. In part (4), I attempt to rebut three objections to this view. Part (5) contains some concluding remarks concerning the normative question of whether advance directives in dementia are morally binding or not – to which my answer is a qualified "No".

I. The Principle of Precedent Autonomy and the "Dominance Thesis"

The principle of precedent autonomy rests on a premiss which I propose to call the "dominance thesis". The dominance thesis holds that in cases of a conflict between two kinds of interests, namely critical and experiential interests, interests of the first kind override or "dominate" those of the second kind. The distinction between critical and experiential interests was famously introduced by Ronald Dworkin.[4] Both kinds of interests, Dworkin argues, are "reasons people have for wanting their lives to go one way rather than another"[5]. Experiential interests are interests whose fulfillment consists in experiences, be it the experience of listening to a Mozart symphony, of enjoying food, of meditating over a complex chess problem or of having sex. These interests are time-sensitive in the sense that a person believes the experience to be desirable only when she actually has the experiential interest. Critical interests, by contrast, stem from judgements about what makes a life valuable. The fulfillment of these interests is not tied to actual experiences. Rather, they are interests that define our life plans and determine how we think we ought to live. They serve to guide and control our experiential interests. A person may have a critical interest in promoting science, in leading a

---

4 Dworkin. *Life's Dominion*, 201–11. For a more detailed discussion of this influential distinction, see, e.g., Dresser. "Dworkin on Dementia," 35–6; Jaworska, Agnieszka. "Respecting the Margins of Agency: Alzheimer's Patients and the Capacity to Value." In: *Philosophy & Public Affairs* 28 (1999): 105–38.

5 Dworkin. *Life's Dominion*, 201.

healthy life, in being useful to her fellow beings, in maximizing her own welfare, in maintaining close friendships or in retaining her sexual purity. These interests are normative in the sense that they relate to projects the person thinks she ought to pursue and which she thinks make her life valuable and worthwhile.

It is possible that a person can lose her ability to form critical interests while still being able to entertain experiential interests. In some stages of dementia, for example, the demented patient can lose the ability to form critical interests, but may still have experiential interests. She may enjoy good food and feel basic pleasures, such as pleasure involved in attempting to communicate or in plays. These experiential interests need not, but may run contrary to the critical interests the once competent person expressed in her advance directive. Whereas the competent person may have expressed the wish that, should she ever be in a state of dementia, life-sustaining treatment ought to be withheld, the experiential interests of the demented patient may be indicative of the wish that life-sustaining treatment should be provided and that she should be given the opportunity to continue her life. In other words, the critical interests she once had as a competent person may clash with the experiential interests she now has as a demented patient.[6]

The dominance thesis claims that, should critical interests collide with experiential interests, the former interests trump the latter ones. Thus, we ought to respect them even at the price of acting against a person's present experiential interests. Evidently, this view has an impact on the question of the validity of advance directives pertaining to a state of dementia. Supposing that the dominance thesis is true, the experiential interests of the demented patient, should they be in conflict with former critical interests expressed in the advance directive, should be accorded less weight than the critical interests. Contravening experiential interests cannot then eliminate the normative authority of critical interests, and when treating the demented patient we ought to respect the preceding autonomous choices of the competent person as expressed in the advance directive. The requirement to respect her precedent autonomy would persist even though she is in a state in which she is no longer capable of making autonomous decisions. Any attempt to

6 This clash does not necessarily imply that the demented patient is no longer identical with the competent person who issued the advance directive. In this paper, I do not enter the complicated debate on advance directives and the personal identity problem. For a detailed discussion of this problem, see, e.g., Buchanan, Allen. "Advance Directives and the Personal Identity Problem." In: *Philosophy & Public Affairs* 17 (1988): 277–302; Buchanan and Brock, *Deciding for Others*, 152–89 (chap. 3); DeGrazia, David. *Human Identity and Bioethics*. Cambridge: Cambridge University Press, 2005, 159–202 (chap. 5).

negate her critical interests on the basis of her experiential interests would, on this reading, be a violation of her autonomy.[7]

II. The Relation between Critical and Experiential Interests – Various Constellations

Is the dominance thesis true? Should we therefore honor the critical interests embodied in advance directives in dementia? I do not think there is a clear-cut yes-or-no answer to these questions. Rather, I will adopt a context-dependent approach: as dementia is a complex phenomenon that comprises different stages,[8] we should allow for the possibility that the dominance thesis holds true in some cases but not in others.[9] It is therefore imperative to take a step back and to disentangle the various ways in which critical and experiential interests may relate to each other. Broadly speaking, we can distinguish between "no-conflict-cases" and "conflict-cases".

(A) *No-conflict-cases*: There are some scenarios in which critical and experiential interests do not conflict at all. In these cases, the dominance thesis, which presupposes such a conflict, is not applicable. We can distinguish between three sub-scenarios:

---

7 Most recently Buller, Tom. "Advance Consent, Critical Interests and Dementia Research." In: *Journal of Medical Ethics* 41 (2015): 701–07, esp. 702, embraces this view.

8 When talking about different stages of dementia, I refer to the "global deterioration scale for assessment of primary degenerative dementia" as developed by Reisberg, Barry, Ferris, Steven, de Leon, Mony and Crook, Thomas. "The Global Deterioration Scale for Assessment of Primary Degenerative Dementia." In: *American Journal of Psychiatry* 139 (1982): 1136–39. Reisberg et al. distinguish between the initial "forgetfulness phase", in which the deficit is primarily subjective but verifiable, the intermediate "confusional phase", in which the deficit is apparent to an objective observer, and the "late dementia phase", in which the patient can no longer survive without assistance. The first phase comprises stages 1 ("no cognitive decline") and 2 ("very mild cognitive decline"), the second stages 3 ("mild cognitive decline") and 4 ("moderate cognitive decline"), the third stages 5 ("moderately severe cognitive decline"), 6 ("severe cognitive decline") and 7 ("very severe cognitive decline") of the disease.

9 For a defence of a context-dependent approach to end-of-life decisions, see also Menzel, Paul, Steinbock, Bonnie. "Advance Directives, Dementia, and Physician-Assisted Death." In: *Journal of Law, Medicine and Ethics* 41 (2013): 484–500, esp. 485; Menzel, Paul, Chandler-Cramer, Colette. "Advance Directives, Dementia, and Withholding Food and Water by Mouth." In: *The Hastings Center Report* 44 (2014): 23–37, esp. 33–34.

(A1) *Concordance*: Critical interests may be consonant with experiential interests. A person may have a critical interest in leading a healthy life and have an experiential interest in eating salads and vegetables. Another person may aspire to leading an ascetic and "pure" life devoted to religious ideals, and this critical interest may coincide with the absence of any sexual desire and an experiential interest in abstaining from sexual relationships. In these cases, it would be inappropriate to talk of critical interests dominating experiential interests. Both kinds of interests match, and the question whether critical interests dominate experiential interests is inapposite.

(A2) *Post-mortem interests*: It may also be the case that there is no conflict between critical and experiential interests because a person's critical interests relate to a state in which she has no interests whatsoever. A person may have a critical interest in increasing the welfare of others and therefore consent to donate her organs to those in need of them after her death. Or she may, in her last will, declare her wish that all her property be given to charity organizations. These interests pertain to states in which the person who holds them will be dead, i.e. will have no interests of any kind. One is inclined to say that in these cases, we ought to respect the person's critical interests after her death. However, it would be wrong to say that her critical interests override her experiential interests, since there are no experiential interests that could be overridden. In the absence of a conflict between critical and experiential interests, the question whether we ought to subordinate experiential interests to critical ones does not arise.

Post-mortem directives of this kind provide an important insight: critical interests do not (necessarily) cease to be authoritative if these interests cease to exist. If there is an obligation to honor them, the mere fact that their fulfillment or non-fulfillment no longer affects the well-being of the subject does not cancel the obligation.[10] With regard to advance directives in dementia, this means that the mere fact that a late stage demented person, having lost competence, no longer has

10 For a defence of this claim, see also McMahan, Jeff. *The Ethics of Killing. Problems at the Margins of Life.* Oxford: Oxford University Press, 2002, 497. Menzel and Steinbock write that critical interests still "exist [...] even after one no longer experiences them" (Menzel, Steinbock. "Advance Directives, Dementia, and Physician-Assisted Death," 489). Buchanan labels these interests "surviving interests" (Buchanan. "Advance Directives and the Personal Identity Problem," 287); see also Buchanan, Brock. *Deciding for Others*, 162–64. According to Davis, interests can "survive" as long as it is nomologically possible for the interest holder to regain competence (Davis. "Precedent Autonomy, Advance Directives, and End-of-Life Care," 367–71). To say that interests still "exist" after the death of the interest holder strikes me as counterintuitive. It would mean that

critical interests does not imply that there is no obligation to respect the critical interests of the once competent person. Rather, additional argument is needed to show that the preceding critical interests of the once competent person ought not to be respected when this person is deprived of her cognitive abilities, i.e. loses her capacity to form critical interests.

(A3) *No contravening interests*: A person's critical interests may relate to a state in which the person, lacking the ability to form critical interests, still has experiential interests, but only experiential interests that do not run contrary to the preceding critical interests. Some advance directives in dementia exemplify this possibility. A person may write an advance directive in which she requests to withhold water and food by mouth in late stage dementia. In that state of advanced dementia, she may either resist eating and drinking – that is, her current interests may align with the directive – or she may not resist eating and drinking but not desire to eat and drink either. The first case is a Concordance Case. In the latter case, her will, based on her experiential interests, is neutral with regard to the will that she expressed in the advance directive. The person's current will does not align with her former critical interest, but it does not run contrary to it either.[11]

For the same reason that I just mentioned with regard to post-mortem directives, there is no compelling argument against respecting advance directives in these cases. As critical interests do not lose their authority simply because they cease to exist, nothing speaks against respecting the former wishes of the competent person as long as the demented patient does not exhibit any signs of an interest that stands in opposition to his former critical interests. If the patient's current interests align with her former critical interests or at least do not run counter to them, we have to respect her former critical interests to the extent that we have to respect her autonomy. Therefore, in the absence of any evidence to the contrary, we ought to honor advance directives that are expressive of these critical interests. Nevertheless, it would be wrong to say that the patient's former critical interests dominate her experiential interests. There is no conflict between these two kinds of interests in the first place, and in the absence of such a conflict, the question whether we ought to subordinate experiential interests to critical ones does not arise.

---

we have no way of setting limits to the persistence of interests. Do we really want to say that Julius Caesar, anno 2015, still has an interest in not being murdered?

11 For a more detailed description of these cases, see Menzel, Steinbock. "Advance Directives, Dementia, and Physician-Assisted Death," 493; Menzel, Chandler-Cramer. "Advance Directives, Dementia, and Withholding Food and Water by Mouth," 25, 27.

(B) *Conflict-cases*: It may be the case that there is a conflict between critical and experiential interests. Two kinds of conflict are possible: the colliding interests may exist contemporaneously or they may exist at different times.

(B1) *Simultaneous conflict*: In cases of a simultaneous conflict, critical and experiential interests exist at the same time. Leading a healthy life may be central to a person's conception of a good life, but while having a critical interest in living healthily she may also have an experiential interest connected to a strong desire to smoke a cigarette. Someone may have a critical interest in being a faithful spouse but also feel strongly tempted to commit an act of adultery and have an experiential interest in doing so. Or someone may have a critical interest in promoting science even at the expense of her personal well-being while having an experiential interest in taking an extended holiday rather than working.

In these cases of a contemporaneous conflict between critical and experiential interests, the authority of critical interests remains untouched by contravening experiential interests. The reason is that critical interests are (in part) *defined* as interests whose function is to control experiential interests. Being normative in nature, they are interests concerning what we ought to do, not interests in pleasurable experiences. To have a critical interest in promoting science means, among other things, to have a (critical) interest in (sometimes) not fulfilling those experiential interests that run contrary it.[12] Therefore, the normative authority of critical interests is not negated by concomitant, but contravening experiential interests. (To say that critical interests retain their normative authority is, of course, not to say that they will necessarily be action-guiding, for cases of weakness of will are always possible.) Since critical interests are those a person thinks she ought to act upon even in the light of contravening experiential interests, it is analytically true that to have a critical interest means to have an interest in not following (some) experiential interests.

(B2) *Non-simultaneous conflict*: There may, however, also be a non-simultaneous conflict between critical and experiential interests: for example, a person may lose her ability to have critical interests, but still have experiential interests, and these latter interests may run contrary to the critical interests the person had when she was a competent person. At an earlier point of time t_1, a person P may have a critical interest that at a later point of time t_2 action A should be performed, while at t_2, P, having lost competence, no longer has any critical interest, but still has an experiential interest, namely the experiential interest that A should *not*

12 See Buller. "Advance Consent, Critical Interests and Dementia Research," 702.

be performed. These kinds of conflict occur when the experiential interests of a demented patient run contrary to the critical interests that she expressed in the advance directive as a competent person. In these cases, it is no longer analytically true that critical interests are more authoritative than experiential ones. Whereas to actually *have* a critical interest means to have an interest that is designed to control our experiential interests, *having had* a critical interest that is in conflict with one's current desires and wishes does not necessarily imply the normative authority of the now lost critical interests over the still existent experiential interests. Do critical interests dominate experiential interests in these cases? To answer this question, another distinction is called for, namely the distinction between a transitory and a permanent loss of competence.

(B2a) *Transitory loss of competence*: A first stage in which a person is competent may be followed by a second stage in which this person loses her competence and then by a third stage in which the person regains her competence. At t_1, a competent person may have the critical interest to lead a healthy and normal life. At t_2, under the influence of severe psychosis or severe depression, she may, deprived of her cognitive capacities, have the experiential interest in injuring herself. At t_3, having regained her competence, she may have a critical interest similar to the one she had at t_1 and therefore be grateful that the experiential interest she had at t_2 was not fulfilled.

A famous example of this constellation is the case of Ulysses: Ulysses, at t_1, has a critical interest in preserving his life and in *not* following the death-bringing chant of the Sirens (which we may take as a metaphor for a temporary psychosis). He therefore orders his mates to tie him to the mast and to ignore his later pleas to release him. At t_2, Ulysses has an experiential interest in following the chant of the Sirens, but, being tied to the mast by his companions, is prevented from fulfilling it. At t_3, Ulysses, now no longer within the reach of the Sirens, regains his critical interest in preserving his life and therefore retrospectively welcomes that at t_2 his mates hindered him from following the chant of the Sirens. Thus, at t_2, Ulysses, having lost his ability to form critical interests, has an experiential interest that runs counter to his former critical interest, while at t_3, having regained his ability to form critical interests, he has a critical interest similar to the one he had at t_1.[13]

13 For a more detailed discussion of the Ulysses scenarios, see Dresser, "Bound to Treatment: The Ulysses Contract"; Quante, *Personales Leben und menschlicher Tod*, 287–90; Davis, "Precedent Autonomy and Subsequent Consent", 288–9; Elster, Jon. *Ulysses Unbound. Studies in Rationality, Precommitment, and Constraints.* Cambridge: Cambridge University Press, 2010; Hallich, Oliver. "Selbstbindungen und medizinischer

Some advance directives in dementia have the structure of Ulysses instructions. More precisely, this characterization applies to advance directives that relate to the early onset stages of dementia, most notably to stage 2 according to the "global deterioration scale" ("very mild cognitive decline"), in which the patient complains of memory deficits but is still clearly a competent person and shows appropriate concern about the symptoms of the disease. Imagine that a fully competent person, having undergone presymptomatic testing which indicates the onset of the disease before its symptoms are manifest,[14] anticipates that in the "phase of forgetfulness" she will show the first symptoms of dementia. She may fear that in this stage she will fail to perform certain tasks, that she will become aggressive because of a loss of impulse control, or that she will misplace an object of value. She may then instruct others to prevent her, if necessary by force, from doing harm in one of the anticipated ways. For example, she may instruct them to place the object of value beyond her reach or to administer, even by force, sedative drugs if she shows signs of aggressive behavior. Later, in a phase of temporarily receding lucidity in which she regains her impulse control and competence, she may welcome that someone hindered her from following her aggressive impulses or from misplacing the object of value in the preceding phase of incompetence.

With regard to these cases, we are inclined to judge that it is morally legitimate, perhaps even morally required, to disregard the demented patient's current experiential interests that run counter to her former critical interests. We usually find it morally unobjectionable and legitimate to override a psychotic patient's interest to injure herself, Ulysses' interest to be released from the mast or the early stage demented patient's impulse to be aggressive or to misplace an object of value. Does this mean that in these cases critical interests dominate later experiential interests?

The answer is in the negative. It is true that, when disregarding the patient's experiential interests at t_2, we act *in accordance* with the critical interest she had at t_1. But acting in accordance with critical interests does not mean that these critical interests are the *justificatory reason* for why we act as we do. Rather, many reasons speak in favor of the view that the justificatory reason for disregarding the experiential interest at t_2 is the subsequent consent of the person who has

---

Paternalismus: Zum normativen Status von 'Odysseus-Anweisungen'." In: *Zeitschrift für philosophische Forschung* 65 (2011): 151–72.

14 For presymptomatic testing of dementia by means of blood tests and biomarkers, see Davis, Dena. "Alzheimer's Disease and Pre-Emptive Suicide." In: *Journal of Medical Ethics* 40 (2014): 543–9, esp. 547–8.

regained her competence.[15] As an analogous example, think of the paternalization of children: we often act paternalistically towards our children when it concerns their later welfare. That is, we disregard their current experiential interests (e.g. their experiential interest to eat ten ice creams and six pieces of candy a day) and act against them in order to promote their well-being. However, we do so not because we respect their preceding preferences – normally, our children do not sign consent forms on Monday authorizing us to disregard their food-preferences on Tuesday – but because we anticipate that they will later retrospectively consent to this treatment. Paternalization of children shows the possibility of legitimately overriding a person's interests in the absence of a directive that explicitly authorizes us to disregard a subject's wishes and interests at a later point of time.

Thus, we cannot invoke Ulysses cases to support the dominance thesis. Even if we think (as we usually do) that we are justified in disregarding a subject's experiential interests that run contrary to preceding critical interests in cases of a transitory loss of competence, this view does not commit us to accepting that we do so because we respect these preceding interests. It does not imply that these critical interests override experiential interests.

(B2b) *Permanent loss of competence*: The loss of competence in cases of a non-simultaneous conflict between critical and experiential interests may also be permanent. The person who has lost her competence may not regain it. This may occur for one of two reasons. The first reason is that the person is in an advanced stage of the disease, more specifically in stage 6 ("severe cognitive decline") or 7 ("very severe cognitive decline") according to the "global deterioration scale". In these stages, the patient is largely unaware of recent events and experiences and of her surroundings. Moreover, she may have lost all verbal abilities and psychomotor skills. Her cognitive capacities have been irrevocably lost. The second possible reason for a permanent loss of competence is the enactment of an advance directive that requires ending the patient's life in a state of incompetence. If a directive – even one that pertains to an earlier stage of dementia in which the patient has only temporarily lost her competence but may still regain it – demands the ending of the patient's life in a state in which she has lost her cognitive skills, the loss of competence *turns out* to be permanent if the directive is enacted. Assume that at t_1, a competent person expresses the wish that, should she be in an early state of dementia at a later point of time t_2, life-sustaining treatment ought to be forgone

15 For a detailed defence of this view, see Hallich. "Selbstbindungen und medizinischer Paternalismus," 159–65. For a discussion of the role of subsequent consent, see also Davis. "Precedent Autonomy and Subsequent Consent."

in, e.g., the case of pneumonia. At t_2, the patient, now being in an early stage of dementia with a temporary loss of competence, appears to take delight in basic pleasures such as eating or quietly sitting in the sunshine. Should she catch pneumonia, fulfilling her current wishes would require keeping her alive, so it would mean ignoring the wishes of the former competent person. By contrast, ignoring her current wishes and honoring the directive would mean bringing about her death. As death brings with it a permanent loss of competence, the loss of competence would then *turn out* to be permanent in the light of the enactment of the directive. This holds true notwithstanding the fact that, without the enactment of the directive, the loss of competence would have been only transitory.

In these cases, unlike in Ulysses cases, it is not an option to justify the disregarding of the patient's experiential interests with reference to subsequent consent. As late dementia or the enactment of an advance directive that requires the termination of the patient's life will be followed by death, not by a state in which competence is regained, we cannot claim that the justificatory reason for disregarding a demented person's interests is that this person will later, in a state of regained competence, consent to it. Rather, a defender of the view that the principle of precedent autonomy authorizes us to act against the demented patient's wishes in these cases has to show that critical interests dominate experiential interests even if the patient has *permanently* lost her cognitive skills (or will lose them if the directive is enacted). In what follows, I will attempt to show that this claim is false. In these cases, or so I argue, experiential interests negate the authority of critical interests.

III. Can Experiential Interests Negate the Authority of Critical Interests?

Critical interests *possess* normative authority insofar as they count as interests that we have to respect to the extent that we have to respect a person's right to autonomy. Accordingly, they lose their normative authority if they cease to have this status, i.e. if they no longer define the set of wishes and desires that we have to honor to the extent that we have to respect a person's autonomy. (Of course, autonomy can be outweighed by other considerations when it comes to decide what we ought to do all things considered. Therefore, critical interests generate only prima facie obligations to respect someone's will.)

How, then, can critical interests be deprived of their normative authority? Examples of a loss of authority of critical interests come to mind easily. Think of a deeply religious person who, in the course of her life, becomes an atheist. At the age of twenty, she defines her goals in life in terms of pleasing God and leading a pure and spiritual life, and she is firmly dedicated to pursuing the ideal of a pious and solitary existence. At forty, she has an interest in worldly pleasures, in promoting her own welfare and in having a family. At twenty, she believes in the sanctity of human life and is convinced that human lives ought to be prolonged at all costs, while at forty, she has come to believe that the prolongation of a life full of pain and dependence on others ought to be avoided. The plans and projects that shaped her life when she was twenty have undergone a complete revision by the time she is forty.

In this case, the former set of preferences has lost its normative authority in the later stages of the person' s life. An advance directive that stems from the religious beliefs and preferences the person had at twenty would no longer be expressive of preferences and wishes that possess normative authority when the person is forty. It would therefore have lost its validity. It is important to be clear about the sense of "valid" that is at stake here: there is *a* sense of "valid" – let us call it the "ethical" sense – in which it is correct to say that an advance directive loses its validity if the preferences to which it gives expression cease to be authoritative. This loss of validity does not preclude the possibility that the directive is still *legally* valid. One can easily imagine advance directives that are legally binding even though they no longer represent the person's current wishes. In this case, the person who made the directive is comparable to someone living in an unhappy and ruined marriage that is still a marriage according to the law: her advance directive has lost its ethical validity, but it is still valid "according to the law". When we talk of advance directives ceasing to be valid because one set of preferences loses its normative authority, we draw on the ethical, not on the legal sense of "valid".

Examples like the one of the believer who becomes an atheist help us bring to light the conditions that have and, even more importantly, those that do not have to be satisfied in order for critical interests to lose their normative authority. What happens in the above example is clear: a set of critical interests is, in the course of time, replaced by another and radically different set of critical interests. Unlike in the *no-conflict-scenarios* of the type (A2) and (A3), critical interests here do not just cease to exist – in which case, as I argued above, they would retain their normative authority – but are rescinded on account of a different set of critical interests that is incompatible with the first. "Incompatible" means that a person could not coherently identify with these two sets of preferences at the same time: one cannot be a deeply religious person while also being a convinced atheist and one cannot have a life plan to lead a solitary life and a life plan to have a family at the same time. Thus, a person' s earlier preferences no longer constitute the set of preferences we have to honor in order to respect her autonomy if another set of preferences that cannot coexist with the first set has eradicated them. This condition of the replacement of one set of preferences by another set that is incompatible with the first – call it the *replacement condition* – is a *necessary* condition for critical interests to lose their normative authority and consequently for the invalidation of an advance directive that is expressive of these critical interests.

In cases of a non-simultaneous conflict between critical and experiential interests, the replacement condition is satisfied. Think, for example, of Dworkin's famous "Margo case":[16] Margo is an intellectually agile person. Dworkin invites us to imagine that in a state of competence, she expresses revulsion at the prospect of becoming demented and being dependent on others. She firmly expresses (perhaps by means of an advance directive) her desire that, should she ever become demented, she would no longer want to be kept alive if she, for example, got pneumonia. Margo then becomes demented, but still seems to be, according to a medical student who regularly visits her, "one of the happiest people I have ever known",[17] who enjoys quietly sitting in the sunshine, caressing animals, or eating peanut-butter-and-jelly sandwiches and who exhibits all signs of joy in life. The demented Margo evidently has an interest to live that runs contrary to her former critical interests. The replacement condition is satisfied: the original set of critical preferences is replaced by another set of preferences.[18] This latter set of preferences stems from experiential interests that are incompatible with the first: it is impossible to honor the competent person's wish that life-sustaining treatment be withheld in a state of dementia and the demented person's interest to live at the same time.

It is also important to highlight the conditions that do *not* have to be satisfied for critical interests to lose their normative authority. First, the loss of authority

16 See Dworkin. *Life's Dominion*, 220–9. The Margo case and Dworkin's normative assessment of the case have become a constant reference point in the literature on advance directives in dementia. It has elicited Dresser's trenchant criticism (see, e.g., Dresser. "Dworkin on Dementia"); for further comments on the Margo case, see, e.g., Jaworska. "Respecting the Margins of Agency"; McMahan. *The Ethics of Killing*, 498–502; Sumner, L.W. *Assisted Death. A Study in Ethics and Law*. New York: Oxford University Press, 2011, 108–17; Menzel, Steinbock. "Advance Directives, Dementia, and Physician-Assisted Death", 489–92; Beauchamp, Childress. *Principles of Biomedical Ethics*, 228–9; Hawkins, Jennifer. "Well-Being, Time, and Dementia." In: *Ethics* 124 (2014): 507–42, esp. 510–19.

17 Dworkin. *Life's Dominion*, 221.

18 For the time being, I ignore the fact that in this case, the original set of critical interests is replaced not by another set of critical interests, but by experiential interests. I address this issue in section IV.

of critical interests does not require a *decision* to change one's preferences. (Let us call this condition the *decision condition.*) The above example illustrates that critical interests may lose their authority as the result of a gradual process that may stretch over a considerable span of time. It will often be impossible to mark a clear turning point that indicates the point of time at which the new preferences were "born": at forty, the person may not be able to say when exactly she lost her faith. It may be just as impossible for her to say when she became a disbeliever as it is impossible for someone to fix the point of time at which her hair turned grey. She may never have willingly made a decision to abandon her faith. There may also be overlapping phases in which the person is still partially religious but has already to a great extent lost her religious beliefs. The loss of normative authority of critical interests may happen by and by.

The impact of this observation on advance directives in dementia is evident: The mere fact that a demented patient has not decided to abandon the preferences that she expressed in the advance directive does not guarantee that these preferences retain their normative authority. It does not rule out the possibility that the advance directive that gives expression to these preferences has become invalid by other means.

Finally, in order to lose its validity, an advance directive need not be *revoked.*[19] (Let us call this condition the *revocation condition.*) A revocation is an overt act by means of which a person gives expression to the withdrawal of a former decision. For example, someone might tear apart a consent form that authorizes others to withhold food and water in late-stage dementia, thereby revoking her former consent. *A revocation is a sufficient but not a necessary condition for an advance directive to lose its validity.* That is, whenever a person revokes an advance directive it ceases to be valid. Nevertheless, it is also possible that the advance directive loses its validity without being revoked because it is possible that the preferences expressed in an advance directive lose their normative authority without being overtly taken back or in any way explicitly disaffirmed. Clearly, an advance directive loses its validity without being revoked if, after a certain time span, it has not been explicitly disaffirmed, but not explicitly renewed either. If a considerable time span has elapsed since the directive has been made and it has not been reaffirmed or renewed since then, we are likely to regard this as sufficient evidence that the advance directive no longer reflects a person's present set of preferences.

19 King. *Making Sense of Advance Directives*, 204–13. According to King, a revocation is the only way of invalidating an advance directive. This claim mirrors the rather loose use of the term 'revocation' in the literature on advance directives. Often, the term is used in a very general sense to cover *all* forms of invalidation of an advance directive.

We would therefore decline to regard it as binding notwithstanding the fact that the patient did not revoke it.

Again, this observation directly bears on advance directives in dementia: since revocation is not a necessary condition for an advance directive to lose its validity, an advance directive in dementia may lose its validity even though it has not been explicitly revoked. In other words, the mere fact that the demented patient has not revoked the advance directive does not guarantee its validity.

In cases of a non-contemporaneous conflict between critical and experiential interests and a permanent loss of competence, the necessary condition for the invalidation of an advance directive, the replacement condition, is fulfilled, while the revocation condition and the decision condition are not fulfilled. However, since the latter two conditions are sufficient, but not necessary conditions for the invalidation of advance directives, the fact that they are not satisfied does not call into question the view that in cases of this kind, experiential interests negate the normative authority of critical interests and invalidate the advance directive. Rather, a preliminary conclusion is as follows: if the basic desires and wishes of the demented patient run contrary to the critical interests of the once competent person, these wishes and desires take over the normative authority of the former critical interests. They then form the set of interests that we have to respect to the extent that we have to respect the person's autonomy. Should the "happy demented" like Dworkin's Margo exhibit all signs of a desire to live, then this desire, stemming from her experiential interests like the interest in enjoying good food or sitting quietly in the sunshine, outweighs the former critical interest that life-sustaining treatment ought to be withheld in a state of dementia. Insofar as the right to autonomy is concerned, this desire, so my tentative conclusion goes, has to be respected notwithstanding the fact that the competent Margo articulated the wish that it be ignored.[20]

---

20 Admittedly, whether the principle of autonomy requires the satisfaction of experiential interests or not is a contested issue. On a broadly Kantian model, one might argue that it is only interests that are based in reason, i.e. critical interests that express our autonomy and that are protected by the right to autonomy, whereas experiential interests based on pleasure or desire are not. However, the main idea of my argument does not hinge on a positive answer to the question of whether the principle of autonomy requires us to respect experiential interests or not. Even if the answer to this question is in the negative, the fact remains that the experiential interests of the demented patient *are* interests that – in the absence of compelling arguments to the contrary – deserve to be respected. One might plausibly argue that a cat's interest not to be exposed to boiling water ought to be respected without invoking the principle of autonomy to ground this

IV. Three Objections

Of course, this cannot be the end of the story. The foregoing argument is likely to elicit the objection that it simply ignores the crucial distinction between critical and experiential interests. It appears to sidestep the question of whether the dominance thesis is true or not by focusing on cases in which the difference between critical and experiential interests is irrelevant. If a religious person becomes an atheist in the course of her life, critical interests lose their authority because other *critical* interests eradicate them. Things seem to look differently if it is *experiential* interests that replace critical interests. Why, for example, should a demented patient's pleasure in good food that gives rise to an experiential interest be on par with the former critical interest of an intellectually agile person that, in a state of dementia, life-sustaining treatment ought to be withheld? In what follows I will examine three lines of argument to support the view that in scenarios of the kind that are now under consideration critical interests are *unlike* experiential interests in that they alone may deprive our former critical interests of their normative authority. All of them, or so I argue, are unpersuasive.

IV.1 Asymmetry of Cognitive Capacities

The first line of argument draws our attention to the fact that there is an asymmetry between the cognitive capacities of the competent person who wrote the advance directive and the demented person who has lost all cognitive skills. This asymmetry, so the objection goes, speaks against the view that preferences that originate from experiential interests may negate preferences that stem from critical interests.[21]

It goes without saying that the asymmetry the objection points to really exists. However, it need not disconcert us. In various contexts, we often place more rigid standards of competence on validly assenting to a procedure than on validly withdrawing from it. For example, in order for a subject to validly consent to participation in a cancer research program, this subject usually has to meet criteria of informed consent, i.e. consenting in light of a full understanding of the procedure

moral obligation. Analogously, as long as the principle of precedent autonomy turns out to be unpersuasive in conflict cases of the kind now under consideration, there is good reason to assume that the experiential interests of the demented patient, be their satisfaction required by the principle of autonomy or not, ought to be honored.

21 See, e.g., King. *Making Sense of Advance Directives*, 204–13. King endorses the view that a valid revocation must exhibit a degree of autonomy similar to the one that is required to make the advance directive valid.

to which she is about to submit herself, an understanding of the relevant information, an awareness of the risk her participation implies etc. In order to take back his consent validly, however, he need not fulfill these conditions: if, in a state of restricted competence, e.g. under the influence of misinformation, he tears apart the consent form, we will accept this as a valid revision of his former decision. The justification for this asymmetry is as follows: higher standards of competence for entering a procedure shield the subject against precipitately taking part in a procedure which may involve serious dangers and risks. Conversely, lower standards of competence for stepping back from it are justified because by stepping back from it the subject merely reenters into the "default position". Under normal circumstances, there is no risk in *not* taking part in a medical experiment. Therefore, the competence requirements for repealing one's consent to participate in a research program are lower than those a subject has to meet for validly entering into it.[22]

Similarly, the competence standards that have to be met in order to *in*validate an advance directive are less rigid than those that have to be met for making a valid advance directive. Someone will not succeed in making a valid advance directive if, on a whim, she formulates her end-of-life directive that artificial nourishment be withheld in a terminal state of a disease. By contrast, if she tears apart the advance directive (and does not renew it) in a freakish or whimsical state of mind, this will be accepted as an invalidation (in this case even as a revocation) of the advance directive. As in the case of consent to participation in a research program, this asymmetry is well justified. Different risks are at stake in making and in repealing an advance directive. By making an advance directive, a person makes a risky decision insofar as she determines her future treatment without being able to completely anticipate the future state of affairs to which her directive relates. Although we usually regard advance directives as a means of reducing the risk of being exposed to life-prolonging measures against our will, the fact remains that we can never know exactly whether our future intentions and desires will match

22 In a similar vein, Buchanan and Brock defend a "sliding-scale account" of competence (Buchanan, Brock. *Deciding for Others*, 17–86 [chap. 1]). They argue that "no single standard of decision-making competence is adequate" (ibd., 52) and that "the standard of competence ought to vary in part with the expected harms or benefits to the patient of acting in accordance with the patient's choice" (ibd., 51). As Beauchamp and Childress have noted, we should not take this claim to mean that competence itself varies in relation to risk, since risky decisions do not require more ability at decision making than less risky ones. Rather, the core idea of the "sliding-scale account" should be that the *evidence* for determining competence varies according to risk; see Beauchamp, Childress. *Principles of Biomedical Ethics*, 119–20.

with the will that guided our decisions when we made the advance directive. It is always uncertain and risky to anticipate one's future will. By contrast, when withdrawing the directive, the subject reenters into the "default position", i.e. a state in which she leaves open how she will be treated in the future. As making an advance directive is a risky decision, whereas repealing it is not, it is reasonable that the standards imposed on validly making an advance directive are more demanding than those imposed on validly withdrawing it.

Hence, the mere fact that a demented patient, having lost competence, is unable to comply with the standards of competence that have to be met for an advance directive to be valid does not imply that the patient is unable to conform to the standards that have to be met to invalidate the advance directive. The asymmetry between the cognitive skills of the competent person and those of the demented patient, undeniable as it is, is not at odds with the view that experiential interests may negate the normative authority of critical interests.

IV.2 Anticipation of Future Preference Changes

A second objection to the view that experiential interests of the demented patient may negate the authority of contravening critical interests of the once competent patient is the following one. When writing an advance directive, the competent patient *foresees* that, when being in a state of dementia, she will have the desire that her physicians and relatives disregard her former critical interests and act upon her later experiential interests. Therefore, so the objection goes, not fulfilling these later experiential interests is exactly the *point* of advance directives in dementia.[23] To bring out the salient point of the objection more clearly, promises provide an illuminating analogy: assume that, when marrying, I promise my wife that I will not betray her. I may, when marrying, foresee that I will later be exposed to temptations in which I will have a strong inclination to become unfaithful. At a later point of time, I may actually be exposed to these temptations. But since not betraying my wife is exactly what I have promised her, it would be absurd to say that my later desire to betray her negates the promise I made to her. The point of the promise is just to make sure that I will not follow my desire; therefore, my having a desire to do what I promised *not* to do does not suspend or negate its binding force. One could argue that, for the same reason, experiential interests cannot negate the normative authority of critical interests in scenarios of the kind now

---

23 Sumner states this point very clearly: "It would be perverse to disregard my earlier directives simply because I am now in the very condition of incapacity I anticipated in recording them" (Sumner. *Assisted Death*, 111).

under consideration. Just as not following my desires is what keeping my promise consists in, acting contrary to the demented patient' s experiential interests is what respecting the person' s autonomy consists in. As Feinberg memorably puts it, the right of autonomy is like the sovereignty of a nation over its territory:[24] it extends over a *sphere* of interests. This sphere comprises those contravening interests that the competent patient who exercises her right to autonomy foresees.[25] Therefore, the objection goes, the principle of autonomy demands negating these foreseen preferences.

Though intriguing, this argument is flawed for at least two reasons. First, we have to take into consideration that we change not only our preferences, but also our evaluations of foreseen changes of preferences. A person who, when making an advance directive, foresees a future change of her preferences, may still, at a later point of time, come to reevaluate this foreseen change of preferences. Often, it will be impossible to decide whether a preference that runs contrary to the one the competent person expressed in the advance directive is exactly the one that the competent patient foresaw or whether it is indicative of a reevaluation of the foreseen change of preferences. If the second alternative obtains, the alteration of the patient's evaluation of the foreseen preference change must be respected as an exercise of personal autonomy.[26]

---

24 Feinberg. *Harm to Self*, 47–51.

25 Davis labels this view the "extension view" of autonomy and plausibly ascribes it to, e.g., Rhoden and Dworkin. Davis. "Precedent Autonomy, Advance Directives, and End-of-Life Care," 365–7; Davis. "Precedent Autonomy and Subsequent Consent", 273–81.

26 This problem vitiates Davis' attempt to base precedent autonomy on a "resolution preference", i.e. an evaluative judgement that is formed in awareness of two conflicting preferences and that is either contemporary with the two conflicting preferences or, if these exist at different times, with one of them, typically the former one. (Davis. "Precedent Autonomy, Advance Directives, and End-of-Life Care," 365–7; Davis. "Precedent Autonomy and Subsequent Consent", 273–81). According to Davis, a resolution preference expresses what a person wants, all things considered. Therefore, to respect his or her autonomy, we must respect his or her resolution preference. However, even resolution preferences may be subject to changes of mind; a person may come to abandon or to alter his or her resolution preference. Similar problems arise with King' s suggestion to incorporate an "antirevocation provision" in advance directives in order to protect the subject against involuntary revocations of his former will (King. *Making Sense of Advance Directives*, 204–13). This antirevocation condition, King suggests, should specify circumstances under which the apparent revocation of an advance directive should not be honored. But again, even the antirevocation provision is prone to changes of will and may therefore become invalid. For the problem of anticipated preference changes, see also Kleinig, John. *Paternalism*. New Jersey: Rowman & Allanheld, 1984,

By way of illustration, the following example might be helpful. A smoker sincerely wants to overcome her addiction. She thinks that she ought to abstain from nicotine because leading a healthy life is more important to her than the fulfillment of short-lived hedonic desires. She foresees that she will soon have a strong desire to smoke a cigarette. She attempts to forestall the fulfillment of this desire by instructing all her friends to make sure that, as soon as the desire arises, she will have no access to nicotine. Later, as was foreseen by her, she has a strong desire to smoke a cigarette. How can we decide whether the desire to smoke a cigarette is exactly the wish that she foresaw and whose fulfillment she tried to forestall or whether it is expressive of a different evaluation of the preference change she foresaw? It seems impossible to exclude the second alternative. The desire to smoke a cigarette may be the result of a revision of the former view that leading a healthy life is more important to the person's life plan than the fulfillment of short-lived desires. For example, the smoker may have come to believe that preserving her health is not that important to her life plan after all or that all the medical reports she read about the lethal consequences of smoking were unfounded. If that is the case, the altered evaluation of the foreseen preference change has to be honored as an expression of the subject's autonomy. Since there is no compelling argument to show that it cannot be the case, the mere fact that the preference change was foreseen does not warrant the claim that the first of the two conflicting preferences ought to be acted upon.

The same problem occurs with advance directives in dementia. A person may issue an advance directive in which she instructs her physicians to forgo life-sustaining treatment when she has become demented. She may foresee that, when being demented, she will strongly want her physicians to disregard her former critical interest and that, contrary to her express wish, she will then demand that life-sustaining treatment be provided. As a demented patient, she may really come to have the wish that life-sustaining treatment be provided. Still, it remains an open question how the demented patient's preference has to be interpreted: is it exactly the preference the competent person foresaw and whose fulfillment she tried to prevent or is it a new preference that gives expression to the reevaluation of the previous wish that the later foreseen preference not be satisfied? Again, as we not only change our preferences, but also our evaluations of foreseen changes of preferences, we cannot rule out the possibility that the later preference indicates that the patient has reevaluated the preference change she (rightly) foresaw as a

---

who rightly states: "consent is not to be construed after the manner of an irrevocable contract but as an ongoing commitment that may be reassessed and given up." (ibid. 57)

competent person. If this is the case, we have to respect this reevaluation as an exercise of personal autonomy.[27]

Second, the possibility of foreseeing a future change of preferences is not specific to the relation between critical and experiential interests. It is true that, as in the case of an advance directive in dementia, someone may have a critical interest that her foreseen contravening experiential interests be negated. But it is also true that someone may have a critical interest that her foreseen future *critical* interests be negated. In this case, however, the later critical interests do *not* lose their authority to negate the former critical interests although these later interests are those whose fulfillment the person tried to prevent. Think of a profoundly religious person who is devoted to leading a pious and pure ascetic life and wishes to bequeath all her property to a religious organization. She may foresee that one day under the influence of a secular environment she will lose her faith. She may try to guard herself against this foreseen change of her (critical) interests and may time and again confirm her last will and her intention to donate her property to the religious organization. Nevertheless, one day it may happen that she actually loses her faith and becomes an atheist. If, in these new circumstances, she distances herself from her former decision and makes clear that she no longer wishes to bequeath her property to the religious organization, this changed preference will be respected notwithstanding the fact that she foresaw and vainly tried to forestall it at an earlier point of time. So the foreseeability of the preference change does not diminish the normative authority of the later preferences. If this is the case, the fact that a person foresaw this change is of no relevance to the authority of her

27 This holds true especially in view of the fact that demented patients do have the capacity to value, as Jaworska has convincingly argued (Jaworska. "Respecting the Margins of Agency"). Referring to Dworkin's distinction between critical and experiential interests, Jaworska points out that this distinction is too coarse and needs to be replaced by a more fine-grained one. She categorizes the valuations of demented patients as critical interests, thereby introducing a sense of "critical interest" that is different from the one that Dworkin draws upon. Whether we follow her in doing so or not seems to me a question of minor terminological importance. Jaworska's crucial insight is that the preferences of demented patients are distinct from mere desires, that they may, at least in the first stages of dementia, still be stable and that, although they do not imply grasp of one's life as a whole, they are expressive of valuations. As valuing involves reflection, the capacity to value, so Jaworska argues, shows that demented patients have not lost their autonomy. For Jaworska's critique of Dworkin's distinction between critical and experiential interests, see also Menzel, Steinbock. "Advance Directives, Dementia, and Physician-Assisted Death," 490–2.

later interests, and this also holds true even in cases in which experiential interests replace former critical interests.

IV.3 Qualitative Difference between Critical and Experiential Interests

A third objection to the view that experiential interests may negate the normative authority of critical interests draws on a value judgement about these two kinds of interests. The objector may contend that there is a *qualitative* difference between them. Critical interests, he might argue, are superior in worth to experiential interests. He could spell out the argument in various ways. First, he could argue that critical interests are superior in worth to experiential interests because they give expression to distinctively *human* capacities. (Animals, though they may have the capacity to form experiential interests, lack the capacity to form critical interests.)[28] Second, the objector might argue that critical interests are superior in worth to experiential interests because they give expression to what constitutes our lives as *persons*. If critical interests, unlike experiential ones, define what it is to be a person, they define the set of preferences that we have to honor to the extent that we have to respect a person's autonomy.[29] Third, in order to justify her claim that critical interests are superior in worth to experiential interests, the objector may adduce the fact that most members of a society *regard* critical interests as superior to non-critical ones.[30] The objection then points to the social fact that there is a prevalent attitude among most members of a society that in cases of a conflict critical interests ought to override experiential interests.

---

28 Dworkin, though not explicitly, embraces this view when he grounds the dominance thesis in considerations concerning human dignity: "I have been arguing that we not only have, in common with all sensate creatures, experiential interests in the quality of our future experiences but also critical interests in the character and value of our lives as a whole. These critical interests are connected, as I said, to our convictions about the intrinsic value – the sanctity or inviolability – of our own lives. [...] Dignity is a central aspect of [...] the intrinsic importance of human life." (Dworkin. *Life's Dominion*, 235–6).

29 Quante defends this view: "To lead one's life as a person means to identify oneself, be it in a positive or in a negative way, with one's future, one's future experiential interests included. If a culture attaches central value to leading one's life as a person, there is a strong reason for acknowledging and respecting those valuations of a person that he or she expresses in an advance directive as an exercise of his or her personal autonomy" (Quante. *Personales Leben und menschlicher Tod*, 286; transl. by author).

30 See the quotation from Quante's *Personales Leben und menschlicher Tod* in the preceding footnote, which allows for this interpretation as well.

I cannot examine these arguments in detail. It suffices to say that more argument would be needed to make them persuasive. As they stand, they appear to rest on a naturalistic fallacy. As is well known, we cannot infer value judgements from purely descriptive premises.[31] Thus, we cannot infer the statement that critical interests are superior in worth to experiential interests from the purely descriptive statement that the capacity to form critical interests is specific for human beings.[32] Similarly, the mere fact that critical interests constitute our lives as persons does not make them superior in worth to experiential interests. Of course, one is free to define "person" as an evaluative concept and to stipulate by definitional fiat that personal interests, *because* they define what a person is, are superior in worth to non-personal ones, thereby avoiding a naturalistic fallacy. However, the argument that critical interests are superior in worth to experiential interests *because* they define our lives as persons then becomes blatantly circular. It boils down to saying that critical interests are superior in worth to other interests because they are superior in worth to other interests. Finally, the mere social fact that most people in a society accept the view that critical interests ought to dominate experiential interests does not validate the value judgement that critical interests are superior in worth to experiential interests either. The majority of members of a society may accept the most absurd views. The mere social fact that people *regard* critical interests as superior to non-critical ones does not warrant the claim that they are right in doing so.

Even leaving these worries aside, the objector faces another problem. Let us, for the sake of the argument, assume that a value judgement about the superior worth of critical over experiential interests is true. Still, its truth does not imply the truth of the normative judgement that in cases of a conflict between the two kinds of interests we *ought* to respect the critical interests even at the price of disregarding the demented patient's current experiential interests. It is a common vice in moral philosophy to overlook the categorical difference between value judgements and "ought" judgements, particularly if both kinds of discourse are lumped together under headings such as "prescriptive language" or, even worse, "moral language". As G.H. von Wright pointed out most forcefully, the proposition that we ought to do what is good does not express a conceptual truth. Value

31 See, e.g., Hare, Richard. *The Language of Morals*. Oxford: Oxford University Press, 1952, 1–55, 79–93 (chap. 1–3, 5). It would be beyond the scope of this paper to go into the details of the discussion of metaethical naturalism. I simply take it for granted that metaethical naturalism cannot be consistently defended.

32 For a classical critique of the "speciecism" that is involved here, see Singer, Peter. *Practical Ethics*. Cambridge: Cambridge University Press, ^{3}2011, 48–70 (chap. 3).

concepts are not intrinsically normative.[33] Therefore, the transition from "This is good" to "This ought to be done" or to "This ought to be realized" is not a logical transition, and the transition from "Interest A is superior in value to interest B" to "In cases of a conflict between A and B, A ought to be respected" is not a logical transition either. The dominance thesis is a *normative* thesis; it is a claim about what kind of interests we *ought* to honor in cases of a conflict between critical and experiential interests. Being normative does not follow from a value judgement about the superior worth of critical over experiential interests.

As all three objections turn out to be unpersuasive, I see no reason to take back the preliminary conclusion that I argued for in the preceding section: in scenarios of a non-contemporaneous conflict between critical and experiential interests, experiential interests can negate the normative authority of critical interests.

V. Concluding Remarks: The Binding Force of Advance Directives in Dementia

The upshot of the argument is as follows: if the experiential interests of the demented patient run contrary to the critical interests of the once competent person that were expressed in the advance directive, the critical interests do *not* dominate the experiential ones. Therefore, the principle of respect for autonomy does *not* commit us to subordinating the interests of the demented patient to those of the competent person. Rather, it speaks in favor of letting experiential interests override critical ones in these cases.

To guard against misunderstandings, I wish to emphasize that this conclusion is not to deny that advance directives are a highly useful tool for guiding medical choices. They are far from being superfluous. This is so for two reasons.

First, the view that experiential interests may negate the authority of critical interests applies only to (some) cases in which these two kinds of interests *collide*. In the absence of a collision of this kind, critical interests retain their authority. As I argued at length with regard to "no-conflict scenarios", the mere fact that critical interests cease to exist does not deprive them of their normative authority. Their

33 See von Wright, Georg Henrik. *The Varieties of Goodness*. Bristol: Thoemmes Press, 1963, 155–7. According to Moore's influential analysis of the relation between 'good' and 'ought', normative concepts like 'ought' and 'duty' can be analyzed in terms of 'good', whereas 'good' itself, being a simple concept, cannot be analyzed in terms of normative concepts; see Moore, George Edward. *Principia Ethica. Revised Edition. With the Preface to the Second Edition and Other Papers*. Cambridge University Press: Cambridge, 1993, 76–8, 196–8 (chap. 1, § 17, chap. 5, § 89).

authority is also left untouched in cases of a simultaneous conflict between critical and experiential interests. Furthermore, in "Ulysses cases" we are justified in acting in accordance with the former critical interests as long as we can reasonably expect the patient's subsequent consent. In sum, should the demented patient not exhibit any signs of a contravening interest, there is no argument against respecting the former wishes of the competent person with regard to how she is to be treated in a state in which competence has been lost.[34]

Second, in cases of a transitory loss of competence, i.e. in cases in which the person regains her competence after a phase in which she is unable to make competent decisions, advance directives help us to rightly anticipate a person's subsequent consent to a treatment she has been subjected to during a phase of incompetence. For example, a person who anticipates that under the influence of a severe psychosis she will want to commit suicide may write an advance directive that authorizes others to prevent her, if necessary by force, from committing suicide in this state of a loss of competence. In this case, the advance directive corroborates the assumption that the patient will most likely consent to having been prevented from committing suicide by force after the phase of incompetence. Similarly, advance directives that pertain to the onset stages of dementia will increase the reliability of judgements about the patient's later consent to a treatment during a preceding phase of a loss of cognitive skills that she is expected to give in a later phase of recurring competence. Thus, insofar as subsequent consent is relevant to justifying a treatment during a phase of a loss of competence, advance directives are an important tool for guiding medical choices because they make judgements about an expected subsequent consent more reliable than they would be without an advance directive.

Bearing these two caveats in mind, can we conclude that in cases of a non-simultaneous conflict between critical and experiential interests and a permanent

---

34 A similar point is made by McMahan. *The Ethics of Killing*, 497–8; Menzel, Steinbock. "Advance Directives, Dementia, and Physician-Assisted Death," 492–3; Menzel, Chandler-Cramer. "Advance Directives, Dementia, and Withholding Food and Water by Mouth," 24–9. Rhoden neglects this important point. She contends that rejecting precedent autonomy implies that the competent patient's right to refuse treatment would be upheld only as long as she remains competent. "Taken to an extreme, this could mean that a Jehovah's Witness could refuse a blood transfusion until he 'bled out' and became incompetent, after which he could be transfused." (Rhoden. "The Limits of Legal Objectivity," 857) However, this counterintuitive consequence follows only if the rejection of the principle of precedent autonomy is extended to no-conflict cases, which it need not be.

loss of competence we ought to disregard the critical interests and act in accordance with the experiential interests? Perhaps surprisingly, the answer is "No". The foregoing argument does *not* rule out the possibility that we should disregard the patient's actual experiential preferences and act in accordance with the competent patient's wishes. It only rules out the possibility that we justify doing so by drawing on the principle of precedent autonomy. There is nothing contradictory in claiming that we are justified in acting *in accordance* with the former interests without resorting to the principle of precedent autonomy, i.e. without claiming that the reason for doing so is that we respect or honor these preceding critical interests. (As I stressed above, "to act in accordance with the former interests" does not mean that these former interests are necessarily the justificatory reasons for acting in accordance with them.)[35] For example, within a utilitarian framework, one might point to the fact that there is a strong societal interest in giving critical interests priority over experiential interests, i.e. that most members of a society have a strong interest in subordinating experience-related desires and wishes to critical interests in cases of a conflict. Impartially universalizing these interests, one might argue, will lead us to prioritize critical over experiential interests because doing so will, in sum and considered from an impartial point of view, maximize the preference satisfaction of all parties involved.

The price to be paid for pursuing this line of argument would be that we openly admit that acting against the demented patient's wishes is not an instance of respecting her precedent autonomy but rather an instance of privileging society's (or the majority of its members') interests. It would require abandoning the pleasant and flattering view that, when acting in accordance with the wishes the patient articulated in the advance directive, we do so for the sake of the patient. It would compel us to accept the less flattering view that when placing critical interests over experiential interests we are not good Samaritans selflessly protecting the patient's autonomy but are simply trying to enforce the implementation

35 E.g., McMahan's sagacious defence of the view that the competent person's preferences ought to be accorded more weight than those of the demented patient is independent of the principle of precedent autonomy. McMahan construes conflict cases as conflicts between two distinct parts of a life, namely between the earlier good of the competent self and that of the later incompetent self. While it may be in the best interest of the demented patient to live, ignoring the directive may retroactively diminish the value of the life prior to the onset of dementia. McMahan argues that physicians should give priority to the earlier part of the life because it is overwhelmingly the dominant part of the life as a whole (McMahan. *The Ethics of Killing*, 498–503). For a detailed discussion of McMahan's position, see Hawkins. "Well-Being, Time, and Dementia," 514–5.

of decision-making standards that most members of a society approve of.[36] If, by contrast, we stipulate that our decision should be guided by the attempt to respect the patient's autonomy, then, contrary to what is often thought, we lack arguments to respect the competent person's will in cases in which the later experiential interests run contrary to the foregoing critical interests. We should then disregard the advance directive.

References

Alzheimer's Society. *Dementia 2014 Report. Statistics.* <http://www.alz.co.uk/research/statistics> (last access 11.10.2015).

Beauchamp, Tom, Childress, James. *Principles of Biomedical Ethics.* Oxford: Oxford University Press, [7]2013.

Buchanan, Allen. "Advance Directives and the Personal Identity Problem." In: *Philosophy & Public Affairs* 17 (1988): 277–302.

Buchanan, Allen, Brock, Dan. *Deciding for Others. The Ethics of Surrogate Decision Making.* Cambridge: University Press, 1990.

Buller, Tom. "Advance Consent, Critical Interests and Dementia Research." In: *Journal of Medical Ethics* 41 (2015): 701–07.

Cantor, Norman. "Prospective Autonomy: On the Limits of Shaping One's Post-competent Medical Fate." In: *Journal of Contemporary Health Law & Policy* 8 (1992): 13–48.

Cantor, Norman. *Making Medical Decisions for the Profoundly Disabled.* Boston/MA: MIT Press, 2005.

Davis, Dena. "Alzheimer's Disease and Pre-Emptive Suicide." In: *Journal of Medical Ethics* 40 (2014): 543–49.

Davis, John. "Precedent Autonomy, Advance Directives, and End-of-Life Care." In: Bonnie Steinbock (ed.). *Oxford Handbook of Bioethics.* Oxford: Oxford University Press, 2009, 349–74.

Davis, John. "The Concept of Precedent Autonomy." In: *Bioethics* 16 (2002): 114–33.

---

36 In the same spirit, Dresser and Robertson object that it is fundamentally dishonest to cloak those value-judgements that underlie the subordination of the demented patient's interests to those of the competent person with labels as self-determination and dignity; see Dresser. "Life, Death, and Incompetent Patients," 389–90; Dresser. "Missing Persons. Legal Perceptions of Incompetent Patients," 647–9; Dresser, Robertson. "Quality of Life and Non-Treatment Decisions for Incompetent Patients," 242–3; Robertson. "Second Thoughts on Living Wills," 9.

Davis, John. "Precedent Autonomy and Subsequent Consent." In: *Ethical Theory and Moral Practice* 7 (2004): 267–91.

DeGrazia, David. *Human Identity and Bioethics*. Cambridge: Cambridge University Press, 2005.

Dresser, Rebecca. "Bound to Treatment: The Ulysses Contract." In: *The Hastings Center Report* 14 (1984): 13–16.

Dresser, Rebecca. "Dworkin on Dementia: Elegant Theory, Questionable Policy." In: *The Hastings Center Report* 25 (1995): 32–38.

Dresser, Rebecca. "Life, Death, and Incompetent Patients: Conceptual Infirmities and Hidden Values in the Law." In: *Arizona Law Review* 28 (1986): 373–405.

Dresser, Rebecca. "Missing Persons: Legal Perceptions of Incompetent Patients." In: *Rutgers Law Review* 46 (1994): 609–719.

Dresser, Rebecca, Robertson, John. "Quality of Life and Non-Treatment Decisions for Incompetent Patients: A Critique of the Orthodox Approach." In: *Law, Medicine & Health Care* 17 (1989): 234–44.

Dworkin, Ronald. *Life's Dominion. An Argument About Abortion, Euthanasia, and Individual Freedom*. New York: Random House, 1994.

Elster, Jon. *Ulysses Unbound. Studies in Rationality, Precommitment, and Constraints*. Cambridge: Cambridge University Press, 2010.

Faden, Ruth, Beauchamp, Tom. *A History and Theory of Informed Consent*. Oxford: Oxford University Press, 1986.

Feinberg, Joel. *Harm to Self. The Moral Limits of the Criminal Law 3*. Oxford: Oxford University Press, 1986.

Hallich, Oliver. "Selbstbindungen und medizinischer Paternalismus: Zum normativen Status von 'Odysseus-Anweisungen.'" In: *Zeitschrift für philosophische Forschung* 65 (2011): 151–72.

Hare, Richard. *The Language of Morals*. Oxford: Oxford University Press, 1952.

Hawkins, Jennifer. "Well-Being, Time, and Dementia." In: *Ethics* 124 (2014): 507–42.

Jaworska, Agnieszka. "Respecting the Margins of Agency: Alzheimer's Patients and the Capacity to Value." In: *Philosophy & Public Affairs* 28 (1999): 105–38.

Jennings, Bruce. "Alzheimer's Disease: Quality of Life and the Goals of Care." In: John Arras, Elizabeth Fenton, Rebecca Kukla (eds.). *The Routledge Companion to Bioethics*. New York/London: Routledge, 2015, 437–48.

King, Nancy. *Making Sense of Advance Directives*. Washington: Georgetown University Press, 2007.

Kleinig, John. *Paternalism*. New Jersey: Rowman & Allanheld, 1984.

McMahan, Jeff. *The Ethics of Killing. Problems at the Margins of Life*. Oxford: Oxford University Press, 2002.

Menzel, Paul, Steinbock, Bonnie. "Advance Directives, Dementia, and Physician-Assisted Death." In: *Journal of Law, Medicine and Ethics* 41 (2013): 484–500.

Menzel, Paul, Chandler-Cramer, Colette. "Advance Directives Dementia, and Withholding Food and Water by Mouth." In: *The Hastings Center Report* 44 (2014): 23–37.

Moore, George Edward. *Principia Ethica. Revised Edition. With the Preface to the Second Edition and Other Papers*. Cambridge University Press: Cambridge, 1993.

Quante, Michael. *Personales Leben und menschlicher Tod. Personale Identität als Prinzip der biomedizinischen Ethik*. Frankfurt: Suhrkamp, 2002.

Rhoden, Nancy. "The Limits of Legal Objectivity." In: *North Carolina Law Review* 68 (1990): 845–65.

Robertson, John. "Second Thoughts on Living Wills." In: *The Hastings Center Report* 21 (1991): 6–9.

Singer, Peter. *Practical Ethics. Third Edition*. Cambridge: Cambridge University Press, 2011.

Sumner, L. W. *Assisted Death. A Study in Ethics and Law*. New York: Oxford University Press, 2011.

The Alzheimer's Association. "Alzheimer's Disease Facts and Figures. Alzheimer's & Dementia 2015." <http://www.alzheimers.org.uk/site/scripts/documents_info.php?documentID=412> (last access 11.10.2015).

von Wright, Hendrik. *The Varieties of Goodness*. Bristol: Thoemmes Press, 1963.

World Health Organisation. *10 Facts on Dementia*. <http://www.who.int/features/factfiles/dementia/en/> (last access 11.10.2015).

Annette Dufner (Münster/Bayreuth)

Releasing Prisoners with Dementia: Could there be a Recollection Requirement for Expressivist and Communicative Justifications of Punishment?

Abstract: This paper asks whether people in the later stages of dementia who committed crimes when they were still healthy should be punished. I will argue that convincing justifications of punishment fail to justify this. Such theories require a capacity for comprehension on the part of the punished, and, under certain narrowly specified conditions, even a capacity to be at least in principle capable of recalling the crime.

What should we do with people in the later stages of dementia who have committed a crime when they were young and healthy? Should they be subject to a punishment for what they did in the past, even if they do not recall the crime and are not able to comprehend the meaning of any humane form of punishment? An answer to this question can be attempted by investigating theories of personal identity across time in order to figure out whether the demented being is still identical to the one who committed the crime.[1] It has also been argued that we need to look at theories of responsibility ascription.[2] However, another important component of a full answer to the question will have to investigate the exact purpose of a punishment – a task that will require an analysis of the various theories of punishment.

This paper argues that a prison is *not* the right place for criminals in the late stages of dementia, and it represents a condensed summary of an earlier article on the issue.[3] There seems to be something the matter with imprisoning human beings who lack most of their memories, who lack a sense of anticipation regarding the future, who are mostly bed-bound and without recollection of how to use

---

1 Of course Derek Parfit has objected with his slogan that 'identity does not matter' to such normative questions since at least the early 1970s. See Parfit, Derek. "Later Selves and Moral Principles." In: Alan Montefiore (ed). *Philosophy and Personal Relations*, London: Routledge, 1973, 135–69.

2 See Shoemaker, David. "Responsibility without Identity." In: *Harvard Review of Philosophy* 18 (2012): 109–32.

3 Compare Dufner, Annette. "Should the Late Stage Demented be Punished for Past Crimes." In: *Criminal Law and Philosophy* 7 (2013): 137–50.

their bodies, and who are therefore isolated in space and time. Punishments such as imprisonment, which are common and comparatively humane, will be the only forms of punishment that I will consider relevant to my discussion. For the purpose of clarity I will focus exclusively on imprisonment. More specifically, I will argue that applicable theories of punishment, especially theories with an appropriate expressivist, or communicative element, fail to justify the imprisonment of the late-stage demented, because this would require a capacity for comprehension on the part of the punished, and, under certain narrowly specified conditions, even a capacity to be at least in principle capable of recalling the crime.

In legal contexts a competency requirement is familiar, while a recollection requirement is not. Competency usually plays a role when determining whether the person was fully accountable at the time of the crime. Competency also usually plays a role when determining whether someone is fit for a trial and, later, fit for punishment. The recollection requirement seems more unusual, and it can generate various problems. The most central problem is the problem of deceivers: most criminals deny that they remember having committed the crime in question. Of course, this is a pragmatic concern, and it applies likewise to competency and claims of insanity – cases that the criminal justice system has been able to accommodate, despite the problem of deceivers. Is there a substantial reason for this asymmetry, or is the problem merely that severe cases of incompetence or insanity manifest themselves more overtly in people's behavior than severe memory loss?

If the worry turns out to be mostly pragmatic, rather than substantial, then it should not be seen as particularly pressing in the case of the late-stage demented. Whether someone is in the late stages of dementia can usually be determined quite accurately. Moreover, it is a condition that is present for years or even decades before the final stages are reached. All one needs for the purpose of the present argument is the position that people who display memory loss *for involuntary, non-instrumentalized and verifiable clinical reasons* should not be held accountable for their crimes anymore. In order to adopt such a policy, one would not need to also introduce a general recollection requirement for all normal cases. In the following I will only be concerned with such requirements for clinical cases that satisfy the aforementioned restrictions.

It might also be worth recalling that the idea of a recollection requirement is not new. One Early Modern thinker, John Locke, notoriously believed that responsibility depends on having the capacity to *remember* the event in question. Although the question of what to do with demented criminals cannot be fully addressed by appealing to traditional philosophical accounts, it is interesting to consider what he wrote:

> For whatsoever any substance has thought or done, which I cannot recollect, and by my consciousness make my own thought and action, it will no more belong to me, whether a part of me thought or did it, than if it had been thought or done by any other immaterial being anywhere existing. (Locke. "On Identity and Diversity," 49)

The qualification "having the capacity" is important here. When healthy people are sleeping or think of something else, they are not actively remembering the past, but the past is nonetheless in principle available to them. The late-stage demented no longer possess the capacity to remember most of their past, even in principle.

According to the widely held retributivist justification of punishment, a criminal simply *deserves* his or her punishment. Retributivism might be a particularly promising candidate for an argument *in favor of* keeping the demented in prison. The reason is that the idea of desert as such might not necessarily require persisting subjective capacities on behalf of the deserving. It is rather hard to establish this conclusively, though. Arguably, desert can decline along with an individual's diachronic psychological conditions. Desert might not in fact be an all-or-nothing relation. Instead, it might depend on the strength and degree of someone's psychological unity across time. Declining cross-temporal psychological relations, such as progressive memory loss, can then be seen as resulting in a declining degree of desert for punishment. This was the upshot of Parfit's proposal in *Reasons and Persons*[4]. His proposal has remained controversial. The concern has always been that it could lead to mind-numbingly implausible excuses: "I don't remember robbing the bank last week, so I don't deserve the punishment…". The severe and irrevocable psychological decline and process of dying in those who suffer from dementia is a more plausible case, though. If desert declines along with their recollective capacities, then the retributive basis for punishing them declines as well. It would then turn out to be unjust to punish the late-stage demented who have irrevocably forgotten their crimes.

However, some retributive accounts have an entirely different upshot according to which a punishment must be intentionally imposed for the right reason, i.e. to correct a wrong that the punished have committed. Under the further assumption that the psychological capacities of the punished do not matter to the degree to which they deserve their punishment, this could constitute a reason for punishing them irrespective of their current mental capacities, as long as the punishment aims at restoring the right or counter-balancing the wrong that has been done. However, the exact meaning of metaphors such as 'restoring' or 'counter-balancing' is notoriously hard to grasp. I take it that some commentators will certainly take it

4 Parfit, Derek. *Reasons and Persons*. Oxford: Oxford University Press, 1984.

to be a matter of brute fact that punishing the late-stage demented in a particular way amounts to restoring the right or counter-balancing the wrong. If one were to try to defend such a position further, though, one would have to give some explicit meaning to these metaphors and argue that leaving the late-stage demented in prison implements what is meant.

What about the idea of a deterrent effect of keeping demented criminals imprisoned? This might be a more interesting route to take, even though it has often been argued that deterrence does not work quite as well as one would hope.[5] It is also often pointed out that basing a justification of punishment on deterrence alone can lead to the implausible consequence that we ought to punish the undeserving, so that the view has to be supplemented by further constraints. But let us assume that these difficulties can be overcome. Would keeping the late-stage demented in prison have a plausible chance of producing such a deterrent effect? I believe it is possible to argue that it would not. Since the late stage demented are not capable of committing any further crimes, the idea of *individual* deterrence runs mute in their case. It can also be argued that a *general* deterrent effect is unlikely (though maybe not entirely impossible): In the late stages of dementia, it is surely not possible anymore to understand that one is in a prison rather than in a caretaking facility. If the late-stage demented do not notice or understand this difference, why should the threat of remaining incarcerated even in late-stage dementia deter a potential criminal in the general public? Or more precisely: If a potential criminal is not already deterred by the idea of losing freedom during a time of full understanding and competency, why should he be deterred by the additional idea of losing it during a time when understanding and competency are lost and the capacity to make use of this freedom is no longer present?

---

5 For example the Panel on Research on Deterrent and Incapacitative Effects by the US National Academy of Sciences thinks that there is more evidence to the effect that there are general deterrent effects of punishment than to the contrary, but at the same time "cannot yet assert that the evidence warrants an affirmative conclusion regarding deterrence". Blumstein, A., Cohen, J., Nagin, D. (eds.). *Deterrence and Incapacitation: Estimating the Effects of Criminal Sanctions on Crime Rates.* Washington, DC: National Academy of Sciences, 1986, 7. Similar points have also been established in a more recent meta study: Dölling, Dieter, Entorf, Horst, Hermann, Dieter, Rupp, Thomas. "Is Deterrence Effective? Results of a Meta-analysis of Punishment." In: *European Journal on Criminal Policy and Research* 15 (2009): 201–24.

This brings me to expressivist and communicative justifications of punishment, as they have been defended, for example, by Joel Feinberg[6] and Antony Duff.[7] According to expressivism, punishment is a reprobative symbol whereby a society is seen to condemn certain kinds of behavior. On the basis of an expressivist account, one could argue that leaving the late-stage demented in prison is a reprobative symbol that condemns the kind of crime they have committed in the past, and further, that imprisonment signals this condemnation in the right kind of way.

My main concern with an expressivist justification is the following: if we accept the idea that punishing the demented still sends the appropriate message of condemning the crime, and does so in the right kind of way, then why do we not continue to punish the corpse of the prisoner as well? Doing so might send the appropriate message as well. The idea seems outlandish at first, but it is actually not. We could punish a dead body by dismembering it, or, more moderately, by burying it in a special prison graveyard, denying it a place among our "righteous" ancestors. Moreover, if punishing the dead sends the right message, despite the fact that they perceive nothing, then punishing humans in a persistent vegetative coma might send the right message as well. It might be too costly to equip an ordinary prison hospital with the necessary life-sustaining technology for the irrevocably comatose, but this might not change the fact that choosing to do so might send the right signal.

Proponents of expressivist accounts could respond that a society should not just send appropriate signals of condemnation, but also signals of humanitarian values and compassion. Diseases and dying are conditions that affect every human being. Respect and compassion for the humanity in everyone might demand exceptions from the rule of legal punishment when people are severely affected by these conditions. Not doing so might indicate that we are ignoring the very same values that we accuse the perpetrator of having ignored. The human rights declaration has long put restrictions on what we may do to prisoners in order to express our condemnation of their acts. Maybe punishing the demented, the comatose, and the dead lies beyond an appropriate threshold as well.

---

6 Feinberg, Joel. *Doing and Deserving. Essays in the Theory of Responsibility*. Princeton: Princeton University Press, 1970, ch. 5: "The Expressive Function of Punishment." Feinberg believes the expression of a community's condemnation to be a widely acknowledged ingredient of punishment. In particular he quotes Hart as already having affirmed this. See Hart, H.L.A. "The Aims of the Criminal Law." In: *Law and Contemporary Problems* 23 (1958): 401–41.

7 See Duff, Antony. *Punsihment, Communication, and Community*. New York: Oxford University Press, 2001.

A communicative account, such as Duff's, can avoid the problem more easily. In fact, cases of dementia or other mental problems seem to be paradigm cases in which the communicative account makes more extensive stipulations than an expressivist one. If a punishment is not only to be seen as a form of expression directed at the criminal, but as an act of communication to which we hope the punished will *react* in some way, then directing legal punishments at the comatose or the dead will be pointless. Instead, the mental capacities of the addressee will enter the picture as a relevant precondition of justified punishment. This means that a communicative account can easily argue that the late stage demented should not be punished anymore, on the ground that they cannot respond to the punishment in the right kind of way anymore.

These considerations do not present the whole story yet. Expressivist accounts will have to make some further stipulations to determine an appropriate threshold that settles whether the demented should be punished at all. Communicative accounts will have to make some further assertions about the kind of reaction that the criminal should be able to give, and under which conditions such a reaction can still be expected. For both purposes, we have various possible cutoff points in an "ordinary" process of dying, for example: the loss of competency as it is usually required in order for someone to count as a fully autonomous agent before the law, the loss of recollection of the crime, the loss of comprehension of the information that (and maybe why) a punishment is being issued, the loss of various bodily functions, the irreversible loss of consciousness or brain death, organic death, the decay of the dead body. I am inclined to think that a cutoff point that still requires some subjective capacities on behalf of the punished is most plausible.

As plausible candidates, I will consider (a) a very strong requirement of mental competency sufficient for being considered a full agent before the law; (b) a very weak requirement of basic consciousness; (c) a comprehension requirement, sufficient for understanding that (and maybe what) one is being punished for; and (d) a recollection requirement, in the sense of having, in principle, the capacity to recall the time of the crime.

I am inclined to argue that a competency requirement would be too strong. Full competency can already be lost in the early or mid stages of the disease, at a time when patients are still able to comprehend their punishment and remember their crimes. As Agnieszka Jaworska argues, in the earlier and mid stages of the disease, patients still possess the capacity to *value*.[8] Given these assumptions, they should

8 Jaworska, Agnieszka. "Respecting the Margins of Agency: Alzheimer's Patients and the Capacity to Value." In: *Philosophy & Public Affairs* 28 (1999): 105–38.

also still possess the capacity to *appreciate* the fact that they are being punished for a particular crime they committed. This can even be the case at a time when their mental condition is such that they would be able to escape a conviction, were they to commit a further criminal offense.

The idea of a basic consciousness requirement lies at the other end of the spectrum. Even the demented in the terminal stages of the disease still possess this capacity in at least the sense of perceiving their surroundings. Jeff McMahan aptly described patients in this condition as "isolated subjects".[9] They possess the capacity for consciousness at all points in time, but they lack comprehension, cannot hold on to any diachronic recollections or intentions for long stretches of time. They possess a center of consciousness, but have lost the comprehension of their diachronic existence and place in time.

Obviously, a merely conscious being cannot be seen as a rational recipient of an expression of condemnation, or an attempt of communication. If an expression implies that one wants to be understood, or even that one is hoping for a comprehensible reaction, then aiming it at a merely conscious person with no capacity for comprehension is futile. Within the context of a merely expressivist account, one could at this point consider the possibility that the central recipient of the expression is not actually the punished criminal, but society at large. But this is an argument in which the criminal falls out of the picture. If the recipient of the value expression is society at large, we may, again, wonder why we stop short of expressing our condemnation by punishing the dead bodies of criminals. Obviously, stopping short of this implies that we either hope that the criminal will experience hard treatment (which human rights considerations prevent in the case of the merely conscious), or that the criminal will *understand* our expression of condemnation. Whether there will be such comprehension might well be irrelevant here. Important is that the criminal should in principle be able to comprehend what is being expressed. Both an expressivist and obviously also a communicative account should therefore contain such a comprehension requirement.

This leaves the more controversial recollection requirement up for debate. I suspect that in most actual cases, these two requirements will practically amount to the same thing. However, the ways in which people lose their mental capacities at the end of life are manifold, and the two capacities do not always disappear at the same time. Dementia patients tend to forget the more recent past while still being able to recall the more distant past. This makes it possible in principle for a person to still recall the rule that it is objectionable to hurt another person, a rule

---

9 McMahan, Jeff. *The Ethics of Killing*. New York: Oxford University Press, 2002, 65.

that was learned fairly early in life, while at the same time having forgotten the criminal assault committed later in life.

A related case in which these two requirements come apart is the case of an otherwise healthy person who does not recall having committed the crime due to amnesia, but is presented with compelling and comprehensible evidence that it must have been him who committed the crime. To make things easier, let us suppose the amnesia in the example *occurred involuntarily, there was no intention to instrumentalize its occurrence, and its cause is provable* (conditions that are usually fulfilled in cases of dementia). Do we find it plausible to punish such people or to hold them criminally responsible, even though they do not recall the deed?[10]

I believe it can be argued that this idea is unsatisfying. Without recollections, someone can only regret that the crime *occurred*, just as every other person could regret that the crime occurred. A genuine subjective appreciation of the fact that it was *oneself* who committed the crime would not be possible.[11] Anyone claiming that justification of punishment requires the criminal to identify, or at least relate in some special intimate way, with the crime cannot be entirely happy about a pure comprehension requirement in the absence of introspective recollective access. As specified before, though, this consideration should only apply in cases of involuntary and clinically provable amnesia in a very restricted range of cases (such as late-stage dementia).

Further reasons speak in favor of this conclusion. Without recollections, a prisoner might well understand that he or she is being accused of a crime and that all available evidence speaks in favor of this verdict, but only recollections would offer the more intimate information about what really happened, what the real intentions were back then, and what went on inside one's head when committing the action. Apart from preventing a full appreciation of the details of the condemned action, which runs counter to conveying the full meaning of the expressed condemnation and communication attempt, there is always a small chance that important evidence that should lead to a change of verdict will never be available, thereby increasing the chance of legal mistakes.

---

10 It is much harder to avoid the problem of deceivers when it comes to cases of amnesia than when it comes to clinical, late-stage dementia. Persons with amnesia can also re-gain their capacities, while this is unlikely and at most sporadic in cases of late-stage dementia. If amnesia patients do re-gain their capacities, this would in principle have to have an impact on the punishment question according to my position.

11 To ensure the possibility of such a subjective appreciation of one's self-involvement, these recollections should of course also be caused in the right kind of way. They should not be a result of hypnosis or some other external induction.

These considerations apply particularly strongly (but not only) in the case of punishment justifications with a communicative element. If the criminal is seen as a participant in a communication process, not merely as an addressee of a value expression, then we have to hope for a reaction of some kind. An attempt to view the punished as a potential respondent to the punishment – for example by expecting him to be a source of an *explanation* – is futile in the case of the late-stage demented. This plays a role even if the victims, or society at large, are not actually interested in hearing an explanation. When suffering from a lack of recollection, criminals cannot even fully *explain* the events *to themselves*. Their full comprehension and adequate psychological reaction to the condemnation would *depend on* recollections.

References

Blumstein, A., Cohen, J., Nagin, D. (eds.). *Deterrence and Incapacitation: Estimating the Effects of Criminal Sanctions on Crime Rates.* Washington, DC: National Academy of Sciences, 1986.

Dölling, Dieter, Entorf, Horst, Hermann, Dieter, Rupp, Thomas. "Is Deterrence Effective? Results of a Meta-analysis of Punishment." In: *European Journal on Criminal Policy and Research* 15 (2009): 201–24.

Duff, Anthony. *Punishment, Communication, and Community.* New York: Oxford University Press, 2001.

Dufner, Annette. "Should the Late Stage Demented be Punished for Past Crimes." In: *Criminal Law and Philosophy* 7 (2013): 137–50.

Feinberg, Joel. *Doing and Deserving. Essays in the Theory of Responsibility.* Princeton: Princeton University Press, 1970.

Hart, H.L.A. "The Aims of the Criminal Law." In: *Law and Contemporary Problems* 23 (1958): 401–41.

Jaworska, Agnieszka. "Respecting the Margins of Agency: Alzheimer's Patients and the Capacity to Value." In: *Philosophy & Public Affairs* 28 (1999): 105–38.

Locke, John. "On Identity and Diversity." In: John Perry (ed.). *Personal Identity.* Berkeley: University of California Press, 1975, 33–52.

McMahan, Jeff. *The* Ethics *of Killing.* New York: Oxford University Press, 2002.

Parfit, Derek. *Reasons and Persons.* Oxford: Oxford University Press, 1984.

Parfit, Derek. "Later Selves and Moral Principles." In: Alan Montefiore (ed). *Philosophy and Personal Relations*, London: Routledge, 1973, 135–69.

Shoemaker, David. "Responsibility without Identity." *Harvard Review of Philosophy* 18 (2012): 109–32.

List of Authors/AutorInnenverzeichnis

Bauer, Katharina, Dr., Visting Researcher an der Rijksuniversiteit Groningen (Feodor-Lynen Fellowship), Habilitation 2016 mit einer Arbeit zu Theorien praktischer Notwendigkeit, Forschungsschwerpunkte: Konzeptionen praktischer Notwendigkeit, Konzeptionen personaler Identität, Ökonomie und Gabe, französische Gegenwartsphilosophie

Dufner, Annette, Prof. Dr., Professorin für Ethik und Medizinethik an der Universität Bonn, aktuelles Forschungsprojekt „Moral Aggregation – Fairness versus Efficiency in Rescue Conflicts", Forschungsschwerpunkte: Normative und angewandte Ethik, personale Identität, britische Moralphilosophie des 19./20. Jahrhunderts

Hallich, Oliver, Prof. Dr., Professor für Philosophie mit dem Schwerpunkt Praktische Philosophie an der Universität Duisburg-Essen, Forschungsschwerpunkte: Angewandte Ethik, besonders Bioethik, Metaethik, Sozialphilosophie, Platon, Schopenhauer und Nietzsche

Lux, Elaine, Ph.D., Professorin am Nyack College Manhattan Center in New York City und Mentorin im Bereich Literatur und kreatives Schreiben am SUNY/Empire State College Newburgh, Forschungsschwerpunkte: Modern British and American Literature, Chaucer, Writing for Healing, Narrative Theory, Trauma and Narrative, Mythic Patterns in Literature, Adult Learning

Malottke, Letizia, M.A., Doktorandin am Deutschen Seminar der Albert-Ludwigs-Universität Freiburg, Promotionsprojekt zum Thema „Demenz erzählen. Darstellungen von Demenz-Erkrankungen in der deutschsprachigen Gegenwartsliteratur"

Mildorf, Jarmila, Dr., Oberstudienrätin im Hochschuldienst am Institut für Anglistik/Amerikanistik der Universität Paderborn, Forschungsschwerpunkte: Narratologie: Audionarratologie, Second-Person Narration, Sozionarratologie, mündliches Erzählen/Alltagserzählungen, Dialog, Soziolinguistik, Sprache und Literatur/Stilistik; Medizin und Literatur/Medical Humanities, Gender Studies

Rabelhofer, Bettina, Prof. Dr., ao. Professorin für Neuere deutsche Literatur am Institut für Germanistik der Karl-Franzens-Universität Graz und Psychoanalytikerin i.A.u.S., Forschungsschwerpunkte: Literatur und Psychoanalyse, Literatur der Moderne, österreichische Gegenwartsliteratur und Interdiskursivität von Literatur und Psychopathologie

Ringkamp, Daniela Dr., Wissenschaftliche Mitarbeiterin im Bereich Philosophie der Otto-von-Guericke-Universität Magdeburg, Habilitationsprojekt zum Thema „Philosophische Grundlagen einer Ethik der Demenz: Personalität und Autonomie", Forschungsschwerpunkte: Politische Philosophie, Philosophie der Menschenrechte, Ethik und Angewandte Ethik, insbesondere Medizinethik sowie ethische Herausforderungen von Demenzerkrankungen

Schmidhuber, Martina, Dr., Wissenschaftliche Mitarbeiterin am Institut für Geschichte und Ethik der Medizin an der Universität Erlangen-Nürnberg und im Emerging Fields Project „Human Rights in Healthcare", Forschungsschwerpunkte: Ethische Aspekte der Alzheimer-Demenz.

Schwieren, Alexander, Dr., studierte Deutsche Literatur, Mathematik, Journalismus und Kommunikationswissenschaften in Berlin. 2013 promovierte er als Stipendiat beim Zentrum für Literatur- und Kulturforschung in Berlin mit einer Arbeit zum Thema „Gerontographien: Eine Kulturgeschichte des Alterswerkbegriffs".

Strauss, Sara, Dr., Wissenschaftliche Mitarbeiterin am Institut für Anglistik/Amerikanistik der Universität Paderborn, Habilitationsprojekt zum Thema narrative Repräsentation von Alter und Demenz in englischsprachiger Literatur und Kultur, Forschungsschwerpunkte: anglophone Gegenwartsliteratur, Narratologie, Intermedialität, Aging Studies, Medical Humanities

Süwolto, Leonie, Dr., Wissenschaftliche Mitarbeiterin am Institut für Germanistik und Vergleichende Literaturwissenschaft der Universität Paderborn, Habilitationsprojekt zum Thema „Ende des Aristotelismus? Gattung und Geschlecht in der Tragödie um 1800", Forschungsschwerpunkte: Alter(n) in Literatur und Film der Gegenwart (abgeschlossenes Promotionsprojekt), Krankheit und Demenz in der Gegenwartsliteratur, Ästhetik des Tabuisierten in Literatur und Kultur

Zeisberg, Johanna, Universitätsassistentin am Fachbereich für Neuere deutsche Literatur an der Karl-Franzens-Universität in Graz, Promotionsprojekt zum Thema „(Alzheimer-)Demenz und Literatur", Forschungsschwerpunkte: Gegenwartsliteratur und Ethik, Literatur und Philosophie

www.ingramcontent.com/pod-product-compliance
Ingram Content Group UK Ltd.
Pitfield, Milton Keynes, MK11 3LW, UK
UKHW041827100926
8556IPUK00002B/58

9 783631 725399